Alternative Mechanisms
of Multidrug Resistance
in Cancer

Alternative Mechanisms of Multidrug Resistance in Cancer

John A. Kellen
Editor

Birkhäuser
Boston • Basel • Berlin

John A. Kellen
Sunnybrook Health Science Center
University of Toronto
Toronto, Canada M4N 3M5

Library of Congress Cataloging-in-Publication Data

Mechanisms and reversal of multidrug resistance in cancer : the other
  alternatives / John A. Kellen, editor.
        p.   cm.
    Includes bibliographical references and index.
    ISBN 0-8176-3775-3 (h : alk. paper). -- ISBN 3-7643-3775-3 (h
: alk. paper).
    1. Drug resistance in cancer cells.   2. Multidrug resistance.
I. Kellen, John A.
    [DNLM: 1.   Neoplasms--drug therapy. 2.   Drug Resistance, Multiple-
-physiology. 3. Antineoplastic Agents, Combined--pharmacology. QZ
    RC271.C5M42   1995   95-1582
    616.99'4061--dc20   CIP
    DNLM/DLC
    for Library of Congress

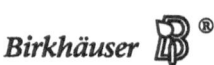

© 1995 Birkhäuser Boston

Softcover reprint of the hardcover 1st edition 1995

Camera-ready text prepared by the editor.

ISBN-13: 978-1-4615-9854-1   e-ISBN-13: 978-1-4615-9852-7
DOI: 10.1007/ 978-1-4615-9852-7

CONTENTS

PREFACE

Nullius in verba...Truth will be tested not by words. Horace (Epistles)

Few read introductions except for book reviewers, who want to take a shortcut and avoid reading the book itself. However, tradition requires that the preface make public why the book was written at all (this is not supposed to include powerful reasons such as augmenting the ego of the editor and authors). Frequently, the inflationary tendency to publish in verbose length is in conflict with market forces and interest.

No doubt, multidrug resistance is a "fashionable" topic, but there are many fashions displayed on the cat-walk of scientific literature. One can rationalize that the forces driving our concern with multidrug resistance reflect the frustration of pharmaceutical companies and oncologists alike: as soon as a new anticancer drug enters clinical trials, cancer cells start eluding extinction with their elaborate and successful mechanisms. Many grants have been awarded and spent, only to confirm the futility of our efforts to defeat this cellular Darwinism. Our medical and scientific training makes it hard, if not impossible, to accept that the survival of a malignant cell, alone or as part of a tissue, is part of the continuance of life. Since exposure to noxious and lethal substances is unavoidable, cells have been forced to develop a multitude of mechanisms to prevent entry or accelerate exit of such materials from intracellular space. The final result from these complex actions is a decrease of intracellular concentrations to tolerable levels, allowing survival of the cell. Cancer cells are no exception; of course, this becomes most undesirable when the cell is malignant and its good housekeeping wards off the effect of cytotoxic drugs.

It is an accepted truism that once we understand the cause of an event, we may prevent, circumvent, or reverse it. Medicine is based on this general tenet. The phenomenon of cross-resistance, whether innate or selected by exposure to one or more drugs, is the result of numerous mechanisms operating in concert; they depend on the level and length of exposure, genetic make-up of the cancer cell, size of the cell population, characteristics of the inducing agent, level of oxygenation, intra- and extracellular pH and probably on many more unknown factors. We are only at the beginning of our insight into this complexity; for every complex question, there is almost certainly a simple answer that is almost always wrong. There are no simple answers for MDR. All biological systems are both capable to defend themselves by the production of toxic substances and possess age-old mechanisms for defending themselves against these. MDR is a problem created by a mixture of variables that affect the outcome of chemotherapy in different and often unpredictable ways. For the clinical oncologist, resistance is synonymous with the fate of the individual patient: what happens to the tumor mass and how it responds to treatment.

Increasing insight into the vulnerability of malignant cells has led to the design of perfectly tailored cytotoxic substances, expected to cause reasonably selective extinction of the cancer cell population. Yet, even the best of such fits allows a critical number of cells to escape and regrow in eventually fatal numbers, as the result of cumulative, cooperative cellular defenses. Perhaps the first stepping stone in our understanding of such defense mechanisms has been the recognition of P-glycoprotein as a general efflux pump. This may be one of the primordial instruments for turfing out unwanted guests, but it does not fulfill our expectations for a single "deus ex machina" which provides all the answers and solves all the problems. P-glycoprotein is considered by some as a "first line of defense," appearing very early in the hierarchy of defense mechanisms, as a normal response to foreign agents and hence inevitable in many, but not all tumors. Introduction of the apparently synonymous terminology: MDR for multidrug resistance and mdr1 for the gene expressing P-glycoprotein, is causing some confusion; MDR in cancer can be caused by a multitude of mechanisms and is a vague term describing the ability of tumor cells to repair sublethal damage caused by structurally unrelated cytotoxic drugs. Acquired multidrug resistance is being extensively studied in rodent and human cell lines, with single or multistep selection, by one or more drugs or other inducers. *In vitro* conditions are ideal for "clean" experiments with a minimum of variables. Clinical studies are more difficult, if not impossible, to compare and evaluate since they differ in treatment protocols, demography as well as methodology and criteria for positivity of the MDR phenotype.

MDR predominantly caused by P-glycoprotein has been coined as "classical," again a term which should be disputed. Binding to P-glycoprotein (as evidenced by photolabelling) is not always synonymous with transport across biomembranes, but reduced drug accumulation in non-Pgp-MDR cells is less well understood. Preoccupation with a single solution has led to the neglect of other explanations. Even more simplistic is the trend to use the term "atypical MDR" for resistance mechanisms involving Topoisomerase II only. Finally, there is a growing grab-bag filled with "non P-glycoprotein mediated" MDR which ranges from other membrane proteins belonging to the ATP-binding cassette (ABC) superfamily to a variety of detoxifying mechanisms, enzymatic and other.

The cooperative effort represented by this book expressed our feelings that we have reached a critical mass of information: within the uncomfortable framework of inherent instability characteristic for the cancer cell, we must accept the continuously adapting and changing complexity of resistance. Some important and some perhaps less important factors have been examined and evaluated. At present, we can not predict which single mechanism will play a leading role — if there is a universal leading role at all; only the passage of time will provide new perspectives.

I had the good fortune to persuade many eminent scientists in the MDR scene to come forward with state of the art reviews in an apparently heterogeneous field. This heterogeneity should not come as a surprise, but as a warning. If clinical researchers wish to more effectively plan treatment with drugs and drug combinations able to circumvent defense mechanisms, they must learn to understand the molecular basis of drug resistance. The gap in our interpretation and application of data are evident and may direct the curious to further analytic and synthetic travail; comprehending the whole as more than the sum of its parts. To quote Galileo: We must look at what others have looked before and see it as no one has seen it before...

John A. Kellen
August 1994

LIST OF CONTRIBUTORS

William T. Bellamy, Ph.D., Arizona Health Science Center, Tucson, Arizona, USA

Pedro J. Beltran, University of Texas M.D. Anderson Cancer Center, Houston, Texas, USA

Diane R. Bielenberg, B.S., University of Texas M.D. Anderson Cancer Center, Houston, Texas, USA

Henk J. Broxterman, Ph.D. Academ. Ziekenhuis, VU Amsterdam, Amsterdam, The Netherlands

Dominic Fan, Ph.D., University of Texas M.D. Anderson Cancer Center, Houston, Texas, USA

Frank Gieseler, M.D., Mediz. Poliklinik de Universität Würzburg, Würzburg, Germany

Karen R. Gravitt, M.Sc., University of Texas M.D. Anderson Cancer Center, Houston, Texas, USA

Krishna P. Gupta, Ph.D., University of Texas M.D. Anderson Cancer Center, Houston, Texas, USA

Cynthia E. Herzog, M.D., University of Texas M.D. Anderson Cancer Center, Houston, Texas, USA

Bridget T. Hill, Ph.D., Ctr. de Recherche Pierre Fabre, Castres, France

Hironori Ishida, M.D., City of Hope Natl. Med. Ctr., Duarte, California, USA

Mohamed Kashani-Sabet, M.D., City of Hope Natl. Med. Ctr., Duarte, California, USA

John A. Kellen, M.D., Ph.D., Sunybrook Health Science Centre, University of Toronto, Toronto, Canada

Hiroshi Kijima, M.D., City of Hope Natl. Med. Ctr., Duarte, California, USA

Robert A. Newman, University of Texas M.D. Anderson Cancer Center, Houston, Texas, USA

Catherine A. O'Brian, Ph.D., University of Texas M.D. Anderson Cancer Center, Houston, Texas, USA

Yukinori Ohta, Ph.D., City of Hope Natl. Med. Ctr., Duarte, California, USA

Robert Radinsky, Ph.D., University of Texas M.D. Anderson Cancer Center, Houston, Texas, USA

John C. Reed, M.D., Ph.D., La Jolla Cancer Research Fnd., La Jolla, California, USA

Kevin J. Scanlon, Ph.D., City of Hope Natl. Med. Ctr., Duarte, California, USA

Teruhiro Utsugi, Ph.D., Taiho Pharm. Co. Ltd., Hanno City, Saitama, Japan

Carolien H.M. Versantvoort, Ph.D., MRC Clinical Oncology and Radiotherapy Unit, MRC Center, Cambridge, U.K.

Yun-Fang Wang, University of Texas M.D. Anderson Cancer Center, Houston, Texas, USA

Nancy E. Ward, M.Sc., University of Texas M.D. Anderson Cancer Center, Houston, Texas, USA

1. MECHANISMS OF MULTIDRUG RESISTANCE

John A. Kellen

The chapter is intended as a basic, orderly listing of what we believe we understand in the all-embracing field of multidrug resistance in cancer. This is in accordance with our expectations that everything we wish to comprehend and manipulate must be reduced to the simplest concepts and categorized. Of course, in the real world, everything is part of continual and complex interrelationships and there are no crisply separated entities. Some philosophers have come to accept that chaos is logical and that to call a concept as "fuzzy" is not pejorative. Most scientists find it very difficult to digest that nature is not Confucian, a harmony of balanced opposites, but a sometimes disconcertingly unclear mixture. Any effort to organize a vast set of categories into a system, simple and with no loose ends, needs both short and tunnel vision; errors and omissions are likely. This never stops list-makers and the tables enumerating resistance mechanisms are becoming longer (Broxterman, 1994). However, it is essential to keep in mind that even the term "multidrug resistance" is a cerebral abstraction, serving the need of satisfying our liking for intellectual frameworks. In reality, the ability to live with poisons is a primordial,ubiquitous phenomenon and is, in essence, the true reason that life is here and has survived. We are (whatever our egotistic delusions of superiority are) part of life and have similar needs and problems as unicellular organisms.

Table 1. Changes associated with or responsible for expression of the MDR phenotype.

Increases in:

Radical scavenging
PKC activity
intracellular calcium concentration
vacuolar H^+-ATPase (concomitant with overexpression of mRNA for subunit C)
intracellular pH
EGF receptor(s)
a 170 kDa membrane-associated serine-threonine kinase
levels of GTP-binding proteins of the ras (p21) family
an unidentified 21 kDa protein
lysosomal accumulation of drug and energy-dependent exocytosis
the MRP protein expression of P190
phosphorylation of a P150 glycoprotein
expression of a 100 kDa protein
cappactin I
a 55 kDa protein, and/or a 36 kDa protein
a VPL-insensitive efflux mechanism
amplification of DHFR gene
rate of drug detoxification

Decreases in:

Cl^- ion conductance
EGF receptor(s)
levels of 72 kDa and 75 kDa proteins

Alterations in:

intracellular distribution of drug(s)
microtubular drug transport
topoisomerases
DNA repair capacity

The ability to survive in an increasingly toxic and dangerous world we find to be admirable and to be encouraged. When all the complex mechanisms which enable survival in adverse conditions are used by the cancer cell to do just that, we immediately isolate the phenomenon and coin a special term, multidrug resistance, to describe it, but with a negative ring to it. This is akin to conceding that gravity is useful - for it permits us to walk comfortably - but it is undesirable in that it causes the smashing of an accidentally dropped crystal ware. Cancer cells too are part of us, though unruly and exuberant. They survive because of a truly functional, evolutionary tested survival system. We are not going to develop effective tools to overcome this if we pretend that they are very distinct from the "normal" or healthy cell.

The sobering fact is that in actual clinical practice, results are grey, not black and white. The understanding of the specifics and characteristics of the cancer cell, at the molecular level, allows us to tailor precisely targeted attack with optimally designed substances. The effect of even the best drugs that interfere with cell proliferation, the ultimate goal in theory, is immediately weakened by the heterogeneity of cancer cells. Some of these are *ab ovo* not vulnerable and others acquire by-pass mechanisms to avoid such lethal interference. We know that even a 99.9% kill is only a passing victory. To ensure a more lasting, if not complete victory, cancer "survival systems" must be understood and bypassed. The usual approach, step by step, is to find appropriate models, mostly rodent or cell cultures and sort out how their resistance comes about, is perpetuated and hopefully modulated.

Drug-resistant variants and sub-populations of cancer cells have been selected *in vitro*, using a wide range of different drugs at different concentrations. Although initially the resistance is highest to the single agent used for selection, variable patterns of cross-resistance are found early or at the very beginning of this process. Observations of single drug resistance, reported in the older literature, are dubious because either cross-resistance was not tested for or the drugs were not available at that time. Difficulties with defining one or more resistance mechanisms are compounded by the fact that *in vitro* selection depends on a multitude of seemingly marginal factors. Experimental conditions differ from the clinical situation in many regards. Actual levels and exposure times of chemotherapeutic agents in cancer patients are really not comparable with the clean-cut models available from cells in culture. The behaviour of different clones and subclones, obtained from originally solid tumors, is not a reflection of the clinical counterpart. Extrapolation of results obtained in cell cultures, when tested for sensitivity, is questionable at best. The factors influencing drug levels achieved *in situ* in malignant growth are numerous and complex; histopathology, grading and even sophisticated molecular markers are not helpful. The local bioavailability of any one substance, at the level of the tumor cell, is the result of numerous variables, starting with the blood supply to the tumor itself (and the declining gradient towards the central parts of growth), the *ad hoc* size of the dormant cellular fraction versus cells undergoing mitosis and the often highly individual metabolism of each drug by the patient. Age, sex, ethnicity, seasonal variations, body weight and the interaction of drug combinations, all play a significant role in the final, critical number of cytotoxic molecules reaching the target cell.

P-GLYCOPROTEIN

For now, the most consistent finding in MDR cancer cells is amplification and/or overexpression of P-glycoprotein, a statement which needs to be qualified: this membrane protein is frequently associated with high-level MDR and with cells *in vitro*. A thing observed is a thing disturbed; cell cultures, out of the context of the variable mix of normal and malignant cells *in vivo*, are not a reliable reflection of "things undisturbed". In fact, *mdr1* amplification *in vivo* has not been observed (Biedler, 1992). The literature about P-glycoprotein is extensive and many exhaustive (and exhausting) reviews are available (Kellen, 1994); since we set out to review non-P-glycoprotein associated MDR, the "classical" efflux pump will be duly mentioned, but not belaboured in any detail. In human lung cancer cell lines (SW-1573), non-P-glycoprotein mechanisms for MDR precede P-glycoprotein expression during *in vitro* selection for doxorubicin resistance (Baas et al., 1990). However, it is necessary to stress that "non-P-glycoprotein" is a misnomer; more often than not, P-glycoprotein is part of multiple resistance mechanisms, may precede them or appear during and following therapy. Reports about its apparent absence in some forms of cancer or in some individual tumor specimens may be flawed by methodological errors, lack of sensitivity of determination or simply because at the time of investigation, positive cells were not present in detectable numbers.

Different mechanisms may underlie the development of acquired MDR, compared to "natural" resistance (in previously untreated cancer cells). However, such a distinction may be an artefact; untreated - with chemotherapy - patients may already have been exposed to other drugs which induced detoxification mechanisms and after exposure to cytostatic or cytotoxic drugs, a selection process, combined with mutations induced by the drugs themselves, may result in a predominantly resistant cell population (Vendrik et al., 1992). There are grounds for suspicion that the MDR and metastatic phenotypes (at least in some tumors) may arise in parallel, perhaps even as the result of similar mechanisms (Jang et al., 1991).

In monolayer culture systems, acquisition of MDR is issually a protracted process; a single exposure to cisplatin or cyclophosphamide *in vitro* of cells growing in three-dimensional aggregates sufficies to induce significant, albeit transient drug resistance. This may represent a typical adaptive mechanism at the multicellular level and a model of the sometimes rapid development of MDR in tumors *in vivo*. Even transient and low levels of MDR may be clinically relevant (Graham et al., 1994). The use of three-dimensional cell culture systems, in compact cell spheroids, improves our understanding of cell differentiation under conditions which are closer to the *in vivo* situation. This model enables us to study the induction of the drug resistance phenotype which may resemble the clinical course in human tumors (Steeg et al., 1994).

Critics of the dogmatic creed about the efflux pump being the main tool of defense have many plausible arguments: significant overexpression of P-glycoprotein can be induced only with high levels of the particular drug or drugs (which do not correspond to clinically achievable levels), there is no exact correlation between clinical resistance and P-glycoprotein expression, resistance to different drugs varies in cell lines expressing comparable levels of P-glycoprotein and many other. Experimentally, the role of P-glycoprotein is well defined, reasonably understood and can be manipulated in a predictable manner; the extent of its contribution to the overall clinical response to chemotherapy is still not clear (Versantvoort et al., 1992).

The selection of resistant malignant cells by various substances usually activates several defense mechanisms, involving drug transport, metabolism and the ability of the drug or drug combinations to reach their respective target sites (Rabier et al., 1991). Cells, selected during relatively short drug exposure *in vitro* routinely express P-glycoprotein; longer exposure at higher drug levels causes additional alterations in the cross-resistance phenotype, modifying or complementing the initial resistance pattern (Devine and Melera, 1994). Higher intracellular substance levels may overcome efflux inhibition by substrate concentration-dependent passive pathways (Wigler, 1994). Again, simple observations based on particular cell lines from tumor models can not be generalized and depend on techniques and conditions of culture. The "well-being" of the cultured cells influences their proliferative activity; a significant correlation has been found in kidney carcinoma cells between cell doubling times and co-expression of P-glycoprotein and Glutathione-

S-Transferase (Efferth et al., 1992).

Absence of prior exposure to a defined inducing agent does not preclude spontaneously arising MDR (Schuetz and Schuetz, 1990), at least in primary rat hepatocytes. Even if this observation has not been tested in various tumor models, it serves as a reminder that alterations of culture conditions (even without drug exposure) can modulate the MDR phenotype. Furthermore, constitutive levels of *mdr1* mRNA (innate or acquired) do not necessarily result in functional expression of the MDR phenotype (Kramer et al., 1993) and the selective pressure by one drug may confer only partial resistance to another, as is the case with mitoxantrone and doxorubicin, whereas resistance selected by doxorubicin confers complete resistance to mitoxantrone (Taylor et al., 1991) in MCF7 human breast cancer cells.

The stability of the MDR phenotype, ie. retention of resistance even after treatment by antineoplastic agents, is another factor which may play a highly individualized role in each patient. The "primitive" (sensitive) phenotype of the tumor changes when exposed to one or more chemotherapeutic substances; the result may be a number of variations in resistance, which in turn gives ris to new variations when treatment is temporarily discontinues (Pauwels et al., 1993).

The stimulating agent itself also plays a role in the type of resistance evoked. For example, fractionated X-irradiation generates a subline of Chinese hamster ovary AuxB1 cells, characterised by overexpression of a functional P-glycoprotein without concomitant increase in Pgp mRNA (Hill and McClean, 1994), with resistance to etoposide and vincristine, but not to Adriamycin. How this model can be applied to the frequent combination of radiation therapy with chemotherapy is difficult to answer and will be discussed in Chapter 8 at greater length. The interpretation of resistance models (because all reproducible data gathered are indeed based on models) requires a correct understanding of the mechanisms involved, in quantitative terms. However, the facts of life or death are never straightforward, even if expressed in exact numbers. A clinically relevant model should exhibit a low level of MDR with resistance induced *in vivo*. The application of experimental data, observed *in vitro*, to clinical situations in order to guide and predict optimal chemotherapy calls for mathematical modelling. This should allow for some "law and order" in seemingly chaotic and hardly reproducible conditions. There have been several efforts to put tumor behaviour into a mathematical straight-jacket; several schools of thought have developed and there is no consensus as to an optimal solution (Goldie, 1988). In general, the chemical control of growth in tumor populations developing drug resistance has been expressed in differential equations (Costa et al., 1992). Formulas for response duration, tumor-doubling times and resistant tumor volume have been designed with some success for acute leukemia (Gregory et al., 1991). Specifically, a model for computer simulation of anthracycline transport in MDR tumor cells has been proposed (Demant et al., 1990), based mainly on drug efflux related to P-glycoprotein.

REFERENCES

Baas F, Jongsma APM, Broxterman HJ, Arceci RJ, Housman D, Scheffer GI, Riethorst A, van Groeningen M, Nieuwint AWM, Joenje H (1990): Non-P-Glycoprotein mediated Mechanism for Multidrug Resistance Precedes P-Glycoprotein Expression during *in Vitro* Selection for Doxorubicin Resistance in a Human Lung Cancer Cell Line. *Cancer Res* 50:5392-5398

Biedler JL (1992): Genetic Aspects of Multidrug Resistance. *Cancer* 70:1799-1809

Broxterman HJ (1994): Personal communication

Costa MIS (1992): Optimal chemical control of populations developing drug resistance. *IMA J Mathemat Appl in Med & Biol* 9:215-226

Demant EJF, Sehested M, Jensen PB (1990): A model for computer simulation of P-glycoprotein and transmembrane Δ pH mediated anthracycline transport in multidrug-resistant tumor cells. *Biochim Biophys A* 1055:117-125

Devine EJF, Melera PW (1994): Diversity of Multidrug Resistance in Mammalian Cells. *J Biol Chem* 269:6133-6139

Efferth T, Mattern J, Volm M (1992): Immunohistochemical detection of P Glycoprotein, Glutathione S Transferase and DNA Topoisomerase II in Human Tumors. *Oncology* 49:368-375

Graham CH, Kobayashi H, Stankiewicz KS, Man S, Kapitain SJ, Kerbel RS (1994): Rapid Acquisition of Multicellular Drug Resistance After a Single Exposure of Mammary Tumor Cells to Antitumor Alkylating Agents. *JNCI* 86:975-982

Goldie JH (1988): Mathematical Models to Predict Behaviour of Tumours? *Eur J Cancer Clin Oncol* 24:587-589

Gregory WM, Richards MA, Slevin NL, Souhami RL (1991): A Mathematical Model Relating Response Durations to Amount of Subclinical Resistant Disease. *Cancer Res* 51:1210-1216

Hill BT, McClean S (1994):   Characterization of a novel multidrug resistant
    subline selected *in vitro* by exposure to fractionated X-irradiation in the
    presence of verapamil. *Proc AACR* 35:343

Jang A, Hill RP (1991):   Drug senisitivty and metastatic ability in B16
    melanoma cells. *Clin Exp Metastasis* 9:393-402

Kellen JA, ed. (1994):   Reversal of Multidrug Resistance in Cancer.   Boca
    Raton: CRC Press

Kramer R, Weber TK, Morse B, Arceci R, Staniunas R, Steel G Jr,
    Summerhayes IC (1993):   Constitutive expression of multidrug
    resistance in human colorectal tumours and cell lines. *Br J Cancer*
    67:959-968

Pauwels O, Kiss R (1993):   Chemoresistant Cell Lines: Morphonuclear
    Characteristics and Chemosensitivity Development During Long-Term
    Culture. *Anticancer Res* 13:1593-1600

Rabier MJ, Bruno NA, Slate DL (1991):   Multifactorial Resistance in LS174T
    Human Colon Carcinoma Cells Selected With Doxorubicin. *Int J
    Cancer* 49:601-607

Schuetz E, Schuetz J (1990): Multidrug resistance arises without prior exposure
    or toxic agents in primary cultures of rat hepatocytes. *Proc AACR*
    31:379

Steeg PS, Alley MC, Grever MR (1994): An Added Dimension: Will Three-
    dimensional Cultures Improve Our Understanding of Drug Resistance?
    JNCI 86:953-955

Taylor CW, Dalton WS, Parrish PR, Gleason MC, Bellamy WT, Thompson FH,
    Roe DJ, Trent JM (1991): Different mechanisms of decreased drug
    accumulation in doxorubicin and mitoxantrone resistant variants of
    MCF7 human breast cancer cell line. *Br J Cancer* 63:923-929

Vendrik CPJ, Bergers JJ, De Jong WH, Steerenberg PA (1992): Resistance to
    cytostatic drugs at the cellular level. *Cancer Chemother Pharmacol*
    29:413-429

Versantvoort HCM, Broxterman HJ, Dekker FH, Kuiper CM, Lankelma J
    (1992):   Probing daunorubicin accumulation defects in non-P-
    glycoprotein expressing multidrug-resistant cell lines using digitonin.
    Int J Cancer 50:906-911

Wigler PW (1994): Reversal of Multidrug Resistance in Cancer Cells. *JNCI*
    86:148

OTHER TRANSPORTERS

Numerous transporters mediate transcellular movement of substances; secretion (generally understood as basal-to-apical transport) across epithelium (i.e. in the intestine and colon) is a function of multiple organic cation transport mechanisms. Many careful studies describe absence of measurable P-glycoprotein expression in cells with distinct MDR and simultaneously increased presence of various membrane proteins. These findings are summed up in Table 2. The functions of sorcin and forscolin remain to be clarified; proteins with kDa below 170 have been reported in an anecdotal manner, even if the respective method of determination appears to be specific and reliable.

The notable exemption is MRP, the multidrug resistance-associated protein, found in various cancers (Table 3). MRP has a minor sequence homology with P-glycoprotein, belongs to the ATP-binding casette transporters and has been identified in resistant tumors in absence of P-glycoprotein (Cole et al., 1992). Frequently, no relationship between *mdr1* expression and MRP mRNA has been observed (Kruh et al., 1994). MRP already has a firm place in the hierarchy of MDR and will be discussed separately in Chapter 4. There are substantial gaps in our understanding of the relation between drug resistance and transport mechanisms (Marquardt et al., 1992). While the amount of information in this field is impressive and growing, some results are contradictory and no common principles have become apparent; results obtained from certain models (mostly *in vitro*) are valid for a particular cell line or lines, at specific culture conditions and for a certain drug or drugs only.

Table 2. Transporters (other than "classical" P-gp 170)

term	kDa	References
Sorcin	22	Meyers, 1989a
Forskolin	35	Wadler et al., 1989
Nuclear protein	38	Ciaccio et al., 1992
"	<45	Mazzoni et al., 1990
Mini-P-gp	65	Kawai et al., 1994
"	85	De La Torre et al., 1993 Sugimoto et al., 1993
"	95	Lee et al., 1994 Chen et al., 1990
LRP	110	Scheper et al., 1993 Broxterman et al., 1994
P150	150	Krishnamachary et al., 1992 Marsh et al., 1987
MRP	190	Cole et al., 1992 Grant et al., 1994 Barrand et al., 1994* Krishnamachary et al., 1993
Co-expressed with P-gp (?):		
--	180	Meyers et al., 1989b
P150, 180, 210	150-210	McGrath et al., 1988

*probably identical with MRP

Table 3. The incidence of MRP in various human tumors and tumor-derived cell lines.

MULTIDRUG RESISTANCE-ASSOCIATED PROTEIN (MRP)

Tumor (cell line)	Reference
Breast Ca (MCF7/VP)	Schneider et al., 1994
Leukemia, hum. (U 937)	Slapak et al., 1994
SCLC (UMCC-1/VP)	Doyle et al., 1994
NSCLC, hum. (SW-1573)	Zaman et al., 1993
HL60/ADR	Kuiper et al., 1994 Krishnamachary et al., 1993 McGrath et al., 1989
H69HR	Grant et al., 1994
NIH3T3	Kruh et al., 1994
Thyroid Ca (anaplastic)	Sugawara et al., 1994
HT1080/DR4	Slovak et al., 1993
H69/AR (human)	Cole et al., 1992

See also Table 2

12   John A. Kellen

REFERENCES

Barrand MA, Heppell-Parton AC, Wright KA, Rabbitts PH, Twentyman PR
    (1994):   A 190-Kilodalton Protein Overexpressed in Non-P-
    Glycoprotein-Containing Multidrug-Resistant Cells and its Relationship
    to the *mrp* Gene. *JNCI* 86:110-117
Booser DJ, Hortobagyi GN (1994):   Anthracycline Antibiotics in Cancer
    Therapy. *Drugs* 47:223-258
Broxterman HJ, Kuiper CM, Schuurhuis GJ, Ossenkoppele GJ, Feller N, Scheper
    RJ, Lankema J, Pinedo HM (1994): Analysis of P-glycoprotein and
    non-Pgp multidrug resistance in acute myeloid leukemia. *Proc AACR*
    35:348
Chen Y-N, Mickley LA, Schwartz AM, Acton EM, Hwang J, Fojo AT (1990):
    Characterization of Adriamycin-resistant Human Breast Cancer Cells
    Which Display Overexpression of a Novel Resistance-related Membrane
    Protein. *J Biol Chem* 265:100073-100080
Ciaccio PJ, Kuzmich S, Stuart JE, Tew KD (1992): Overexpression of a 38kD
    nuclear protein in ethacrynic acid-resistant HT29 cells. *Proc AACR*
    33:412
Cole SPC, Bhardwaj G, Gerlach JH, Mackie JE, Grant CE, Almquist KC,
    Stewart AJ, Kurz EU, Duncan AM, Geeley RG (1992): Overexpression
    of a Transporter Gene in a Multidrug-Resistant Human Lung Cancer
    Cell Line. *Science* 258:1650-1652
De La Torre M, Hao X-Y, Larsson R, Nygren P, Tsuruo T, Mannervik B, Bergh
    J (1993): Characterization of Four Doxorubicin Adapted Human Breast
    Cancer Cell Lines with Respect to Chemotherapeutic Drug Sensitivity,
    Drug Resistance Associated Membrane Proteins and Glutathione
    Transferases. *Anticancer Res* 13:1425-1430
Doyle LA, Kaufman SH, Fojo AT, Bailey ChL, Gazdar AF (1993): A novel 95
    kilodalton membrane polypeptide associated with lung cancer drug
    resistance. *Lung Cancer* 9:317-326
Doyle LA, Ross DD, Ordonez JV, Yang W, Gao Y, Tong Y, Belani CP, Gutheil
    JC (1994): An etoposide-resistant small cell lung cancer subline
    overexpresses the MRP gene. *Proc AACR* 35:467
Grant CE, Valdimarsson G, Hipfner DR, Almquist KC, Cole SPC, Deeley RG
    (1994): Overexpression of Multidrug Resistance-associated Protein
    (MRP) Increases Resistance to Natural Product Drugs. *Cancer Res*
    54:357-361
Kawai K, Kusano I, Ido M, Sakurai M, Shiraishi T, Yatani R (1994):
    Identification of a P-glycoprotein-related protein (mini-P-glycoprotein)
    which is overexpressed in multidrug-resistant cells. *BBRC* 198:804-810

Krishnamachary N, Center MS (1992): Detection and Characterization of Membrane Protein Changes in Multidrug Resistant HL-60 Cells. *Oncology Res* 4:23-28

Krishnamachary N, Center MS (1993): The MRP Gene Associated with a Non-P-glycoprotein Multidrug Resistance Encodes a 190-kDa Membrane Bound Glycoprotein. *Cancer Res* 53:3658-3661

Kruh GD, Chan A, Gaughan K, Meyers K, Breuninger L, Miki T, Aaronson SA (1994): Expression cDNA library transfer establishes *mrp* as a multidrug resistance gene. *Proc AACR* 35:343

Kuiper CM, Broxterman HJ, Eekman JK, Ruhdal KAB, Versantvoort CHM, Pinedo HM, Lankelma J (1994): Functional detection of MRP overexpressing tumor cell lines using flow cytometry and laser scan microscopy. *Proc AACR* 35:348

Lee JS, Dickstein B, Bates SE (1994): Reduced drug accumulation without P-glycoprotein (Pgp) expression in MCF-7 AdrVp cells. *Proc AACR* 35:357

Marsh W, Center MS (1987): Adriamycin resistance in HL60 Cells and Accompanying Modification of a Surface Membrane Protein Contained in Drug-sensitive Cells. *Cancer Res* 47:5080-5086

Mazzoni A, Trace F, Russo P, Nicolin A, Rustum YM (1990): Generation and Characterization of a Low-Degree Drug-Resistant Human Tumor Cell Line. *Oncology* 47:488-494

McGrath T, Center MS (1988): Mechanisms of Multidrug Resistance in HL60 Cells: Evidence That a Surface Membrane Protein Distinct from P-Glycoprotein Contributes to Reduced Cellular Accumulation of Drug. *Cancer Res* 48:3959-3963

McGrath T, Latoud Ch, Arnold ST, Safa AR, Felsted RL, Center MS (1989): Mechanisms of Multidrug Resistance in HL60 Cells. *Biochem Pharmacol* 38:3611-3619

Meyers BM (1989): Sorcin is a Cardiac Calcium-Binding Protein. *Proc AACR* 30:505

Oesterreich S, Weng Ch-N, Qiu M, Hilsenbeck SG, Osborn CK, Fuqua SAW (1993): The Small Heat Shock Protein hsp27 Is Correlated with Growth and Drug Resistance in Human Breast Cancer Cell Lines. *Cancer Res* 53:4443-4448

Scheper RJ, Broxterman HJ, Scheffer GL, Kaaijk P, Dalton WS, van Heijningen THM, van Kalken CK, Slovak ML, de Vries EGE, van der Valk P, Meijer ChJLM, Pinedo HM (1993): Overexpression of a M_r 110,000 Vesicular Protein in Non-P-Glycoprotein-mediated Multidrug Resistance. *Cancer Res* 53:1475-1479

Schneider E, Horton JK, Yang Ch-H, Nakagawa M, Cowan KH (1994): Multidrug Resistance-associated Protein Gene Overexpression and Reduced Drug Sensitivity of Topoisomerase II in a Human Breast Carcinoma MCF7 Cell Line Selected for Etoposide Resistance. *Cancer Res* 54:152-158

Slapak CA, Mizunuma N, Kufe DW (1994): Overexpression of the multidrug resistance associated protein without gene amplification in doxorubicin selected U937 cells. *Proc AACR* 35:342

Slovak ML, Ho JP, Bhardwaj G, Kurz EU, Deeley RG, Cole SPC (1993): Localization of a Novel Multidrug Resistance-associated Gene in the HT1080/DR4 and H69AR Human Tumor Cell Lines. *Cancer Res* 53:3221-3225

Sugawara I, Arai T, Yamashita T, Hasumi K, Masunuga A, Itoyama S, Obara T (1994): Expression of multidrug-related protein (MRP) mRNA in anaplastic thyroid carcinoma. *Proc AACR* 35:343

Sugimoto Y, Hamada H, Tsukahara S, Noguchi K, Yamaguchi K, Sato M, Tsuruo T (1993): Molecular Cloning and Characterization of the Complementary DNA for the M_r 85,000 Protein Overexpressed in Adriamycin-resistant Human Tumor Cells. *Cancer Res* 53:2538-2543

Wadler S, Thompson D, Wiernik PH (1989): Forskolin phosphorylates a 35 kD protein in multidrug resistant variants of murine sarcoma S180 cells. *Proc AACR* 30:506

Zaman GJR, Versantvoort CHM, Smit JJM, Eijdems EWHM, de Haas M, Smith AJ, Broxterman HJ, Mudler NH, de Vries EGE, Bass F, Borst P (1993): Analysis of the Expression of *mrp*, the Gene for a New Putative Transmembrane Drug Transporter, in Human Multidrug Resistant Lung Cancer Cell Lines. *Cancer Res* 53:1747-1750

INTRACELLULAR COMPARTMENTALIZATION

Contemporary chemotherapy is aimed at various intracellular targets; all other conditions being equal (i.e. the numbers of drug molecules penetrating the cell membrane), the cell kill achieved should be comparable, either from direct cytotoxicity (interference with vital pathways of the cell) or facilitation of inhibited apoptotic programes. The latter is in fact a restoration of the natural mortality of the cells. Our preoccupation with efflux mechanisms overshadows information on various characteristic structural alterations of the cancer cell, such as differences in vesicles and microtubule architecture, distribution and kinetics.

Cells have the ability to expel drugs by vesicular transport. Vesicle formation starts at the perinuclear region, with some regions preferentially involved. Resistant cells are often described as being more vesicular (Sehested et al., 1991) with endosomal drug trapping and vesicular extrusion increased (Sehested et al., 1987) and enhanced sequestration of some cytostatic drugs in cytoplasmic vesicles (Sognier et al., 1992). Intracytoplasmic vesicles are held responsible for mitoxanrone resistance in EPG85-257RNOV cells, by keeping the drug from its target sites and serving as an export system via exocytosis. These organelles have been found filled with anticancer compounds (by light or fluorescence microscopy) and participate in unidirectional transport to the cell periphery. Migration is directed by or at least associated with the microfilament tubulin, aided by motor molecules (perhaps kinesin, dynein or other) (Vichi and Tritton, 1992). The distribution of microtubules is frequently of higher density in resistant cancer cells when compared to sensitive cells (Dietel, 1993). The intracellular vesicular transport of many compounds is partly controlled by cytoskeletal filaments (tau-proteins). By scanning electron microscopy, differences in the distribution of microtubules between sensitive and resistance human gastric carcinoma cells have been found. The tubular network was denser in MDR cells. Some routinely used cytostatic drugs, such as vincristine, induce a perturbation of the cytoskeleton which alters the microtubule organization and remodels the nucleus (Huang, 1994).

Based on observation showing modifications of cytokeratin by mitoxantrone, studies by Bauman et al. (1994) indicate that the expression of cytokeratins 8 and 18 confers a MDR phenotype on cells exposed to mitoxantrone, doxorubicin, methotrexate, colcemid and vincristine. This drug resistance could not be attributed to altered drug accumulation of efflux. It appears that cytokeratin filaments alter the survival response of cells to chemotherapy (but not to ionizing radiation).

Cell membrane modifications result in decreased drug uptake and retention; gel electrophoresis of cytoplasmic membrane proteins point to differences between sensitive and resistant cells (A 2780 human ovarian cancer cells, Mazzoni et al., 1990). Also specific reduction of nuclear uptake for Adriamycin has been reported (in human colon carcinoma clones, Yang et al., 1989). Resistance to Adriamycin in HL60 cells is related to a mechanism by which the drug is first transported to the nucleus but thereafter rapidly exported to the extracellular space, by a transport pathway as yet unknown (Marquardt et al., 1992). A similar situation has been reported for daunorubicin (Remnick et al., 1989); intracellular distribution of this drug by altered binding or exocytosis protects putative nuclear targets.

The binding of many anticancer drugs depends on intracellular pH and their accumulation within the tumor cell can be affected by transmembrane gradients. For ex., the highest concentrations of doxorubicin and daunomycin were found in lysosomes, the most acidic compartments; drug accumulation is reversed by alkaline shifts (Simon et al., 1994).

There is no reliable evidence that decreased drug accumulation is found in non-P-glycoprotein expressing MDR cells. The lack of uniform characteristics among various resistant cancer cell lines and solid tumors is easily explained being the immense heterogeneity of malignant growth.

REFERENCES

Bauman PA, Dalton WS, Anderson JM, Cress AE (1994): Expression of cytokeratin confers multiple drug resistance. *Proc Natl Acad Sci USA* 91:5311-5314
Dietel M (1993): Meeting Report: 2nd Internatl Symposium on Cytostatic Drug Resistance. *Cancer Res* 53:2683-2688
Domènech C, Fierro-Durán G, Rodríguez L, Grau-Oliete MR, Rivera-Fillat MP (1993): Vincristine cellular pharmacokinetic changes associated with multidrug resistance. *Eur J Pharmacol* 248:49-58
Huang J, Leung MF, Sweet P, Slaeter LM (1994): Differential expression of microtubule-associated proteins in vincristine-induced multidrug resistant leukemia cells. *Proc AACR* 35:9
Marquart D, Center MS (1992): Drug Transport Mechanisms in HL60 Cells Isolated for Resistance to Adriamycin: Evidence for Nuclear Drug Accumulation and Redistribution in Resistant Cells. *Cancer Res* 52:3157-3163
Mazzoni A, Trave F, Russo P, Nicolin A, Rustum YM (1990): Generation and Characterization of a Low-Degree Drug-Resistant Human Tumor Cell Line. *Oncology* 47:488-494
Remnick RA, Gervasoni JE, Hindenburg AA, Lutzky J, Krishna S, Rosado M, Taub RN (1989): The subcellular distribution of daunorubicin in drug resistant cell lines that do or do not overexpress the P-glycoprotein. *Proc AACR* 30:511

Sehested M, Skovsgaard T, van deurs B, Winther-Nielsen H (1987): Increased plasma membrane traffic in daunorubicin-resistant P388 leukaemic cells. Effect of daunorubicin and verapamil. *Br J Cancer* 56:747-751

Sehested M, Friche E, Demant EJF, Jensen PB (1991): Drug transport across biomembranes. *J Cancer Res Clin Oncol* 117:89

Simon S, Roy D, Schindler M (1994): Intracellular pH and the control of multidrug resistance. *Proc Natl Acad Sci USA* 91:1128-1132

Sognier MA, Zhang Y, Eberle RL, Belli JA (1992): Characterization of Adriamycin-resistant and radiation-sensitive Chinese hamster cell lines. *Biochem Pharmacol* 444:1859-1868

Vichi P, Tritton TR (1992): Adriamycin: Protection from Cell Death by Removal of Extracellular Drug. *Cancer Res* 52:4135-4138

Yang LY, Trujillo JM (1990): Different mechanisms for multidrug resistance in two models of adriamycin-resistant subclones drived from a human colon carcinoma cell line. *Proc AACR* 30:576

ENZYMES AND DETOXIFICATION

The role of ubiquitous, "physiological" enzyme systems as part of non-specific, highly efficient MDR mechanisms has been acknowledged, but never duly exploited. Numerous reports are collated in Table 4; many avenues have not been pursued further. Xenobiotic metabolizing enzymes function both as activators and detoxifiers of agents involved in cancerogenesis and in chemotherapy. General metabolic pathways are often involved in both and may cause structural and morphological changes in resistant cancer cells (Dufer et al., 1993). Alterations in these pathways may facilitate the breakdown of certain agents or groups of agents into innocuous products, operating in concert with or independently of efflux and transport mechanisms (Bellamy et al., 1988). Enzyme systems can be activated or repressed by various mechanisms; *in vivo*, the effect of dietary fats on a variety of enzyme activities may indirectly influence MDR (Shao et al., 1994). Also, the omnipresent protein phosphorylation systems appear to be altered in MDR (Meyers, 1989).

Enzymes or groups of enzymes are involved in single drug resistance (i.e. not in MDR in its strictest sense); enzyme activities result in metabolic defects in the activation of drugs to cytotoxic compounds. On the other hand, increased enzyme expression augments detoxification (Vendrik et al., 1992) or protects against DNA damage (Fornace et al., 1990). Dietary, hormonal and genetic actors may decisively influence an individual patient's ability to metabolize chemotherapeutic agents. Furthermore, previous or simultaneous treatment with other medications (independent of cancer chemotherapy) may induce drug metabolizing enzyme production in the liver.

Extensive attention is being paid to the glutathione-S-transferases, which are the subject of a separate chapter (2). Multiple families of GST exist and various isoenzymes participate in a broad repertoire of detoxification pathways.

Table 4. Enzyme systems involved in MDR

Enzyme	References
Cytochrome P450 superfamily (CYP)	Wilkinson, 1994
N-acetyltransferases	Wilkinson, 1994
Antioxidant enzymes	Zwelling et al., 1990
Se-dependent gluta- thione peroxidase	Mazzanti et al., 1994
Cytochrome P450IA1	Anttila et al., 1993
NADPH cytochrome P450 reductase	Xu et al., 1994
Superoxide dismutase	Yang et al., 1993 Kramer et al., 1989
Carboxylesterases	Markovic et al., 1993
Thymidylate synthase	Volm et al., 1992
Thymidine kinase sulfatase ß-glucuronidase	Wu et al., 1994
UDP-glucuronyl transferase	Albin et al., 1993
NADH: cytochrome b_5 reductase	Hodnick et al., 1993
Alkylguanine transferase	Kuzmich et al., 1991
Metallothioneins	Kuzmich et al., 1991
Aldehyde dehydrogenases	Kuzmich et al., 1991
O^6-alkylguanine-DNA- alkyltransferase	Joncourt et al., 1991
H^+-ATPase (vacuolar)	Ma et al., 1992
DT diaphorase	O'Dwyer et al., 1992
O^6-methylguanine-DNA- methyl-transferase	Fornace et al., 1990

REFERENCES

Albin N, Massaad L, Toussaint C, Mathieu M-C, Morizet J, Parise O, Gouyette A, Chabot GG (1993): Main Drug-metabolizing Enzyme Systems in Human Breast Tumours and Peritumoral Tissues. *Cancer Res* 53:3541-3546

Anttila S, Horvonen A, Vainio H, Husgafvel-Pursiainen K, Hayes JD, Ketterer B (1993): Immunohistochemical Localization of Glutathione S-Transferases in Human Lung. *Cancer Res* 53:5643-5648

Bellamy WT, Dorr RT, Dalton WS, Alberts DS (1988): Direct Relation of DNA Lesions in Multidrug-resistant Human Myeloma Cells to Intracellular Doxorubicin Concentration. *Cancer Res* 48:6360-6364

Dufer J, Broglio C, Devie-Hubert I, Hennequin E, Delvincourt C, Jardillier JC (1993): Evaluation by image analysis of nuclear changes in multidrug resistant human tumor cells. In: *Biologie prospective* (eds. MM Galteau, G Siest, J Henny), pp 447-450. Paris: John Libey Eurotex

Fornace AJ, Papathanasiou MA, Hollander MCh, Yarosh DB (1990): Expression of the 0^6-Methylguanine-DNA Methyltransferase Gene *MGMT* in MER$^+$ and MER$^-$ Human Tumor Cells. *Cancer Res* 50:7908-7911

Hodnick WE, Sartorelli AC (1993): Reductive Activation of Mitomycin C by NADH: Cytochrome b_5 Reductase. *Cancer Res* 53:4907-4912

Joncourt F, Redmond S, Buser K, Fey M, Tobler A, Brunner K, Gratwohl A, Cerny T (1991): Parallel assessment of several drug resistance parameters in patients with hematological malignancies. *J Cancer Res Clin Oncol* 117:114

Kramer RA, Zahker J (1989): Characterization of intrinsic mechanisms of drug resistance in human colorectal carcinoma cell lines. *Proc AACR* 30:520

Kuzmich S, Tew KD (1991): Detoxification Mechanisms and Tumor Cell Resistance to Anticancer Drugs. *Med Res Rev* 11:185-217

Ma L, Center MS (1992): The Gene Encoding Vacuolate H$^+$-ATPase Subunit C is Overexpressed in Multidrug-Resistant HL60 Cells. *BBRC* 182:675-681

Markovic O, Markovic N (1993): Are Esterases Involved in Multidrug Resistance? *JNCI* 85:1693

Mazzanti R, Fantappie O, Fabrizio P, Pacini S, Ruggiero M (1994): Conferring multiple drug resistance by *mdr1* gene transfection increases susceptibility of irradiation and lipid peroxidation. *Proc AACR* 35:10

Meyers MB (1989): Protein Phosphorylation in Multidrug Resistance Chinese Hamster Cells. *Cancer Comm* 1:233-241

O'Dwyer PJ, Perez RP, Clayton M, Godwin AK, Hamilton TC (1992): Increased DT diaphorase activity and cross-resistance to mitomycin C in a series of cisplatin-resistant human ovarian carcinoma cell lines. *Proc AACR* 33:510

Pfeil D, Bergman J, Fichtner I, Stein U, Hentschel M, Rothe I, Goan S-R (1994): Multidrug Resistance of Murine Leukemia Cells Characterization and Correlation with Cytochrome P-450 Dependent Activities, Cytosolic Calcium and Cell Cycle State. *Anticancer Res* 14:571-576

Sampson KE, McCroskey MC, Abraham I (1993): Identification of a 170 kDa Membrane Kinase with Increased Activity in KB-V1 Multidrug Resistant Cells. *J Cell Biochem* 52:384-395

Shao Y, Pardini RS (1994): Relations between the response of human mammary carcinoma to mitomycin-C and dietary fat in athymic nude mice. *Proc AACR* 35:470

Tagger AY, Wright JA (1988): Molecular and cellular characterization of drug resistant hamster cell lines with alterations in ribonucleotide reductase. *Int J Cancer* 42:760-766

Toussaint C, Albin N, Massaad L, Grunenwald D, Parise O, Morizet J, Gouyette A, Chabot GG (1993): Main Drug- and Carcinogen-metabolizing Enzyme Systems in Human Non-Small Cell Lung Cancer and Peritumoral Tissues. *Cancer Res* 53:4608-4612

Vendrik CPJ, Bergers JJ, De Jong WH, Steerenberg PA (1992): Resistance to cytostatic drugs at the cellular level. *Cancer Chemother Pharmacol* 29:413-429

Volm M, Mattern J (1992): Elevated Expression of Thymidylate Synthase in Doxorubicin Resistant Human Non Small Cell Lung Carcinoma. *Anticancer Res* 12:2293-2296

Wilkinson GR (1994): Xenobiotic metabolism as a factor in individual susceptibility to cancer and treatment. *Proc AACR* 35:698

Wu SJ, Liu XP, Kwock R, Solorzano MM, Avramis VI (1994): Development of azidothymidine resistance in Jurkat T-cells associated with decreased expression of the thymidine kinase gene probably due to hypermethylation of the TK 5' end. *Proc AACR* 35:343

Xu BH, Gupta V, singh SV (1994): Mechanism of differential sensitivity of human bladder cancer cells to mitomycin C and its analogue. *Brit J Cancer* 69:242-246

Yang M, Jiang XR, Blake DR, Zhang Z, Macey MG, Newland AC, Morris CJ (1993): Involvement of anti-oxidant enzymes in multiple drug resistance in a human T-lymphoblastic leukaemia cell line which over-expresses P-glycoprotein. *Int J Oncol* 3:99-104

Zwelling LA, Slovak ML, Doroshow JH, Hinds M, Chan D, Parker E, Mayes J, Sie KL, Meltzer PA, Trent JM (1990): HT1080/DR4: A P-Glycoprotein-Negative Human Fibrosarcoma cell Line Exhibiting Resistance to Topoisomerase II-Reactive Drugs Despite the Presence of a Drug-Sensitive Topoisomerase II. *JNCI* 82:1553-1561

TOPOISOMERASES

Multidrug resistance associated with alterations in DNA topoisomerase II (topo II) activity or amount has been termed atypical MDR by some (Beck, 1989). Because we still do not understand the hierarchy of MDR mechanisms, the time sequence of appearance and their relative importance (which may change in single tumors and vary between different tumors), this term is unjustified. There is as yet no "typical" and therefore no atypical resistance as a defined entity; MDR is multifactorial, if we only look for various mechanisms. Topoisomerases are nuclear enzymes involved in certain phases of DNA metabolism which require topological modifications (Giaccone, 1994). They are both the target of several groups of anticancer drugs (anthracyclines, podophyllotoxines and mitoxantrone) and their alterations are associated with resistance to these drugs.

Alterations in Topo II (and probably other topoisomerases) contribute, directly or indirectly, to MDR (Zwelling et al., 1989) and to transcriptional control of single genes and gene programs (Gieseler et al., 1990). A significant relationship exists between *in vitro* resistance, over-expression of P-glycoprotein and down-regulation of Topo II (Volm et al., 1992). The binding of ATP with topo II may be altered in drug resistant cells (in human leukemia VM-26 cells, Danks et al., 1989). In P388 leukemia cells, topo II catalytic and drug-stimulated cleavage activities are significantly reduced in nuclear extracts from MDR cells (Deffie and Goldenberg, 1989). Frequently, decreased susceptibility to drug-induced DNA damage and reduced levels of Topo II are related (Cole et al., 1991), but a decrease of the latter can not explain the extent of resistance to drugs such as Vinca alkaloids.

In rat glioblastoma cells, sensitive and MDR, low levels of exposure to doxorubicin, etoposide and amsacrine achieves comparable low levels of DNA damage in both cell variants; higher exposure causes the resistant cells to tolerate the drugs, due either to protection of genomic sites sensitive to Topo II interference, alterations in Topo II or alterations of the molecular events leading to cell death after occurence of DNA breaks (Tinguy-Moreaud et al., 1994). The action of drugs on Topo II and the response of the cancer cell is complex; drug-resistant human small cell lung lines (which do not overexpress P-glycoprotein or MRP) contain isoforms of Topo II, which can be distinguished by their M_r and altered subcellular distribution (Feldhoff et al., 1994). Resistant NCI-H69 cells (derived from a small cell lung cancer) may express, in

addition to the "normal" Topo II, an altered enzyme possibly encoded by
a 7.4-kb mRNA, as compared to the usual 6.2-kb mRNA (Binaschi et al.,
1991). On the other hand, in HN_2-resistant Burkitt's lymphoma cells,
topo II activity was reported to be increased (Yalowich and Clariette,
1989); these cells exhibited increased sensitivity to topo II inhibitors.

Chinese hamster lung cells, resistant to 9-OH-ellipticine, contain
a Topo II with "altered" activity, which is stable even in absence of the
drug for over one year (Larsen and Jacquemin-Sablon, 1989).
Adriamycin resistance has been observed in the GLC_4 cell line, attributed
to "changes" in Topo II (again without P-glycoprotein amplification or
overexpression, de Jong et al., 1989). Quantitative differences have been
reported in HCT116 human colon carcinoma and human A549 lung
adenocarcinoma cells, with lower Topo II mRNA levels and decreased
enzyme activitity in the resistant variants (Long et al., 1989). The above
is but a smattering of data which are difficult to constrain to a single
denominator. Reviews of the role of topoisomerases in MDR can be
found in Chapters 5 and 6.

REFERENCES

Beck (1989): Unknotting the Complexities of Multidrug Resistance: The
    Involvement of DNA Topoisomerases in Drug Action and Resistance.
    JNCI 81:1683-1697
Binaschi M, Giaccone G, Gazdar AF, De Isabella P, Astaldi-Ricotti GCB,
    Capranico G, Zunino F (1992): Characterization of a Topoisomerase II
    Gene Rearrangement in a Human Small-Cell Lung Cancer Cell Line.
    JNCI 84:1710-1716
Cole SPC (1991): Non-P-glycoprotein-mediated drug resistance in a lung cancer
    cell line. Presented at the 34th Ann Meet Can Fed Biol Soc (Kingston,
    Ont Canada, June 1991)
Cole SPC, Chanda ER, Dicke FP, Gerlach JH, Mirski SEL (1991): Non-P-
    glycoprotein-mediated Multidrug Resistance in a Small Cell Lung
    Cancer Cell Line: Evidence for Decreased Susceptibility to Drug-
    induced DNA Damage and Reduced Levels of Topoisomerase II.
    Cancer Res 51:3345-3352
Danks MK, Schmidt CA, Deneka DA, Beck WT (1989): Altered interaction of
    ATP with DNA topoisomerase II from VM-26-resistant CEM cells.
    Proc AACR 30:524
Deffie AM, Goldenberg GJ (1989): Altered levels of expression of DNA
    Topoisomerase II in ADR-sensitive and -resistant P388 murine leukemia
    cells. *Proc AACR* 30:514

de Jong S, Zijlstra JG, de Vries EGE, Mulder NH (1989): Reduced drug-induced topoisomerase II-mediated DNA cleavage in an adriamycin resistant cell line. *Proc AACR* 30:526

Feldhoff PW, Mirski SEL, Cole SPC, Sullivan DM (1994): Altered Subcellular Distribution of Topoisomerase IIalpha in a Drug-resistant Human Small Cell Lung Cancer Cell Line. *Cancer Res* 54:756-762

Giaccone G (1994): Small Cell Lung Cancer and Topoisomerases. *Anticancer Res* 14:269-276

Gieseler F, Boege F, Clark M (1990): Alteration of Topoisomerase II Action Is a Possible Molecular Mechanisms of HL-60 Cell Differentiation. *Env Health Perspect* 88:183-185

Larsen AK, Jacquemin-Sablon A (1989): Multiple Resistance Mechanisms in Chinese hamster cells resistant to 9-hydroxy-ellipticine. *Proc AACR* 30:509

Long BH, Wang L, Lorico A, Brattain MG, Casazza AM (1989): Mechanisms of resistance to etoposide (VP16) and tenniposide (VM26) in acquired resistant human colon and lung carcinoma cell line. *Proc AACR* 30:507

Tinguy-Moreaud, de E, Purquier P, Montaudon D, Robert J (1994): Relationships between DNA Damage and Growth Inhibition Induced by Topoisomerase II-Interfering Drugs in Doxorubicin-Sensitive and -Resistant Rat Glioblastoma Cells. *Anticancer Res* 14:99-104

Volm M, Mattern J, Efferth T, Pommerenke EW (1992): Expression of Several Resistance Mechanisms in Untreated Human Kidney and Lung Carcinoma. *Anticancer Res* 12:1063-1068

Yalowich JC, Clariette H (1989): Alkylating agent activity in Etoposide resistant K562 cells containing lower DNA Topoisomerase II activity. *Proc AACR* 30:523

Zwelling L, Slovak M, Chan D, Hinds M, Parker E, Sie KL, Mayes J, Radcliffe A, Trent J (1989): A Novel Topoisomerase II-Associated Resistance Mechanism in Human Fibrosarcoma Cells. *Proc AACR* 30:500

PROTEIN KINASE C

Protein phosphorylation is an essential event in cellular transmembrane signal transduction. Signalling directs diverse and often complex processes, including cellular growth. Numerous enzymes, including the large and still growing family of protein kinases, participate in the control of phosphorylation (Dekker and Parker, 1994).

Signal transduction also plays a role in modulating MDR, perhaps by boosting positive mitogenic pathways that stimulate growth (Posada et al., 1989). Indeed, many MDR cell lines show considerable increase in protein kinase C (PKC), localized entirely in the cytosol (Fine et al., 1993). Another explanation for the mode of action of PKC in multidrug resistance is its regulatory function on P-glycoprotein phosphorylation (Sachs et al., 1994). Transport by P-glycoprotein is a dynamic process, modulated by phosphorylation (Bates et al., 1993). However, overexpression of PKC (in MDR rat fibroblasts) has been reported that was not associated with P-glycoprotein increase but was caused by a decreased rate of drug uptake by the cells (Fan et al., 1992). Other observations found good correlation between P-glycoprotein and PKC activity (Ohkawa et al., 1994). Transfection with PKC cDNA successfully transfers resistance in drug sensitive cells (Gupta et al., 1994b). The assumed regulatory role of PKC in the MDR phenotype has also conflicting aspects: in MOLT-3 human acute lymphoblastic leukemia, MDR cells was found to be down-regulated; this change was localized mainly in the membrane fraction (Schwartz et al., 1989).

Manipulation of PKC by activators and inhibitors have clinical potential as anticancer agents per se or in conjunction with other MDR mechanisms. On Table 5 a brief review of such agents is listed, without claim to be complete. The importance of PKC is reflected in the need for Chapter 9 devoted to this topic.

Table 5. Manipulation of PKC activity by various compounds with the goal to influence MDR.

Compound	Effect	References
Bryostatin 1	activator	Prendville et al., 1994
CGP 41251 (staurosporin derivative)		Fan et al., 1994
antisense PKCO cDNA	inhibitor	Ahmad et al., 1994
UCN-01	inhibitor	Kawakami et al., 1994 Okabe et al., 1994
N-myristolated peptides	competitor	Gupta et al., 1994a Ward et al., 1994

REFERENCES

Ahmad S, Mineta T, Martuza RL, Glazer RI (1994): Antisense expression of protein kinase C alpha inhibits the growth and tumorigenicity of human glioblastoma cells. *Proc AACR* 35:445

Bates SE, Le JS, Dickstein B, Spolyar M, Fojo AT (1993): Differential Modulation of P-Glycoprotein Transport by Protein Kinase Inhibition. *Biochemistry* 37:9156-9164

Dekker LV, Parker PJ (1994): Protein kinase C - a question of specificity. *TIBS* 19:343-435

Fan D, Fidler IJ, Ward NE, Seig Ch, Earnest LE, Housey GM, O'Brian CA (1992): Stable Expression of a cDNA Encoding Rat Brain Protein Kinase C-betaI Confers a Multidrug-Resistant Phenotype on Rat Fibroblasts. *Anticancer Res* 12:661-668

Fan D, Regenass U, Kaufmann H, Beltran PJ, Campbell TE, Fidler IJ (1994):
    The protein-kinase C inhibitor staurosporin derivative CGP 41251
    enhances the in vitro cytotoxicity of doxorubicin against multidrug
    resistant murine fibrosarcoma, murine colon carcinoma and human
    breast carcinoma cells. The 8th NCI-EORTC Symposium on New
    Drugs in Cancer Therapy, p 98, Amsterdam, Netherlands, March 15-18
Fine RL, Sachs CW, Blobe GC, Ahn CH, Hannun YA (1993): Pattern and
    Function of Protein Kinase C isoenzymes in MDR. *Proc AACR* 34:314
Gupta KP, Ward NE, Gravitt KR, O'Brian CA (1994a): Restoration of Drug
    Accumulation in Multidrug-Resistant Human Breast Cancer MCF7 Cells
    by an N-Myristoylated Pseudosubstrate Peptide and an N-myristoylated
    Peptide Substrate Analog of Protein Kinase C. *Proc AACR* 35:445
Gupta S, Kim Ch, Qin Y, Gollapudi S (1994b): Expression of protein kinase C
    isoenzymes in multidrug resistant murine leukemia P388/ADR cells. *Int
    J Oncol* 4:311-315
Kawakami K, Futami H, Hitomi J, Yamaguchi K (1994): Effect of a selective
    protein kinase inhibitor UCN-01 on cell cycle progression of A549 lung
    carcinoma cells. *Proc AACR* 35:445
Ohkawa K, Hatano T, Isonishi S, Takasa K, Joh K, Matsuda M (1994):
    Doxorubicin enhances transient expression of P-glycoprotein and
    modulates activity and isoform expression of protein kinase C in AH66
    rat hepatoma cells. *Int J Oncol* 4:655-659
Okabe M, Akinaga S, Nomura K, Shimizu M, Gomi K (1994): Different cell
    cycle effect of UCN-01 from staurosporine against epidermoid
    carcinoma A431. *Proc AACR* 35:445
Posada J, McKeegan EM, Morin MJ, Tritton TR (1989): Protein kinase C in
    multidrug resistance. *Proc AACR* 30:525
Prendville J, Gescher A, Dickson A, McGown A, Fox B, Crowther D, Courage
    C, Pettit G (1994): Cytosolic PKC receptor levels and whole cell PKC
    isoenzyme expression in a bryostatin-1 resistant cell line. The 8th NCI-
    EORT Symposium on New Drugs in Cancer Therapy. Amsterdam,
    Nethlands, March 15-18
Sachs CW, Blobe GC, Rao US, Fabbro D, Scarborough GA, Hannun YA, Fine
    RL (1994): Phosphorylation of P-glycoprotein by Protein Kinase C
    Isoenzymes beta$_I$ and $_{II}$ Inhibits Drug-stimulated ATPase Activity *in
    vitro*. *Proc AACR* 35:352
Schwartz GK, Arkin H, Holland JF, Ohnuma T (1989): Protein kinase C
    activity and the effects of staurosporine in a multidrug-resistant human
    acute lymphoblastic leukemia cell line. *Proc AACR* 30:531
Ward NE, O'Brian CA (1994): Mechanism of Protein Kinase C Inhibition by
    N-myristoylated peptide Substrate Analogs: Potent and Selective PKC
    Inhibitors with MDR Reversal Activity. *Proc AACR* 35:445

MISCELLANEOUS

Cancer cells appear to respond to suboptimal conditions with defense mechanisms which decrease their vulnerability and permit survival until "things improve". A successful maneuvre is the decrease in doubling time, the result of a low percentage of cells in S-phase and an increasing proportion of the dormant phase of the cell cycle. Many different factors contribute to such a response, which entails not only simple survival in an adverse environment, but also drug resistance.

Hypoxia is such a resistance-inducer (Sakata et al., 1991) in EMT6/Ro mammary tumor cells; these cells, when returned to normal oxygen tension, loose their resistance (which is not related to P-glycoprotein). Chinese hamster ovary cells exposed to short-term and long-term hypoxia develop ADR resistance at different levels; recovery in air before drug exposure resulted in loss of resistance (Wilson et al., 1989).

The growth conditions of cultured cells play a distinctive role in the appearance of the MDR phenotype. When cells are grown in monolayers, drug resistance in EMT-6 murine mammary tumor cells is not expressed. Deductions made from cell cultures, both from normal or tumor cells (heterogeneous or cloned) are weakened by the fact that - at least in some tumor models - drug-resistant phenotypes are not (fully?) expressed when the cells were grown in monolayer cultures. Expression of MDR, similar to the situation observed *in vivo*, was obtained when the cells were grown under three-dimensional conditions. Once cells are grown as multicellular tumor spheroids, typical patterns of cross-drug resistance can be observed (Kobayashi et al., 1993). This is by no means a general phenomenon. In B16-F-10 melanoma cells, levels of *mdr1* mRNA and P-glycoprotein were higher in sparse cultures and, when injected subcutaneously in mice, in cells from small tumors. The relative *mdr1* expression is influenced by cell density and was found to be down-regulated in the CT-26 murine colon and KM12 human colon cancer cells (Yoon et al., 1994, Fan et al., 1994).

Activation of growth factor pathways in MDR cells may enhance drug resistance or provide mitogenic stimuli for MDF-7 cells to recover after drug exposure (Dickstein et al., 1993). An increase in the expression of EGF receptors occured early in the selection for drug resistance. Transferrin also belongs among the growth promoting factors; most, if not all, tumor cells have up-regulated or overexpressed transferrin receptors. Drug resistant cells (such as HL60-R and K562-R) have been found to manifest more receptors than their drug-sensitive counterparts (Barabas and Faulk, 1993). There was no correlation between P-glycoprotein and transferrin receptor overexpression. Some cell lines show the characteristic MDR phenotype, but do not over-express the *mdr1* gene and do not exhibit a significant intracellular drug retention. In the search for a substance which would reverse or at least modify this "atypical" MDR< tyrosine-kinase inhibitors (such as genistein) have been found effective in K562/ADM cell cultures (Takeda et al., 1994).

In actinomycin D-resistant Chinese hamster lung cells (DC-3F/AD X), there is an increase in epidermal growth factor receptor numbers with increased P-glycoprotein expression; it appears that the latter may be modulated by the signalling system transduced by ligand-activated EGF receptors (Meyers et al., 1993). NIH3T3 fibroblasts have been investigated for MDR after transfection with fibroblast growth factor (bFGF), which lacks a conventional signal sequence for secretion. Aberrant growth factor expression regulates gene amplification and can markedly alter drug resistance (Huang and Wright, 1994).

Heat shock proteins (hsp27) are thought to protect cells from various external toxic agents. When induced by elevated temperatures, cultured breast cancer cells display resistance to Doxorubicin (but not to other commonly used chemotherapeutic agents). A MCF-7 mammary carcinoma line with amplified endogenous hsp27 was also found to be higly resistant to Doxorubicin; these cells, when transfected with an antisense hsp27 construct become sensitive again (Oesterreich et al., 1993). Inhibition of cell-surface proteinases (for ex. with alpha-1-anti-trypsin) can negatively influence the growth of many normal and malignant cells in culture. In a human colon carcinoma (JACC 19) and a melanoma cell line (MM96), various degrees of sensitivity and the reversible appearance of resistant cultures have been described (Scott and Tse, 1994).

The relationship between cell membrane permeability and specific chemotherapeutic drugs is far from being completely understood. By definition, MDR is basically cross-resistant to multiple lipophilic compounds and decreased drug accumulation in the target cell can be the result of impaired transport into the cell; the role of membrane lipid constituents may be underestimated. Differences in the content of some lipid membrane components between drug sensitive cells and their MDR sublines have been described (Biedler and Meyers, 1988). Drug influx might be altered by modifications of membrane lipids; changes in cholesterol or the cholesterol:phospholipid ratio are related to reduced drug entry in some MDR cells. Cholesterol depletion in VCR/P60 and VCR/P200 murine leukemic cells resulted in an increase of vincristine uptake (Pallarés-Trujillo et al., 1993). It appears that increased levels of cholesterol/phospholipid at least partially account for lower vincristine accumulation in MDR cells.

In an indirect way, some gene products associated with the blockage of apoptosis play a role in drug resistance by cancer cells. Expression of the *bcl-2* gene can protect cells from a variety of apoptotic stimuli; *bcl-2* products selectively interact with other family members and with many cellular proteins, via homodimer/multimer formation. While the exact mechanisms of action are not understood, high levels of *bcl-2* protein may result from loss of transcriptional repression by the wild tumor supressor p53. In general, failure of cells to die when they should may contribute to malignant growth. If this programmed death of cells which are aging, superfluous or diseased is prevented, immortalization may occur; such cells may tolerate otherwise lethal substances and may remain, in large numbers, in a growth-arrested state - which in turn makes them less vulnerable to a variety of drugs (Chiou et al., 1994). The emerging role of *bcl-2* in multidrug resistance is discussed in Chapters 10 and 11.

REFERENCES

Barabas K, Faulk PW (1993): Transferrin receptors associated with drug resistance in cancer cells. *BBRC* 197:702-708

Biedler JL, Meyers MB (1988): Multidrug resistance (vinca alkaloids, actinomycin D, and anthracycline antibiotics). In: *Drug Resistance in Mammalian Cells* (Ed. Gupta RS) Vol II pp 57-88 CRC Press, Boca Raton

Chiou S-K, Rao L, White E (1994): Bcl-2 Blocks p53-Dependent Apoptosis. *Mol Cell Biol* 14:2556-2563

Dickstein B, Valverius EM, Wosikowski K, Saceda M, Pearson JW, Martin MB, Bates SE (1993): *J Cell Physiol* 157:110-118

Huang A, Wright JA (1994): Fibroblast growth factor mediated alterations in drug resistance, and evidence of gene amplification. *Oncogene* 9:491-499

Kobayashi H, Man S, Graham CH, Kapitain SJ, Teicher BA, Kerbel RS (1993): Acquired multicellular-mediated resistance to alkylating agents in cancer. *Proc Natl Acad Sci* 90:3294-3298

Meyers MB, Yu P, Mendelsohn J (1993): Crosstalk between epidermal growth factor receptor and P-glycoprotein in actinomycin D - resistant Chinese hamster lung cells. *Biochem Pharmacol* 46:1841-1848

Oesterreich S, Wing Ch-N, Qiu M, Hilsenback SG, Osborne CK, Fuqua SAW (1993): The Small Heat Shock protein hsp27 is Correlated with Growth and Drug Resistance in Human Breast Cancer Cell Lines. *Cancer Res* 53:4443-4448

Pallares-Trujillo J, Domenech C, Grau-Oliete MR, Rivera-Fillat MP (1993): Role of cell cholesterol in modulating vincristine uptake and resistance. *Int J Cancer* 55:667-671

Sakata K, Kwok TT, Murphy BJ, Laderoute KR, Gordon GR, Sutherland RM (1991): Hypoxia-induced drug resistance: comparison to P-glycoprotein-associated drug resistance. *Br J Cancer* 64:809-814

Scott KG, Tse CA (1994): Changes in sensitivity of human tumour cells to growth inhibition by proteinase inhibitors. *Cell Biol Internatl* 18:89-93

Takeda Y, Nisho K, Niitani H. Saijo N (1994): Reversal of Multidrug Resistance by tyrosine-kinase inhibitors in a non-P-glycoprotein-mediated Multidrug-Resistant cell line. *Int J Cancer* 57:229-239

Wilson RE, Keng PC, Sutherland RM (1989): Drug Resistance in Chinese Hamster Ovary Cells During Recovery From Severe Hypoxia. *JNCI* 81:1235-1240

Yoon SS, Dong Z, Fan D, Bucana CD, Fidler IJ (1994): *Mdr1* and P-glycoprotein expression levels are regulated by tumor cell density and tumor size. *Proc AACR* 35:346

2. THE ROLE OF GLUTATHIONE S-TRANSFERASES IN DRUG RESISTANCE

William T. Bellamy

Chemotherapy, in specific clinical settings, is an effective modality of cancer chemotherapy. Failure of a chemotherapeutic regimen to induce a response may be due to many different factors. Foremost among these is the inability of the drugs to reach the critical cellular target. In this regard, physiological factors may play a large role in the successful outcome of therapy: absorption, distribution, metabolism, and elimination are key principles in successful cancer chemotherapy. Whether the resistance is intrinsic or acquired, it is necessary to understand the underlying molecular mechanisms in order to devise rational therapeutic approaches aimed at circumventing the resistance. Studies carried out using cultured tumor cell models and other systems have established that a variety of mechanisms can contribute to drug resistance (Bellamy et al., 1994; Woolley and Tew, 1988). The glutathione S-transferases (GSTs) may play an important role in protecting the cell from the toxic effects of a wide variety of electrophilic compounds including herbicides, insecticides, and carcinogens as well as antineoplastic agents (Beckett and Hayes, 1993; Hayes and Wolf, 1988). This chapter will focus on our current understanding of the involvement of these enzymes in drug resistance and as tumor markers. In addition, potential means of manipulating these proteins in order to affect the outcome of cancer chemotherapy will be discussed.

PROPERTIES OF GST

The glutathione S-transferases (EC.2.5.1.18) were first described by Booth et al. (1961). They are present in bacteria, yeast, nematodes, insects, fish, birds, and mammals and constitute a complex supergene family that collectively metabolizes chemotherapeutic drugs, carcinogens, environmental pollutants, and a broad spectrum of electrophilic compounds. Both cytosolic and membrane-bound forms exist in mammalian cells. One of their major functions is to catalyze conjugation reactions between glutathione (GSH) and a variety of electrophilic, organic molecules. The result of this reaction is the conversion of these lipophilic compounds into more polar glutathionyl conjugates which are, in most cases, inactivated and excreted. For a more through discussion of the properties of the glutathione S-transferases, the reader is referred to several recent reviews on the subject (Beckett and Hayes, 1993; Hayes et al., 1993; Mannervik et al., 1993).

Table 1. Biophysical Properties of Cytosolic GST Subunits

Subunit	Class	Isoelectric Point	M_r (kDa)	Substrates
A1	α	8.9	25.9	Cumene hydroperoxide
A2	α	8.4	25.9	Cumene hydroperoxide
M1a one;	μ	6.1	26.7	trans-4-Phenyl-3-buten-2-trans-stilbene oxide
M1b one;	μ	5.5	26.6	trans-4-Phenyl-3-buten-2-trans-stilbene oxide
M2	μ	5.3	26.0	1,2-Dichloro-4-nitrobenzene
M3	μ	5.0	26.3	4-hydroxynon-2-enal
Pi	π	4.7	24.7	Ethacrynic acid; acrolein
T1	θ	---	---	1,2-Epoxy-3-(p-nitrophenoxy) propane
T2	θ	25.1	---	Menaphthyl sulfate

(adapted from Mannervik 1985 and Beckett and Hayes 1994)

STRUCTURE

The cytosolic GSTs are homo- or hetero-dimers composed of subunits with a molecular weight of 23- to 29-kD (Mannervik and Jensson, 1982). Individual isoenzymes within a given GST family may share a common subunit and that the overlapping activities of distinct isoenzymes are often due to the presence of a specific subunit common between two, or more, GSTs. The membrane-bound microsomal GSTs differ from their cytosolic counterparts in that they appear to form functional trimers composed of identical 17-kD subunits (Morgenstern et al., 1985). Reinemer et al. (1991) were the first to report on the 3-D structure of glutathione S-transferase. Their report described the atomic detail of GST-π and at the present time there is at least one representative structure of each of the three major cytosolic classes (Ji et al., 1992; Johnson et al., 1993; Reinemer et al., 1991). An overall structural similarity exists between the GST-π, μ and α classes (Sinning et al., 1993). The active site contains two distinct functional regions: a hydrophilic G-site which binds glutathione; and an adjacent hydrophobic H-site which binds the electrophilic substrate (Dirr et al., 1994). For a more through discussion of the x-ray crystal structures of the glutathione S-transferases see Dirr et al. (1994).

NOMENCLATURE

In all mammalian species the GST are represented by a large number of isoenzymes. Initial attempts to classify the enzymes by the chemical structure of the electrophilic substrates resulted in the use of such terms as aryl transferase, alkyl transferase, aralkyl transferase, alkene transferase, and epoxide transferase. Such a scheme was found to be inadequate as it became clear that there were overlapping activities of the various GST isoenzymes. Subsequent nomenclature has relied on physical and structural properties and, more recently, a genetic classification to reflect subunit composition (Jakoby et al., 1984). In an attempt to unify the GST nomenclature, Mannervik et al. (1992) have proposed a species-independent system in which each genetically distinct subunit has its own designation and is classified by gene family. Most importantly, the designations given to individual isoenzymes in this system reflect their subunit composition, and allelic variants, encoded at the same gene locus, are distinguished by letters.

Table 2. Human GST Nomenclature

Class	Subunit Designation	Greek Letter	Genetic Designation	Current Nomenclature*
Alpha	B_1B_1	ϵ	GST2, type 1	A1-1
Alpha	B_1B_2	δ	GST2, type 1-2	A1-2
Alpha	B_2B_2	$\alpha,\ \beta,\ \gamma$	GST2, type 2	A2-2
Mu	$N_{1a}N_{1a}$	μ	GST1, type 2	M1a-1a
Mu	$N_{1a}N_{1b}$		GST1, type 1-2	M1a-1b
Mu	$N_{1b}N_{1b}$	ψ	GST1, type 1	M1b-1b
Mu	$N_{1a}N_2$			M1a-2
Mu	$N_{1b}N_2$			M1b-2
Mu	N_2N_2		GST4	M2-2
Mu	N_2N_3			M2-3
Mu	N_3N_3	ϕ	GST5	M3-3
Pi	YfYf	π	GST3	P1-1
Theta	T_1T_1	θ		T1-1
Theta	T_2T_2			T2-2
Microsomal				
Microsomal				

*According to the system proposed by Mannervik et al. (1992)
(Based on Beckett and Hayes, 1994)

GENETICS AND REGULATION

The cloning of the GST genes has resulted in a substantial advance in our understanding of the structure and genetic diversity of these enzymes. GST 1, GST 2, and GST 3, which are the loci encoding enzymes of the mu-class, alpha-class, and pi-class GST, respectively (Board 1981; Strange et al., 1984). There are at least three more gene loci, termed GST 4, GST 5, and GST 6 (Laisney et al., 1984; Suzuki et al., 1987). A new class of human GST has been described (Hiratsuka et al., 1990; Hussey and Hayes, 1992; Meyer et al., 1991) which is catalytically and structurally distinct from alpha-, mu-, and pi-classes and has been designated theta. The alpha-, mu-, pi-. and theta-class GSTs share some homology and hence appear to have arisen from a common ancestral gene. Amino acid sequencing and cDNA cloning have demonstrated that the microsomal GST shares no homology with the cytosolic enzymes (DeJong et al., 1988).Thus, there are at least four gene families encoding the cytosolic transferases and an additional one encoding the microsomal form.

The regulation of GST is complex as they are subject to both developmental control and tissue specific expression. Pickett and his colleagues have identified cis-acting elements in the 5' flanking region of the rat Ya subunit gene. One of these elements is located between nucleotides -722 and -682 and responds to planar aromatic compounds such as β-napthoflavone and 3-methylcholanthrene (Rushmore et al., 1991). This site is distinct from the xenobiotic responsive element (XRE) found in the cytochrome P450 1A1 gene and has been designated the antioxidant responsive element (ARE) (Rushmore et al., 1990, 1991). An additional regulatory element responsive to planar aromatic compounds was found and determined to be identical to the XRE in the P4501A1 gene (Rushmore et al., 1990). Friling et al. (1990, 1992) have identified an additional cis-acting element in the 5' flanking region of the murine Ya subunit which was designated the electrophilic-responsive element (EpRE). It is related to the AP-1 binding site and is activated by a Fos/Jun heterodimeric complex (Friling et al., 1992). In addition to activation of EpRE, Bergelson et al. (1994) have demonstrated that, in the rat, the ARE is also activated by Fos/Jun. Induction of the GST Ya by phenobarbital is mediated by the regulatory elements EpRE and ARE (Pinkus et al., 1993).

Regulation of the rat pi-class GST gene has been studied by Muramatsu and his colleagues, who have identified several regulatory elements (Okuda et al., 1987; Sakai et al., 1988). Two enhancers were located 2.5 and 2.2 kb upstream form the transcription start site and have been designated GST-P enhancers I and II (GPEI and GPEII). GPEI contains an AP-1 binding site while GPEII contains two of the SV40 and one of the polyoma virus enhancer sequences. The rat pi gene also contains a silencing element approximately 400 bp upstream from the cap site (Imagawa et al., 1991). It binds at least two nuclear proteins, one of which has been designated SF-A (silencing factor A). This element has been found not only in the rat but in human and mouse cell lines suggesting that it acts as a general regulator of basal expression (Imagawa et al., 1991). Promoter analysis of the human GST-π gene revealed a TATA box, two G/C boxes, and putative phorbol ester and ras -responsive elements (Cowell et al., 1988). GST-π appears to be ras-responsive as it can be induced in rat liver epithelial cells transformed with N-ras (Power et al., 1987) or following he expression of an inducible Ha-ras gene (Li et al., 1988).

Little is known about the regulation of the mu, theta, or microsomal GSTs. In humans, the mu class displays a polymorphic expression with 50-55% of individuals expressing this isoenzyme (Hussey et al., 1987; Seidegard et al., 1985; Zhong et al., 1991). The cloning and sequencing of the GST-mu gene (GSTM1) has led to the discovery that its polymorphic expression is due to a deletion of the entire GSTM1 locus (Seidegard et al., 1988). Recent work with the theta class has revealed that it to is expressed in a polymorphic manner (Pemble et al., 1994).

GST ACTIVITIES

The multiple isozymes of GST have been found to catalyze reactions of a very diverse group of electrophilic, hydrophobic compounds (Mannervik 1985). Within the same isozyme class, the properties of the GST isoenzymes are highly conserved across species; however, between isozyme classes they diverge significantly, even within the same species. The fundamental catalytic action of GST is to facilitate the formation of the thiolate anion, GS-, which can, in turn, attack an electrophilic center forming a GS-conjugate. Although reactions of this general type may occur non enzymatically, the rates are significantly increased through GST catalysis. GST is believed to play an important role in the protection of cells from reactive epoxides by catalyzing the addition of GSH to the epoxide group. One of the most important naturally occurring hepatocarcinogens, aflatoxin B1, is metabolized to a carcinogenic 8,9-epoxide metabolite which may be detoxified by GST (Ramsdell and Eaton 1990). Benzo[a]pyrene, benz[a]anthracene, and 2-acetylaminofluorene are additional carcinogens which may form GSH conjugates (Ramsdell and Eaton 1990; Warholm et al., 1983). Although the GSTs are generally viewed as playing a protective role in the cell, they may also catalyze reactions leading to increased toxicity. Two examples of such a reaction are the metabolism of 1,2-dibromoethane and 1,2-dichloroethane which are biotransformed to reactive sulfur mustards (Igwe 1986).

Through its peroxidase activity, GST serves to protect the cell from reactive oxygen species, such as superoxide anion, hydrogen peroxide, and the hydroxyl radical, which are continuously produced during normal aerobic metabolism and through the metabolism of quinone-containing xenobiotic compounds (Ketterer et al., 1990).

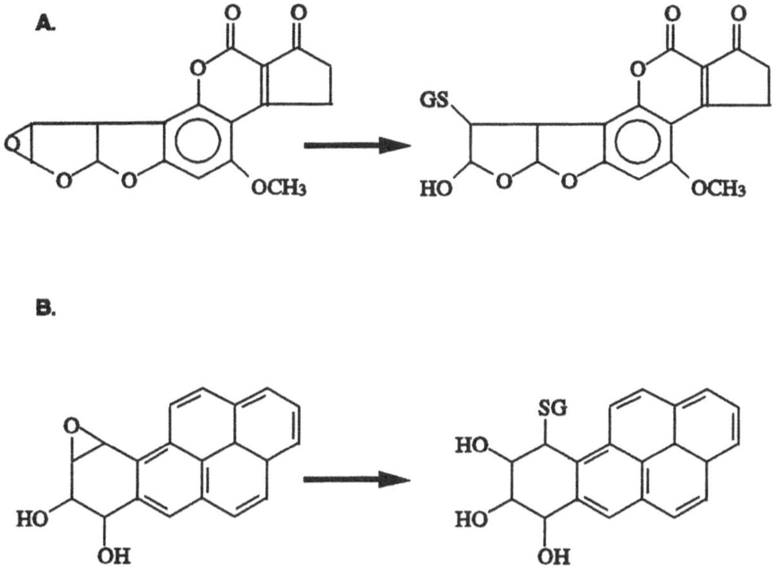

Figure 1. Example of GST-mediated detoxification reaction showing the formation of glutathionyl conjugates of epoxide-containing carcinogenss. (a) aflatoxin B1 8,9-epoxide; (b) benzo[a]pyrene-7,8-diol-9,10-oxide.

Originally referred to as "ligandins", the glutathione S-transferases possess a hydrophobic domain which binds numerous xenobiotic as well as endogenous ligands. This binding function appears to be extremely important in the storage of xenobiotics, including many drugs, as well as heme and bile acids (Hayes et al., 1979). Most of these ligands are hydrophobic and are bound noncovalently by GST. However, a number of reactive metabolites formed from carcinogens are bound covalently by GST. Cytosolic GSTs are not alone in their ability to bind compounds as the microsomal GSTs have been shown to bind metabolites of benzo[a]pyrene, *trans*-stilbene oxide, and phenol (Morgenstern et al., 1987). The binding properties of the transferases have led to the suggestion that GST may act as intracellular transporter of proteins or receptors.

Thus, the GSTs may protect a cell from toxic insults via several mechanisms including the formation of mercapturic acids, the detoxification of reactive peroxides, and the binding and sequestration of reactive compounds.

EXPRESSION OF GST ISOENZYMES

GST Alpha

Expression of the various GST isoenzymes reveals a developmental and tissue-specific pattern. The liver contains the highest level of GST activity and within the liver, the basic or GST alpha-class predominates. In addition to the liver, GST-α is expressed in the kidney, testis and adrenal gland (Aceto et al., 1989; Meikle et al., 1992; Tateoka et al., 1987). Immunohistochemistry has demonstrated that the tissue distribution of the GST-α is similar in both fetal and adult livers. Most hepatocytes have been shown to express the GST-α but Kupffer cells, biliary epithelia, and the biliary canaliculi are generally negative (Hiley et al., 1988; Strange et al., 1989). In the kidney, the expression of the B1 and B2 subunits show a pattern similar to that found in the liver, with lower levels being observed in the fetal period than in the adult. In the lung, expression of GST-α does not appear to be altered during development (Beckett et al., 1990).

GST Mu

Kamisaka et al. (1975) first identified a neutral GST isolated from human liver in 1980. Warholm et al. (1980) subsequently showed that this isoenzyme was distinguished by its high activity toward the substrate trans-4-phenyl-3-buten-2-one. GST mu isoenzymes have been isolated and purified from several extrahepatic tissues including skeletal muscle, brain, heart and aorta (Board et al., 1988; Suzuki et al., 1987; Tsuchida et al., 1990). A distinguishing feature of the GST-μ class is its marked polymorphic expression as mentioned previously. This observation has taken on an added significance in light of the observation that many carcinogens are detoxified by the mu-class isoenzyme.

GST Pi

In humans, the pi class of GST is widely distributed and represents the most thoroughly characterized of all extrahepatic GSTs. It has been purified from a number of sources, including placenta, lung and erythrocytes (Guthenberg et al., 1979; Koskelo et al., 1981; Marcus et al., 1978). Expression of this isoenzyme has been shown to decrease significantly in the liver during development with adult levels much lower than those found in the fetus (Strange et al., 1989). Although hepatocytes display a progressively lower level of GST-π expression during development, the bile duct epithelia remain strongly positive even in the adult (Strange et al., 1990). Renal expression of pi-class GST is similar to that of the GST-α class. GST-π is, quantitatively, the most predominant GST isoenzyme in the lung, but as in the liver, the level of expression is higher in the fetal period than in the adult (Beckett et al., 1990). There has been considerable interest in the overexpression of this particular GST isoenzyme in drug resistant human tumors, particularly in relation to the multidrug resistance phenotype.

GST Theta

The existence of a fourth class of cytosolic GST, known as the theta class, has been discovered (Hiratsuka et al., 1990; Meyer et al., 1991), and the gene cloned (0gura et al., 1991). The isolation of rat and human cDNA clones encoding the theta-class GSTs has unequivocally demonstrated that these enzymes represent a separate family of cytosolic GST (0gura et al., 1991; Pemble et al., 1994). It is not known how many theta-class GST exist in the human. They are involved in the conjugation of halomethanes with glutathione, a reaction which leads to the production of reactive, genotoxic sulfur mustards (Meyer et al., 1991). As with the mu class, there is a polymorphic expression of the theta, with 70% of the population classified as "conjugators" and 30% as "non-conjugators" (Pemble et al., 1994). The consequence of this polymorphism is not known at the present.

Microsomal GST

The isolation and purification of a unique membrane-bound GST in rat liver preparations has been reported by several groups (Morgenstern et al., 1982; Kraus and Gross 1979). This GST isoenzyme has specific activity toward the substrate 1-chloro-2,4-dinitrobenzene which can be increased following exposure to with N-ethylmaleimide (Morgenstern and DePierre, 1983). The cytosolic GSTs are not induced by this agent, but rather, are inactivated by it and it was this observation that led to the recognition of the existence of the microsomal GST. Microsomal GSTs have been implicated in the metabolism of the antineoplastic agent mitoxantrone (Wolf et al., 1986).

GST AS A TUMOR MARKER

Expression of GST isozymes has attracted considerable attention in human tumors because of its potential usefulness as a marker of malignant transformation with particular emphasis placed on the pi and mu classes.

GST-π

GST-pi has been demonstrated to be expressed in malignant tumors derived from colon, kidney, breast, lung, uterus, ovary, stomach, and skin and has been observed to be elevated in tumors relative to the surrounding normal tissue (Clapper et al., 1991a; Dillio et al., 1985; Eimoto et al., 1988; Harrison et al., 1989; Howie et al., 1990b; Kantor et al., 1991; Kodate et al., 1986; Niitsu et al., 1989; Shea et al., 1988; Sasano et al., 1993; Tsuchida et al., 1989; Tsutsumi et al., 1987). Using immunohistochemistry, Kodate et al. (1986) observed that GST-pi was overexpressed in 88% of colonic carcinomas, including both differentiated and undifferentiated adenocarcinomas as well as in 47% of adenomas. Normal colonic epithelia was not found to express this isoenzyme. Tsutsumi et al (1987) made similar observations in a study of 100 gastric carcinoma patients. They found the pi isoenzyme was expressed at high levels in the tumor while normal parietal cells showed only a slight staining. Sasano et al. (1993) found an increased expression of GST-π in 6 of 17 patients with esophageal carcinoma but found no correlation between the amount or pattern of GST-π expression and the clinical findings in these cases, thus suggesting that in patients with esophageal carcinoma, GST-π may be a marker of increased carcinogen exposure rather than of developed esophageal carcinoma. Shiratori et al. (1987) reported strong immunohistochemical staining for GST-π in over 90% of invasive uterine carcinomas. A subsequent study by Riou et al. (1991), also demonstrated an elevation in the expression of GST-π in cervical carcinoma but they did not find a correlation with clinical progression. Howie et al (1990b) found an approximately 2-fold elevation in GST-π expression in carcinomas of the lung, colon and stomach as compared to matched normal tissues,

Table 3. Human tumors with elevated GST-π expression

Tumor	Reference
Breast	Di Illo et al. 1985
Colon	Kodate et al. 1986;
	Howie et al. 1990b;
	Clapper et al. 1991a;
	Kantor et al. 1991
Esophagus	Sasano et al. 1993
Kidney	Harrison et al. 1989
Lung	Howie et al. 1990b;
	Hida et al. 1994
Melanocytes	Kantor et al. 1991
Stomach	Tsutsumi et al. 1987;
	Howie et al. 1990b
Uterus	Shiratori et al. 1987;
	Riou et al. 1991

but did not observe any alteration in its expression in the kidney or liver.

It has been suggested that the measurement of serum GST-π concentration might provide a useful measure for various solid tumors. Several groups have reported elevated serum GST-π concentrations in a number of gastrointestinal cancers (Niitsu et al., 1989; Tsuchida et al., 1989). Hida et al. (1994) have suggested that not only is serum GST-π a good marker for non-small cell lung carcinoma, but that pretreatment values may be predictive of successful therapy with alkylating agents such as cisplatin. Howie et al. (1988) however, have shown that during the normal clotting process, platelets released large amounts of GST-π into the serum which resulted in significant changes in serum GST-π values. They concluded that serum was inappropriate for measuring GST-π and suggested that plasma may be a more suitable matrix. Measurement of GST α and π levels in bronchoaveolar lavage fluid obtained from patients undergoing broncopscopy may have some diagnostic importance as suggested by Howie et al. (1990a). They reported that in patients with benign lesions of the lung, the concentrations of the B1, B2, and pi GST subunits in lavage fluid were not significantly different between normal and diseased lung but in patients with bronchogenic cancer the concentrations of these three subunits were significantly higher in fluid obtained from the malignant area than in that obtained from a normal area of the same lung.

GST-μ

As mentioned in the previous section, GST-μ is expressed in approximately 50% -55% of the human population (Board et al., 1990; Strange et al., 1984). A characteristic feature of this class of GST isoenzymes is a relatively high activity toward mutagenic epoxides, such as benzo[a]pyrene-4,5-oxide and styrene-7,8-oxide. This has led to the suggestion that individuals lacking expression of this isoenzyme may be more susceptible to the toxic effects of such compounds. Using the substrate *trans*-stilbene oxide as a measure of GST-μ activity, Seidegard et al. (1986, 1990) demonstrated significant differences between the distribution of this isoenzyme in populations of control smokers and in lung cancer patients. Other studies carried out in smokers have also observed an increased risk for lung cancer in those individuals who lacked GST-μ expression (Nakachi et al., 1993; Nazar-Stewart et al., 1993). Strange et al. (1991) found similar results when they examined the expression of GST-μ in a group of patients with adenocarcinoma of the stomach or colon. Bell et al. (1993) have suggested that lack of GST-μ expression was attributable to perhaps 25% of bladder carcinomas. Confirming the findings of Bell, Chern et al. (1994), also studying bladder cancer, found that the lack of GST-μ expression correlated with grade III disease but not with grade I or II. Findings such as these have led to the suggestion that expression of mu-class GST may be used as a marker for susceptibility of an individual to various cancers. Not all studies support these findings however, and there are several reports in the literature containing contradictory evidence concerning the expression of mu-class GST and the increased risk of cancer (Brockmoller et al., 1993, Peters et al., 1990; Zhong et al., 1991). The reasons for discrepancies in the findings of these studies is not clear at the present. Many of the studies of the GSTM1 null phenotype have examined its effect on the risk of lung cancers. Tobacco smoke contains many carcinogens, including the polyaromatic hydrocarbons, which can potentially be detoxified by the glutathiones transferases. In the lung, the GST-π isoenzyme predominates and, as discussed by Ketterer (1994), if the detoxification of polycyclic aromatics is occurring promimally in the lung, then the lack of the GST-μ expression should have little effect. It has been hypothesized that the effect observed in individuals with the null phenotype may be the result of diol epoxide metabolites which have been generated in the liver, where the lack of GST-μ expression would allow for the build up and escape of these metabolites into the general circulation where they could thus exert a site-specific carcinogenic effect.

GST AND DRUG RESISTANCE

The GSTs are involved in the metabolism of several antineoplastic agents including the nitrogen mustards, BCNU, and cyclophosphamide and generally results in the inactivation of the drug. With compounds such as the nitrogen mustards, the reaction proceeds by GSH displacement of chloride via an aziridine intermediate, resulting in the inactivation of the compound. Melphalan and chlorambucil have both been shown to form GSH conjugates (Bolton et al., 1991; Ciaccio et al., 1990; Dulik et al., 1986, 1987). Melphalan has been observed to be converted to its mono- and di-glutathionyl conjugates in a reaction catalyzed by sepharose-bound liver cytosolic GST, although under the conditions of this study it was not possible to discern which isoenzyme was responsible for carrying out the reaction (Dulik et al., 1986). In mouse liver preparations, Bolton et al. (1991) found that the GST-α isoenzyme was responsible for conjugating melphalan with GSH and that the GST-π or GST-μ had little effect. The denitrosation of the nitrosourea BCNU is also catalyzed by GST and may occur either by direct denitrosation through the formation of S-nitroso glutathione (Williams 1985) or by indirect denitrozation proceeding through GSH

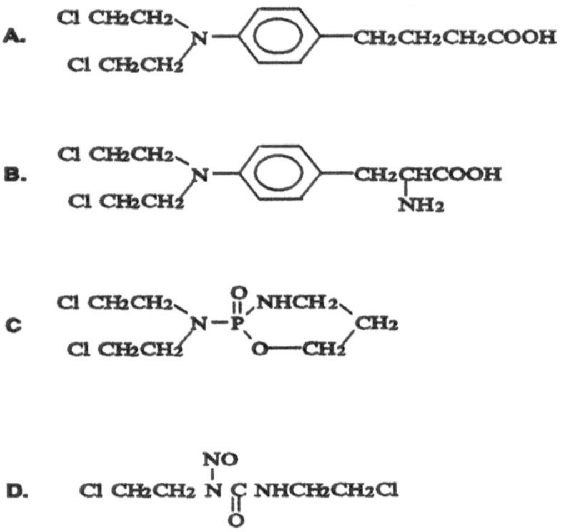

A. Cl CH₂CH₂\N—⟨benzene ring⟩—CH₂CH₂CH₂COOH
   Cl CH₂CH₂/

B. Cl CH₂CH₂\N—⟨benzene ring⟩—CH₂CHCOOH
   Cl CH₂CH₂/   NH₂

C. Cl CH₂CH₂\   O NHCH₂\
         N—P   CH₂
   Cl CH₂CH₂/   O—CH₂/

D.   NO
   Cl CH₂CH₂ N C NHCH₂CH₂Cl
              ‖
              O

Figure 2. Alkylating agents known to serve as substrates for GST. (a) chlorambucil; (b) melphalan; (c) cyclophosphamide; (d) BCNU

conjugation to one of the chloro-bearing carbon atoms with subsequent loss of the nitroso group (Talcott and Levin 1983). GST may protect against the toxic side effects of cyclophosphamide by conjugating GSH with acrolein, the metabolite of cyclophosphamide which has been associated with hemorrhagic cystitis due to this drug (Berhane and Mannervik 1990).

A number of alkylator-resistant sublines have been shown to overexpress GST activity (Buller et al., 1987; Carmichael et al. 1988; Evans et al., 1987; Howie et al., 1990b; Hao et al., 1994; Lewis et al., 1989; Robson et al., 1987; Satoh et al., 1985; Shea et al., 1988; Wang

and Tew 1985). Clapper et al. (1991b) have demonstrated that certain members of the GST alpha family can be selectively induced by alkylating agents. In a series of four human melanoma cell lines, each selected for resistance to a different alkylating agent, Wang et al. (1989) found an overexpression of GST-π isoenzyme. However, there was a lack of cross resistance among these four cell lines to the different alkylating agents used in the study, thus causing them to conclude that, while GST-π may be contributing somewhat, it was not the predominant mechanism of resistance in any of these cells. The evidence to date suggests that the alpha class of GST plays an important role in determining the sensitivity or resistance of cells to alkylating agents such as melphalan and the nitrogen mustards while the rodent GST-μ class isoenzymes have been shown to possess the greatest activity towards BCNU as a substrate (Smith et al., 1989). Because rodents and humans share a different GST isoenzyme profile, it is difficult to extrapolate results obtained in rodent cell lines to human cells, even if the GSTs belong to the same class (Burgess et al., 1989). Thus, the observed denitrosation of BCNU by a rat GST-μ isoenzyme (Smith et al., 1989) does not imply that the same detoxification is catalyzed by human GST-μ, despite the 80% amino acid sequence identity between these protein families (Seidergard et al., 1988).

Batist et al. (1986) reported the elevation of a GST-π isoenzyme in a human MCF-7 breast cancer cell line selected for resistance to doxorubicin. This isoenzyme was elevated approximately 45-fold and found to possess an organic peroxidase activity. This cell line, MCF/Adr[R], also expressed the P-glycoprotein and this observation led to the speculation that GSTs were playing a role in the multidrug resistance phenotype, at least as it related to doxorubicin resistance. While other investigators have reported elevations in both GST-π and glutathione peroxidase activity in MDR cell lines (Chao et al., 1991; Cole et al., 1989; Raghu et al., 1993), its expression appears to be the exception rather than the rule in MDR cell lines.

Although there have numerous reports demonstrating elevated GST in tumor cell lines, such observations are still merely correlations and are not positive proof of the involvement of a particular isoenzyme in the detoxification of a given drug. The ultimate proof for such an activity is through the use of transfection studies of full-length cDNA clones of the various GST isoenzymes. Moscow et al (1989) cloned a full length GST-π gene and transfected it into human MCF-7 breast cancer cells. They observed a 15-fold increase in GST-π activity over the wild-type MCF-7 cells but the transfectants were not resistant to doxorubicin, melphalan or cisplatin. The question as to whether GST-π was interacting with the MDR-1 gene to confer resistance was addressed by transfection studies wherein both the GST-π and MDR-1 genes were co-transfected into MCF-7 cells (Fairchild et al., 1990) As in the previous transfection, the results of this study did not indicate that GST-π was contributing to resistance of doxorubicin in the MDR phenotype. Thus, GST π is unlikely to catalyze the intracellular

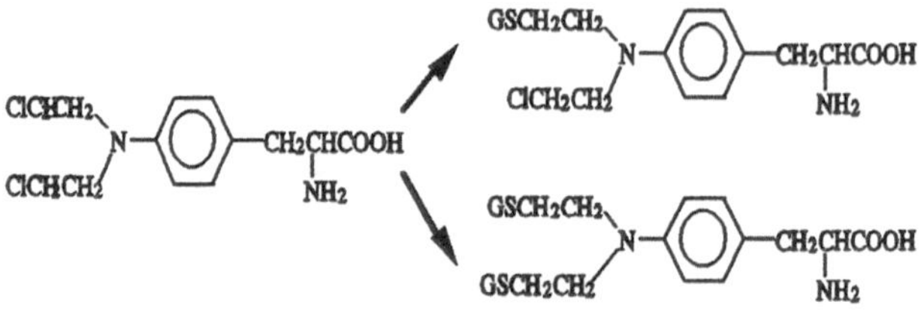

$ClCH_2CH_2$—N—⟨ ⟩—$CH_2CHCOOH$ | NH_2, with $ClCH_2CH_2$

→ $GSCH_2CH_2$, $ClCH_2CH_2$—N—⟨ ⟩—$CH_2CHCOOH$ | NH_2

→ $GSCH_2CH_2$, $GSCH_2CH_2$—N—⟨ ⟩—$CH_2CHCOOH$ | NH_2

Figure 3. Metabolism of melphalan by GST. The GST-catalyzed formation of the mono- and di-glutathionyl conjugates.

conjugation of GSH to these anticancer alkylating agents at rates thatimpact on drug cytotoxicity. Transfection of GST-α however, has been observed to confer resistance to alkylators. Black et al. (1990) transfected GST-α into yeast cells and demonstrated a 2- to 8-fold increase in resistance to chlorambucil. Using a transient transfection system, Pulchalski and Fahl (1990) transfected the rat GST Ya into COS cells and observed a 1.8-fold increase in GST expression and a 1.5-fold level of resistance to cisplatin and 2.9-fold level of resistance to chlorambucil. When evaluating the results of such transfection experiments, the question arises as to what level of resistance is sufficient? Although the increase in resistance obtained in the transfection experiments described above is low, it is of the same magnitude as observed in the clinic (generally less than 10-fold). Conceivably, with the exception of the setting of bone marrow transplantation, a two-fold level of resistance would be sufficient to result in the patient's eventual demise, as the dose of many agents in current use can not be doubled without substantial toxicities.

Studying patients with chronic lymphocytic leukemia, Schisselbauer et al. (1990) found that resistance to nitrogen mustards was associated with a twofold increase in GST activity. Phase II clinical studies are now underway at several institutions to assess the GST inhibitor ethacrynic acid in combination with alkylating agents such as chlorambucil in this disease. In a study of 36 previously untreated non-small cell lung cancer patients, Volm et al. (1992) found a positive correlation between GST-π expression as determined by immunohistochemistry and in vitro resistance to doxorubicin. The significance of these findings are unclear due to the fact that all of the patients in this study were treated surgically and it is not known whether or not they would have responded to chemotherapy. In a series of 41 non-Hodgkin's lymphoma patients the co-expression of MDR-1 and GST-π was associated with a significantly worse outcome than when either was expressed alone (Rodriguiz et al. 1993).

Although the evidence is still limited, there is a general pattern of GST isoenzyme specificity with regard to *in vitro* resistance to individual classes of drugs. As stated above, the alpha class is most likely to be associated with resistance to nitrogen mustard and melphalan while the mu form of GST has been shown to be elevated in a nitrosourea resistance. In theclinical setting, it is unclear which GST isoenzymes are responsible for a particular reaction.

GLUTATHIONE AND DRUG RESISTANCE

Glutathione is a thiol tripeptide, γ-glutamylcsteinylglycine, which is present in virtually all animal cells in millimolar concentrations. It is the predominant nonprotein sulfhydryl compound. For a more detailed review of GSH metabolism, the reader is referred to Fahey and Sunquist (1992) and Meister (1994).

As with the GSTs, glutathione appears to play a role in the detoxification and repair of cellular injury by resulting from alkylating agents and quinone containing compounds such as doxorubicin and mitoxantrone. GSH also participates in the formation of toxic metabolites of several antineoplastic agents including azathioprine (De Miranda et al., 1973) and bleomycin (Caspary et al., 1981) and it may affect the cellular uptake of other agents, such as methotrexate (Leszczynska and Pfaff, 1982). The ability of alkylating agents such as the nitrogen mustards to react with a variety of cellular nucleophiles, including sulfhydryl groups, has long been recognized and analyses of the sulfhydryl content of murine and human tumor cell lines have revealed significant correlations between the GSH content and the level of resistance to these drugs. Early reposts by Calcutt and Connors (1963) and Ball et al. (1966) revealed increased GSH levels in alkylator-resistant tumor cell lines. Since these initial reposts, numerous studies now fill the literature correlating increased GSH and alkylator resistance (See reviews by Meister, 1991 and 1994 for a more through discussion of the role of GSH in resistance).

While the role of GSH in alkylator resistance is well documented, there is also controversy as to whether it is playing a role in doxorubicin resistance in tumor cells. In contrast to studies such as those by Raghu et al. (1993), we had previously demonstrated that in the MDR human multiple myeloma cell line, there was no difference in overall GST activity between the drug-sensitive and -resistant cells nor was there an overexpression of the GST-πisoenzyme discussed in the previous section. These cells did however have elevated levels of nonprotein thiols (Bellamy et al., 1989). When the GSH levels in this cell line were reduced to those of the drug-sensitive parental line, either by pharmacological manipulations using BSO or by placing the cells in a drug-free medium, there was no alteration in the level of doxorubicin resistance. These findings suggested that the elevation in nonprotein thiol content observed in this cell line was an epiphenomenon associated with the resistance selection and maintenance procedures.

GSH may also be responsible for protecting cells against several important toxic side effects of antineoplastic agents. Gurtoo et al. (1981) have demonstrated significant dose-dependent depletion of hepatic NPSH in mice by both cyclophosphamide and acrolein, but not phosphoramide mustard. They demonstrated that cyclophosphamide-induced inhibition of weight gain in rats was enhanced by the depletion GSH by diethyl maleate. Adams et al. (1985) found that, following cyclophosphamide treatment in mice, there was a depletion of both GSH content and GST activity in the bone marrow. There was a subsequent rebound of both which correlated with the ability of the animals to survive a normally lethal dose of the drug (Carmichael et al., 1986). Several reports have indicated an important role for GSH in protecting the cardiac cells from doxorubicin-induced oxygen free radical intermediates (Doroshow et al., 1980; Revis and Marusic, 1978).

Thus, a role for GSH as a determinant of therapeutic efficacy has been demonstrated for a number of antineoplastic agents. The observation that a reduction in intracellular GSH levels may result in the sensitization of drug-resistant tumor cells has led to the initiation of approaches to modulate GSH levels in aneffort to improve the therapeutic efficacy of drugs such as alkylating agents.

CLINICAL ROLE OF GST

In vitro and preclinical studies suggest that modulation of drug resistance can be accomplished through alterations in either GSH pools through the use of agents such as buthionine sulfoximine or GSHmonoethyl ester; or by altering GST activity with a variety of agents designed to inhibit these enzymes. Modulation chemotherapy based on the GSH or GST systems could be directed towards decreasing host toxicity or, alternatively, enhancing drug sensitivity of tumors that are otherwise resistant to classical chemotherapeutic treatment regimens. However, as observed in the multidrug resistance arena, cellular resistance may be multifactorial and therefore to in some systems modulators could have a substantial biochemical effect on GST activity or GSH levels and yet provide only limited useful modulation.

Modulation of GSH

Reduction in cellular GSH levels can be achieved by treatment with BSO. This irreversible inhibitor of γ-glutamyl cysteine synthetase has been demonstrated to reduce cellular GSH levels by as much as 95% (Ozols et al., 1988) and has been found to be able to sensitize resistant cells to a number of anticancer drugs including nitrogen mustards, melphalan, cisplatin and cyclophosphamide (Anderson et al., 1990; Bellamy et al., 1991; Green et al., 1984; Pendyala et al., 1994; Suzukake et al., 1982). Modulation of cellular GSH in this manner can lead to a substantial reversal of alkylating agent resistance in drug-resistant tumor cells, while increasing the sensitivity of some alkylating agent-sensitive cell lines. The sensitizing effect of BSO has also been observed in animal models (Ishikawa et al., 1989; Ozols et al., 1987; Rosenberg et al., 1989; Suzukake et al., 1983) and has set the stage for its evaluation in the clinic. In a phase I trial carried out at the Fox Chase Cancer Center, O'Dwyer et al. (1992), examined the effects of BSO administration prior to the administration of melphalan. BSO, at a dose of 1500 mg/m^2, resulted in glutathione depletion in both normal and tumor tissues. There was no dose escalation of BSO in this study. Patients displayed minimal toxicity to BSO alone and experienced neutropenia and thrombocytopenia following the administration of both BSO and melphalan. While these are both expected side effects of melphalan administration, there was some concern that these toxicities may have been potentiated by the addition of BSO. GSH levels in peripheral mononuclear cells were reduced to less than 20% of normal values although there was considerable patient variation. The rate of depletion was also observed to vary among the patients in this study and recovery was observed within 120 hours of cessation of BSO administration in most patients. As studies such as this move into phase II trials, it will be necessary to demonstrate that depletion of GSH is yielding a therapeutic benefit as suggested by the animal models. The extent and variability of GSH depletion will affect the scheduling of multiple BSO and alkylating agent administrations and it may prove necessary to individualize treatment scheules.

Modulation of GST Activity

One approach to the modulation of GST activity has been through the use of GST inhibitors (Benz et al., 1990; Hall et al., 1989; Tew et al., 1988). Numerous inhibitors of GST have been identified and include both competitive and non-competitive inhibiotrs, true substrates and ligand binding proteins. Many of these inhibitors however are not suitable for the clinic because of their toxicities. Particular interest has been placed on two compounds, the diuretic agent ethacrynic acid and the prostaglandin I, analogue piriprost. Tew et al. (1988) demonstrated that a rat breast carcinoma cell line resistant to nitrogen mustards and two human colon carcinoma cell lines were sensitized to the cytotoxic effects of chlorambucil with the addition of relatively nontoxic concentrations of either ethacrynic acid or piriprost. The precise isoenzymes which these two compounds are affecting is not known.

Table 4. Examples of GST inhibitors

Class	Example
Glutathione derivatives	s-hexylglutathione
Steroid hormones	Estradiol-17-sulfate
Bile acids	Deoxycholate
Anti-inflammatory agents	Indomethacin; piriprost
Diuretics	Ethacrynic acid
Metal salts	Mercuric chloride
Dyes	Cibacron blue

adapted from Tew et al. 1993

Ethacrynic acid is a competitive inhibitor which is conjugated to GSH in a reaction catalyzed by all three major cytosolic GST classes. Studies carried out in a SCID mouse-xenograft model revealed a modest delay in tumr growth in the presence of melphalan and ethacrynic acid (Clapper et al., 1990). In their phase I study, O'Dwyer et al. (1991) examined the combination of ethacrynic acid with the alkylator thiotepa in a series of 27 previously treated patients with advanced cancer. At each dose level studied, they observed a decrease in GST activity which recovered within 6 hours of administering ethacrynic acid. The maximally tolerated dose of ethacrynic acid was determined to be 75 mg/m^2 based on the development of marked diuresis and other metabolic abnormalities. At 50 mg/m^2 the diuresis was considered manageable and myelosuppression was determined to be the most important toxicity of the combination. When thiotepa was combined with ethacrynic acid, the thiotepa plasma clearance was approximately one-half of that measured at equivalent thiotepa doses in a single agent arm of the study. Even with this alteration in thiotepa pharmacokinetics, the toxicity of this drug combined with ethacrynic acid did not appear to be increased over that observed with thiotepa as a single agent. The efficacy of ethacrynic acid is currently being evaluated in a phase II trial in patients with chronic lymphocytic leukemia A novel approach has been through the use of isoenzyme specific modulation. Utilizing information on the crystal structure of GST a series of isoenzyme selective inhibitors have been developed which have an improved potency over previously described GST inhibitors (Morgan et al., 1994). These compounds have been shown to be effective potentiators of alkylating agent cytotoxicity both in tumor cell lines as well as in in vivo tumor models in mice and may prove to be of clinical benefit.

CONCLUSION

As discussed in this chapter, the multiple isoenzymes of GST play many roles in protecting the cell from a wide range of toxic insults. In the case of carcinogens, this level of protection is beneficial to the normal tissue but in the case of malignant tumors, it may confer drug resistance which can further limit the effective use of antineoplastic agents. GST-π expression appears to be a useful marker of a number of human neoplasms including gastrointestinal, uterine and lung carcinomas. GST-μ displays a polymorphic expression with those individuals having the "null "phenotype perhaps at an increased risk for the development of bladder or lung carcinomas. Several promising strategies to overcome drug resistance due to overexpression of the GSTs are emerging from basic and preclinical studies and have led to the initiation of several phase I and phase II clinical trials designed to modulate these enzymes in an attempt to improve cancer chemotherapy.

REFERENCES

Aceto A, C. D, Angelucci S, Tenaglia R, Zezza A, Caccuri AM, Federici G (1989): Glutathione-related enzyme activities in testis of patients with malignant diseases. *Clin Chim Acta* 183:83-86

Adams KJ, Carmichael J, Wolf CR (1985): Altered mouse bone marrow glutathione and glutathione transferase levels in response to cytotoxins. *Cancer Res* 45:1669-1673

Anderson ME, Naganuma A, Meister A (1990): Protection against cisplatin toxicity by administration of glutathione ester. *Faseb J* 4:3251-3255

Ball CR, Connors TA, Double JA, Ujhazy V, Whisson ME (1966): Comparison of nitrogen-mustard-sensitive and -resistant Yoshida sarcomas. *Int J Cancer* 1:319-327

Bass NM, Kirsch RE, Tuff SA, Marks I, Saunders SJ (1977): Ligandin heterogeniety: Evidence that the two non-identical subunits are the monomers of two distinct proteins. *Biochim Biophys Acta* 492:163-175

Batist G, Tulpule A, Sinha BK, Katki AG, Myers CE, Cowan KH (1986): Overexpression of a novel anionic glutathione transferase in multidrug-resistant human breast cancer cells. *J Biol Chem* 261:15544-15549

Beckett GJ, Howie AF, Hume R, Matharoo B, Hiley C, Jones P, Strange RC (1990): Human glutathione S-transferases: radioimmunoassay studies on the expression of alpha-, mu- and pi-class isoenzymes in developing lung and kidney. *Biochim Biophys Acta* 1036:176-182

Beckett GJ, Hayes JD (1993): Glutathione S-transferases: biomedical applications. *Adv Clin Chem* 30:281-380

Bell DA, Taylor JA, Paulson DF, Robertson CN, Mohler JL, Lucier GW (1993): Genetic risk and carcinogen exposure: a common inherited defect of the carcinogen-metabolism gene glutathione s-transferase M1 (GSTM1) that increases susceptibility to bladder cancer. *J Natl Cancer Inst* 85:1159-1164

Bellamy WT, Dalton WS, Meltzer P, Dorr RT (1989): Role of glutathione and its associated enzymes in multidrug-resistant human myeloma cells. *Biochem Pharmacol* 38:787-793

Bellamy WT, Dalton WS, Gleason MC, Grogan TM, Trent JM (1991): Development and characterization of a melphalan-resistant human multiple myeloma cell line. *Cancer Res* 51:995-1002

Bellamy WT, Dalton WS (1994): Multidrug resistance in the laboratory and clinic. *Adv Clin Chem* 31: In press

Benz CG, Keniry MA, Ford JM, Townsend AJ, Cox FW, Palayoor S, Matlin S, Hait WN, Cowan KH (1990): Biochemical correlates of the antitumor and antimitochondrialproperties of gossypol enantiomers. *Mol Pharmacol* 37:840-847

Bergelson S, Pinkus R, Daniel V (1994): Induction of AP-1 (Fos/Jun) by chemical agents mediates activation of glutathione S-transferase and quinone reductase gene expression. *Oncogene* 9:565-571

Berhane K, Mannervik B (1990): Inactivation of the genotoxic aldehyde acrolein by human glutathione transferases of classes alpha, mu, and pi. *Mol Pharmacol* 37:251-254

Black SM, Beggs JD, Hayes JD, Bartoszek A, Muramatsu M, Sakai M, Wolf CR (1990): Expression of human glutathione S-transferases in Saccharomyces cerevisiae confers resistance to the anticancer drugs adriamycin and chlorambucil. *Biochem J* 268:309-315

Board PG, Suzuki T, Shaw DC (1988): Human muscle glutathione S-transferase (GST-4) shows close homology to human liver GST-1. *Biochim Biophys Acta* 953:214-217

Board P, Coggan M, Johnston P, Ross V, Suzuki T, Webb G (1990): Genetic heterogeneity of the human glutathione transferases: a complex of gene families. *Pharmacol Ther* 48:357-369

Bolton MG, Colvin OM, Hilton J (1991): Specificity of isoenzymes of murine glutathione s-transferase for the conjugation of glutathione with L-phenylalanine mustard. *Cancer Res* 51:2410-2415

Booth J, Boyland E, Sims P (1961): An enzyme from rat liver catalysing conjugations with glutathione. *Biochem. J.* 79:516-524

Brockmoller J, Kerb R, Drakoulis N, Nitz M, Roots I (1993): Genotype and phenotype of glutathione s-transferase class mu isoenzymes in lung cancer patients and controls. *Cancer Res* 53:1004-1011

Buller AL, Clapper ML, Tew KD (1987): Glutathione S-transferases in nitrogen mustard-resistant and -sensitive cell lines. *Mol Pharmacol* 31:575-578

Burgess JR, Chow NW, Reddy CC, Tu CP (1989): Amino acid substitutions in the human glutathione S-transferases confer different specificities in the prostaglandin endoperoxide conversion pathway. *Biochem Biophys Res Commun* 158:497-502

Calcutt G, Connors TA (1963): Tumour sulfhydryl levels and sensitivity to the nitrogen mustard merophan. *Biochem Pharmacol* 12:839-845

Carmichael J, Adams DJ, Ansell J, Wolf CR (1986): Glutathione and
    glutathione transferase levels in mouse granulocytes following
    cyclophosphamide administration. *Cancer Res* 46:735-739
Carmichael J, Forrester LM, Lewis AD, Hayes JD, Hayes PC, Wolf CR
    (1988): Glutathione S-transferase isoenzymes and glutathione peroxidase
    activity in normal and tumour samples from human lung. *Carcinogenesis*
    9:1617-1621
Caspary WJ, Lanzo DA, Niziak C (1981): Intermediates in the ferrous oxidase
    cycle of bleomycin. *Biochemistry* 20:3868-3875
Chao CC, Huang YT, Ma CM, Chou WY, Chao SL (1991): Overexpression
    of glutathione s-transferase and elevation of thiol pools in a multidrug-
    resistant human colon cancer cell line. *Mol Pharmacol* 41:69-75
Chern HD, Romkes-sparks M, Hu JJ, Persad R, Sibley GA, Smith PJ, Branch
    RA (1994): Homozygous deleted genotype of glutathione s-transferase M1
    increases susceptibility to agressive bladder cancer. *Proc Amer Assoc
    Cancer Res* 35:285
Ciaccio PJ, Tew KD, LaCreta FP (1990): The spontaneous and glutathione S-
    transferase-mediated reaction of chlorambucil with glutathione. *Cancer
    Commun* 2:279-285
Clapper, ML, Hoffman SJ, Tew KD (1990): Sensitization of human colon
    tumor xenografts to L-phenylalanine mustard using ethacrynic acid. *J Cell
    Pharmacol* 1:71-78
Clapper ML, Hoffman SJ, Tew KD (1991a): Glutathione S-transferases in
    normal and malignant human colon tissue. *Biochim Biophys Acta*
    1096:209-216
Clapper ML, Seestaller LM, Tew KD (1991b): Induction of glutathione -s-
    transferase alpha RNA in tumor cells following exposure to chlorambucil.
    Proc Amer Assoc Cancer Res 32:361
Cole SP, Downes HF, Mirski SE, Clements DJ (1989): Alterations in
    glutathione and glutathione-related enzymesin a multidrug-resistant small
    cell lung cancer cell line. *Mol Pharmacol* 37:192-197
Cowell IG, Dixon KH, Pemble SE, Ketterer B, Taylor JB (1988): The
    structure of the human glutathione S-transferase pi gene. *Biochem J*
    255:79-83
De Miranda P, Beachman L, Creagh TH, Elion GB (1973): The metabolic
    fate of the methylnitroimidazole moiety of azathioprine in the rat. *J
    Pharmacol Exp Ther* 187:588-601
DeJong JL, Morgenstern R, Jornvall H, DePierre JW, Tu CP (1988): Gene
    expression of rat and human microsomal glutathione S-transferases. *J Biol
    Chem* 263:8430-8436

Di Ilio C, Sacchetta P, Del Boccio G, La Rovere G, Federici G (1985): Glutathione peroxidase, glutathione S-transferase and glutathione reductase activities in normal and neoplastic human breast tissue. *Cancer Lett* 29:37-42

Dirr H, Reinemer P, Huber R (1994): X-ray crystal structures of cytosolic glutathione S-transferases. Implications for protein architecture, substrate recognition and catalytic function. *Eur J Biochem* 220:645-61

Doroshow JH, Locker GY, Myers CE (1980): Enzymatic defenses of the mouse heart against reactive oxygen metabolites: alterations produced by doxorubicin. *J Clin Invest* 65:128-135

Dulik DM, Fenselau C, Hilton J (1986): Characterization of melphalan-glutathione adducts whose formation is catalyzed by glutathione transferases. *Biochem Pharmacol* 35:3405-3409

Dulik DM, Fenselau C (1987): Conversion of melphalan to 4-(glutathionyl)phenylalanine. A novel mechanism for conjugation by glutathione-S-transferases. *Drug Metab Dispos Biol Fate Chem* 15:195-199

Eimoto H, Tsutsumi M, Nakajima A, Yamamoto K, Takashima Y, Murayama H, Konishi Y (1988): Expression of glutathione s-transferase placental form in human lung carcinomas. *Carcinogenesis* 9:2325-2327

Evans CG, Bodell WJ, Tokuda K, Doane-Setzer P, Smith M (1987): Glutathione and related enzymes in rat brain tumor cell resistance to 1,3-bis(2-chloroethyl)-1-nitrosourea and nitrogen mustard. *Cancer Res* 47:2525-2530

Fahey RC, Sundquist AR (1991): Evolution of glutathione metabolism. *Adv Enzymol* 64:1-53

Fairchild CR, Moscow JA, O'Brien EE, Cowan KH (1990): Multidrug resistance in cells transfected with human genes encoding a variant P-glycoprotein and glutathione S-transferase-pi. *Mol Pharmacol* 37:801-809

Friling RS, Bensimon A, Tichauer Y, Daniel V (1990): Xenobiotic-inducible expression of murine glutathione S-transferase Ya subunit gene is controlled by an electrophile-responsive element. *Proc Natl Acad Sci U S A* 87:6258-6262

Friling RS, Bergelson S, Daniel V (1992): Two adjacent AP-1-like binding sites form the electrophile-responsive element of the murine glutathione S-transferase Ya subunit gene. *Proc Natl Acad Sci USA* 89:668-672

Godwin AK, Meister A, O'Dwyer PJ, Huang CS, Hamilton TC, Anderson ME (1992): High resistance to cisplatin in human ovarian cancer cell lines is associated with marked increase of glutathione synthesis. *Proc Natl Acad Sci U S A* 89:3070-3074

Green JA, Vistica DT, Young RC, Hamilton TC, Rogan AM, Ozols RF (1984): Potentiation of melphalan cytotoxicity in human ovarian cancer cell lines by glutathione depletion. *Cancer Res* 44:5427-5431

Gurtoo HL, Hipkins JH, Sharma CD (1981): Role of glutathione in the
    metabolism-dependent toxicity and chemotherapy of cyclophosphamide.
    Cancer Res 41:3584-3591

Guthenberg C, Akerfeldt K, Mannervik B (1979): Purification of glutathione
    s-transferase from human placenta. *Acta Chem Scand* B33:595-596

Habig WH, Pabst MJ, Jakoby WB (1974): Glutathione S-transferases. The
    first enzymatic step in mercapturic acid formation. *J Biol Chem* 249:7130-
    7139

Habig WH, Pabst MJ, Jakoby WB (1976): Glutathione S-transferase AA from
    rat liver. *Arch Biochem Biophys* 175:710-716

Hall A, Robson CN, Hickson ID, Harris AL, Proctor SJ, Cattan AR (1989):
    Possible role of inhibition of glutathione S-transferase in the partial
    reversal of chlorambucil resistance by indomethacin in a Chinese hamster
    ovary cell line. *Cancer Res* 49:6265-6268

Hao XY, Widersten M, Ridderstrom M, Hellman U, Mannervik B (1994): Co-
    variation of glutathione transferase expression and cytostatic drug
    resistance in HeLa cells: establishment of class Mu glutathione transferase
    M3-3 as the dominating isoenzyme. *Biochem J* 297:59-67

Harrison DJ, Kharbanda R, Bishop D, McLelland LI, Hayes JD (1989):
    Glutathione S-transferase isoenzymes in human renal carcinoma
    demonstrated by immunohistochemistry. *Carcinogenesis* 10:1257-1260

Hayes JD, Strange RC, Percy-Robb IW (1979): Identification of two
    lithocholic acid-binding proteins: separation of ligandin from glutathione s
    transferase. *Biochem J* 181:699-708

Hayes JD, Wolf CR (1988): Role of glutathione transferase in drug resistance.
    In: *Glutathione Conjugation*,   Sies H, Ketterer B, eds.   New York:
    Academic Press

Hayes JD, Judah DJ, Ellis EM, McLellan LI, Neal GE (1993): Role of
    glutathione s-transferase and aldehyde reductase in resistance to aflatoxin
    B1. In: *Structure and Function of Glutathione Transferases*,   Tew KD,
    Pickett CB, Mantle TJ, Mannervik B, Hayes JD, eds.   Boca Raton: CRC
    Press

Hida T, Kuwabara M, Ariyoshi Y, Takahashi T, Sugiura T, Hosoda K, Niitsu
    Y, Ueda R (1994): Serum glutathione S-transferase-pi level as a tumor
    marker for non-small cell lung cancer: Potential predictive value in
    chemotherapeuti c response. *Cancer* 73:1377-1382

Hiley C, Fryer A, Bell J, Hume R, Strange RC (1988): The human
    glutathione S-transferases. Immunohistochemical studies of the
    developmental expression of Alpha- and Pi-class isoenzymes in liver.
    Biochem J 254:255-259

Hiratsuka A, Sebata N, Kawashima K, Okuda H, Ogura K, Watabe T, Satoh K, Hatayama I, Tsuchida S, Ishikawa T, et al (1990): A new class of rat glutathione S-transferase Yrs-Yrs inactivating reactive sulfate esters as metabolites of carcinogenic arylmethanols. *J Biol Chem* 265:11973-11981

Howie AF, Hayes JD, Beckett GJ (1988): Purification of acidic glutathione S-transferases from human lung, placenta and erythrocyte and the development of a specific radioimmunoassay for their measurement. *Clin Chim Acta* 177:65-75

Howie AF, Bell D, Hayes PC, Hayes JD, Beckett GJ (1990a): Glutathione S-transferase isoenzymes in human bronchoalveolar lavage: a possible early marker for the detection of lung cancer. *Carcinogenesis* 11:295-300

Howie AF, Forrester LM, Glancey MJ, Schlager JJ, Powis G, Beckett GJ, Hayes JD, Wolf CR (1990b): Glutathione S-transferase and glutathione peroxidase expression in normal and tumour human tissues. *Carcinogenesis* 11:451-458

Hussey AJ, Hayes JD, Beckett GJ (1987): The polymorphic expression of neutral glutathione S-transferase in human mononuclear leucocytes as measured by specific radioimmunoassay. *Biochem Pharmacol* 36:4013-4015

Hussey AJ, Hayes JD (1992): Characterization of a human class-Theta glutathione S-transferase with activity towards 1-menaphthyl sulphate. *Biochem J* 286:929-935

Igwe O (1986): Biologically active intermediates generated by reduced glutathione conjugation pathway. *Biochem Pharmacol* 35:2987-2994

Imagawa M, Osada S, Okuda A, Muramatsu M (1991): Silencer binding proteins function on multiple cis-elements in the glutathione transferase P gene. *Nucleic Acids Res* 19:5-10

Ishikawa M, Takayanagi Y, Sasaki K (1989): Modification of cyclophosphamide-induced urotoxicity by buthionine sulfoximine and disulfiram in mice. *Res Commun Chem Pathol Pharmacol* 65:265-268

Jakoby WB, Ketterer B, Mannervik B (1984): Glutathione transferases: nomenclature. *Biochem Pharmacol* 33:2539-2540

Ji X, Johnson WW, Sesay MA, Dickert L, Prasad SM, Ammon HL, Armstrong RN, Gilliland GL (1994): Structure and function of the xenobiotic substrate binding site of a glutathione S-transferase as revealed by X-ray crystallographic analysis of product complexes with the diastereomers of 9-(S-glutathionyl) -10-hydroxy-9,10-dihydrophenanthrene. *Biochemistry* 33:1043-1052

Johnson WW, Liu S, Ji X, Gilliland GL, Armstrong RN (1993): Tyrosine 115 participates both in chemical and physical steps of the catalytic mechanism of a glutathione s-transferase. *J. Biol Chem* 268:11508-11511

Kamisaka K, Habig WH, Ketley JN, Arias M, Jakoby WB (1975): Multiple forms of human glutathione S-transferase and their affinity for bilirubin. *Eur J Biochem* 60:153-161

Kantor R, Giardina S, Bartolazzi A, Townsend A, Myers CE, Cowan KH, Longo DL, Natali P (1991): Monoclonal antibodies to glutathione s-transferas pi-immunohistochemical analysis of human tissues and cancers. *Int J Cancer* 47:193-201

Ketterer B, Meyer DJ, Taylor JB, Pemble S, Coles B, Fraser G (1990): Glutathione s-transferases and protection against oxidative stress. In: *Glutathione S-transferases and drug resistance*,   Hayes JD, Pickett CB, Mantle TJ, eds.   London: Taylor and Francis

Ketterer B (1994): The glutathione transferases: role in protection and susceptibility to cancer. *Proc Amer Assoc Cancer Res* 35:694-695

Kodate C, Fukushi A, Narita T, Kudo H, Soma Y, Sato K (1986): Human placental form of glutathione S-transferase (GST-pi) as a new immunohistochemical marker for human colonic carcinoma. *Jpn J Cancer Res* 77:226-229

Koskelo K, Valmet E, Tenhunen R (1981): Purification and characterization of an acid glutathione S-transferase from human lung. *Scand J Clin Lab Invest* 41:683-689

Kraus P, Gross B (1979): Particle-bound glutathione-S-transferases. *Enzyme* 24:205-208

Laisney V, Nguyen VC, Gross MS, Frezal J (1984): Human genes for glutathione S-transferases. *Hum Genet* 68:221-227

Leszczynska A, Pfaff E (1982): Activation by reduced glutathione of methotrexate transport into isolated rat liver cells. *Biochem Pharmacol* 31:1911-1918

Lewis AD, Hickson I, Robson CN, Harris AL, Hayes JD, Griffiths SA, Manson MM, Hall AE, Moss JE, Wolf CR (1987): Amplification and increased expression of alpha class glutathione s-transferase-encoding genes associated with resistance to nitrogen mustards. *Proc Natl Acad Sci USA* 85:8511-8515

Li Y, Seyama T, Godwin AK, Winokur TS, Lebovitz RM (1988): MTrasT24, a metallothionein-ras fusion gene, modulates expression in cultured rat liver cells of two genes associated with in vivo liver cancer. *Proc Natl Acad Sci USA* 85:344-348

Mannervik B, Jensson H (1982): Binary combinations of four protein subunits with different catalytic specificities explain the relationship between six basic glutathione S-transferases in rat liver cytosol. *J Biol Chem* 257:9909-9912

Mannervik B (1985): The isoenzymes of glutathione transferase. *Adv Enzymol Relat Areas Mol Biol* 57:357-417

Mannervik B, Awasthi YC, Board PG, Hayes JD, Di IC, Ketterer B,
    Listowsky I, Morgenstern R, Muramatsu M, Pearson WR, et al (1992):
    Nomenclature for human glutathione transferases. *Biochem J* 282:305-306

Mannervik B, Berhane K, Bjornestedt R, Board PG, Jones TA, Kolm RH,
    Olin B, Sinning I, Sroga GE, Stenberg G, Tardioli S, Widersten M
    (1993): Structural and functional characterization of the binding sites for
    glutathione (G-site) and the hydrophobic electrophilic substrate (H-site) in
    glutathione transferases. In: *Structure and Function of Glutathione
    Transferases*, Tew KD, Pickett CB, Mantle TJ, Mannervik B, Hayes JD,
    eds. Boca Raton: CRC Press

Marcus CJ, Habig WH, Jakoby WB (1978): Glutathione transferase from
    human erythrocytes. Nonidentity with the enzymes from liver. *Arch
    Biochem Biophys* 188:287-293

Meikle I, Hayes JD, Walker SW (1992): Expression of an abundant alpha-
    class glutathione S-transferase in bovine and human adrenal cortex tissues.
    J Endocrinol 132:83-92

Meister A (1991) Glutathione deficiency produced by inhibition of its
    synthesis and its reversal: applications in research and therapy *Pharmacol
    Ther* 51:155-194

Meister A (1994): Glutathione, ascorbate, and cellular protection. *Cancer Res*
    54: 1969s-1975s

Meyer DJ, Coles B, Pemble SE, Gilmore KS, Fraser GM, Ketterer B (1991):
    Theta, a new class of glutathione transferases purified from rat and man.
    Biochem J 274:409-414

Morgan AS, Ciaccio PJ, Tew KD, Schmidt DE, Kelley MK, Flatgaard JE,
    Villar HO, Lyttle MH, Kauvar LM (1994): Isozyme specific modulation
    of glutathione s-transferase in cancer therapy. *Proc Amer Assoc Cancer
    Res* 356:376

Morgenstern R, Guthenberg C, Depierre JW (1982): Microsomal glutathione
    S-transferase. Purification, initial characterization and demonstration that it
    is not identical to the cytosolic glutathione S-transferases A, B and C. *Eur
    J Biochem* 128:243-248

Morgenstern R, DePierre JW (1983): Microsomal glutathione transferase.
    Purification in unactivated form and further characterization of the
    activation process, substrate specificity and amino acid composition. *Eur J
    Biochem* 134:591-597

Morgenstern R, DePierre JW, Jornvall H (1985): Microsomal glutathione
    transferase. Primary structure. *J Biol Chem* 260:13976-13983

Morgenstern R, Wallin H, DePierre JW (1987): Mechanisms of activation of
    the microsomal glutathione transferase. In: *Glutathione S-transferases and
    Carcinogenesis*, Mantle TJ, Pickett CB, Hayes JD, eds. London: Taylor
    and Francis

Moscow JA, Townsend AJ, Cowan KH (1989): Elevation of pi class
    glutathione S-transferase activity in human breast cancer cells by
    transfection of the GST pi gene and its effect on sensitivity to toxins. *Mol
    Pharmacol* 36:22-28

Nakachi K, Imai K, Hayashi S, Kawajiri K (1993): Polymorphisms of the
    CTP1A1 and glutathione s-transferase genes associated with susceptibility
    to lung cancer in relation to cigarette dose in a japanese population.
    Cancer Res 53:2994-2999

Nazar-Stewart V, Motulsky A, Eaton DL, White E, Hornung S, Leng Z,
    Stapelton P, Weiss N (1993): The glutathione s-transferase mu
    polymorphism as a marker for susceptibility to lung carcinoma. *Cancer
    Res* 53:2313-2318

Niitsu Y, Takahashi Y, Saito T, Hirata Y, Arisato N, Maruyama H, Kohgo Y,
    Listowsky I (1989): Serum glutathione-S-transferase-pi as a tumor marker
    for gastrointestinal malignancies. *Cancer* 63:317-323

O'Dwyer PJ, LaCreta F, Nash S, Tinsley PW, Schilder R, Clapper ML, Tew
    KD, Panting L, Litwin S, Comis RL, et al (1991): Phase I study of
    thiotepa in combination with the glutathione transferase inhibitor
    ethacrynic acid. *Cancer Res* 51:6059-6065

O'Dwyer PJ, Hamilton TC, Young RC, LaCreta FP, Carp N, Tew KD,
    Padavic K, Comis RL, Ozols RF (1992): Depletion of glutathione in
    normal and malignant human cells in vivo by buthionine sulfoximine:
    clinical and biochemical results [see comments]. *J Natl Cancer Inst*
    84:264-267

Ogura K, Nishiyama T, Okada T, Kajital J, Narihata H, Watabe T, Hiratsuka
    A, Watabe T (1991): Molecular cloning and amino acid sequencing of rat
    liver class theta glutathione S-transferase Yrs-Yrs inactivating reactive
    sulfate esters of carcinogenic arylmethanols. *Biochem Biophys Res
    Commun* 181:1294-1300

Okuda A, Sakai M, Muramatsu M (1987): The structure of the rat glutathione
    S-transferase P gene and related pseudogenes. *J Biol Chem* 262:3858-3863

Ozols RF, Louie KG, Plowman J, Behrens BC, Fine RL, Dykes D, Hamilton
    TC (1987): Enhanced melphalan cytotoxicity in human ovarian cancer in
    vitro and in tumor-bearing nude mice by buthionine sulfoximine depletion
    of glutathione. *Biochem Pharmacol* 36:147-153

Ozols RF, Hamilton TC, Masuda H, Young RC (1988): Manipulation of
    cellular thiols to influence drug resistance. In: *Mechanisms of Drug
    Resistance in Neoplastic Cells,* Woolley PV, Tew KD, eds. New York:
    Academic Press

Pemble SE, Schroeder KR, Taylor JB, Spencer SR, Meyer DJ, Hallier E, Bolt
    HM, Ketterer B (1994): Human glutathione transferase theta: cDNA
    cloning and the demonstration of a null polymorphism by PCR. *Proc
    Amer Assoc Cancer Res* 35:123

Pendyala L, Creaven P, Weinstein A, Zdanowicz J, Molnar M (1994): Effect of glutathione depletion on the cytotoxicity of iproplatin and cisplation in a melanoma cell line SK-MEL-2. *Proc Amer Assoc Cancer Res* 35:434

Peters WH, Kock L, Nagengast FM, Roelofs HM (1990): Immunodetection with a monoclonal antibody of glutathione S-transferase mu in patients with and without carcinomas. *Biochem Pharmacol*; 39591-39597

Pinkus R, Bergelson S, Daniel V (1993): Phenobarbital induction of AP-1 binding activity mediates activation of glutathione s-transferase and quinone reductase gene expression. *Biochem J* 290:637-640

Power C, Sinha S, Webber C, Manson MM, Neal GE (1987): Transformation related expression of glutathione-s-transferase P in rat liver cells. *Carcinogenesis* 8:797-801

Puchalski RB, Fahl WE (1990): Expression of recombinant glutathione S-transferase pi, Ya, or Yb1 confers resistance to alkylating agents. *Proc Natl Acad Sci U S A* 87:2443-2447

Raghu G, Pierre-Jerome M, Dordal MS, Simonian P, Bauer KD (1993): P-glycoprotein and alterations in the glutathione/glutathione-peroxidase cycle underlie doxorubicin resistance in HL-60-R, a subclone of the HL-60 human leukemia cell line. *Int J Cancer* 53:804-811

Ramsdell HS, Eaton DL (1990): Mouse liver glutathione s-transferase isoenzyme activity toward aflatoxin B1-8,9-epoxide and benzo[a]pyrene-7,8-9,10-epoxide. *Toxicol Appl Pharmacol* 105:216-225

Reinemer P, Dirr HW, Ladenstein R, Schaffer J, Gallay O, Huber R (1991): The three-dimensional structure of class pi glutathione S-transferase in complex with glutathione sulfonate at 2.3 A resolution. *Embo J* 10:1997-2005

Revis NW, Marusic N (1978): Glutathione peroxidase activity and selenium concentration in the hearts of doxorubicin-treated rabbits. *J Mol Cell Cardiol* 10:945-951

Riou G, Barrois M, Zhou D (1991): Expression of anionic glutathione s transferase (GST-p) gene in carcinomas of the uterine cervix and in normal cervices. *Br J Cancer* 63:191-194

Robson CN, Lewis AD, Wolf CR, Hayes JD, Hall A, Proctor SJ, Harris AL, Hickson ID (1987): Reduced levels of drug-induced DNA cross-linking in nitrogen mustard-resistant Chinese hamster ovary cells expressing elevated glutathione S-transferase activity. *Cancer Res* 47:6022-6027

Rodriguiz C, Commes T, Robert J, Rossi J (1993): Expression of P-glycoprotein and anionic glutathione s-transferase genes in non-Hodgkin's lymphoma. *Leuk Res* 17:149-156

Rosenberg MC, Colvin OM, Griffith OW, Bigner SH, Elion GB, Horton JK, Lilley E, Bigner D, Friedman HS (1989): Establishment of a melphalan-resistant rhabdomyosarcoma xenograft with cross-reistance to vincristine and enhanced sensitivity following buthionine sulfoximine-mediated glutathione depletion. *Cancer Res* 49:6917-6922

Rushmore TH, King RG, Paulson KE, Pickett CB (1990): Regulation of glutathione S-transferase Ya subunit gene expression: identification of a unique xenobiotic-responsive element controlling inducible expression by planar aromatic compounds. *Proc Natl Acad Sci U S A* 87:3826-3830

Rushmore TH, Morton MR, Pickett CB (1991): The antioxidant responsive element. Activation by oxidative stress and identification of the DNA consensus sequence required for functional activity. *J Biol Chem* 266:11632-11639

Sakai M, Okuda A, Muramatsu M (1988): Multiple regulatory elements and phorbol 12-O-tetradecanoate 13-acetate responsiveness of the rat placental glutathione transferase gene. *Proc Natl Acad Sci USA* 85:9456-9460

Sasano H, Miuazaki S, Shiga K, Goukon Y, Nishihira T, Nagura H (1993): Glutathione s-transferase in human esophageal carcinoma. *Anticancer Res* 13:363-368

Satoh K, Kitahara A, Soma Y, Inaba Y, Hatayama I, Sato K (1985): Purification, induction, and distribution of placental glutathione transferase: a new marker enzyme for preneoplastic cells in the rat chemical hepatocarcinogenesis. *Proc Natl Acad Sci USA* 82:3964-3968

Schisselbauer JC, Silber R, Papadopoulos E, Abrams K, LaCreta FP, Tew KD (1990): Characterization of glutathione S-transferase expression in lymphocytes from chronic lymphocytic leukemia patients. *Cancer Res* 50:3562-3568

Seidegard J, Pero RW (1985): The hereditary transmission of high glutathione transferase activity towards trans-stilbene oxide in human mononuclear leukocytes. *Hum Genet* 69:66-68

Seidegard J, Pero RW, Miller DG, Beattie EJ (1986): A glutathione transferase in human leukocytes as a marker for the susceptibility to lung cancer. *Carcinogenesis* 7:751-753

Seidegard J, Vorachek WR, Pero RW, Pearson WR (1988): Hereditary differences in the expression of the human glutathione transferase active on trans-stilbene oxide are due to a gene deletion. *Proc Natl Acad Sci U S A* 85:7293-7297

Seidegard J, Pero RW, Markowitz MM, Roush G, Miller DG, Beattie EJ (1990): Isoenzyme(s) of glutathione transferase (class Mu) as a marker for the susceptibility to lung cancer: a follow up study. *Carcinogenesis* 11:33-36

Shea TC, Kelley SL, Henner WD (1988): Identification of an anionic form of glutathione transferase present in many human tumors and human tumor cell lines. *Cancer Res* 48:527-533

Shiratori Y, Soma Y, Maruyama H, Sato S, Takano A, Sato K (1987): Immunohistochemical detection of the placental form of glutathione S-transferase in dysplastic and neoplastic human uterine cervix lesions. *Cancer Res* 47:6806-6809

Sinning I, Kleywegt GJ, Cowan SW, Reinemer P, Dirr HW, Huber R, Gilliland GL, Armstrong RN, Ji X, Board PG, et al (1993): Structure determination and refinement of human alpha class glutathione transferase A1-1, and a comparison with the Mu and Pi class enzymes. *J Mol Biol* 232:192-212

Smith MT, Evans CG, Doane SP, Castro VM, Tahir MK, Mannervik B (1989): Denitrosation of 1,3-bis(2-chloroethyl)-1-nitrosourea by class mu glutathione transferases and its role in cellular resistance in rat brain tumor cells. *Cancer Res* 49:2621-2625

Strange RC, Faulder CG, Davis BA, Hume R, Brown JA, Cotton W, Hopkinson DA (1984): The human glutathione s-transferases: Studies on the tissue distribution and genetic variation of the GST1, GST2 and GST3 isozymes. *Ann Hum Genet* 48:11-20

Strange RC, Howie AF, Hume R, Matheroo B, Bell J, Hiley C, Jones P, Beckett GJ (1989): Radioimmunoassay studies of the developmental expression of alpha, mu and pi class glutathione s-transferases in the developing liver. *Biochim Biophys Acta* 993:186-190

Strange RC, Fryer AA, Hiley C, Bell J, Cosser D, Hume R (1990): Developmental expression of GST in human tissues. In: *Glutathion S-transferases and Drug Resistance*, Hayes JD, Mantle TJ, Pickett CB, eds. London: Taylor and Francis

Strange RC, Matharoo B, Faulder GC, Jones P, Cotton W, Elder JB, Deakin M (1991): The human glutathione S-transferases: a case-control study of the incidence of the GST1 0 phenotype in patients with adenocarcinoma. *Carcinogenesis* 12:25-28

Suzukake K, Petro BJ, Vistica DT (1982): Reduction in glutathione content of L-PAM-resistant L1210 cells confers drug sensitivity. *Biochem Pharmacol* 31:121-124

Suzuki T, Coggan M, Shaw DC, Board PG (1987): Electrophoretic and immunological analysis of human glutathione S-transferase isozymes. *Ann Hum Genet* 51:95-106

Talcott RE, Levin VA (1983): Glutathione-dependent denitrosation of N,N'-bis(2-chloroethyl)N-nitrosourea (BCNU): nitrite release catalyzed by mouse liver cytosol in vitro. *Drug Metab Dispos Biol Fate Chem* 11:175-176

Tateoka N, Tsuchida S, Soma Y, Sato K (1987): Purification and characterization of glutathione S-transferases in human kidney. *Clin Chim Acta* 166:207-18

Tew KD, Bomber AM, Hoffman SJ (1988): Ethacrynic acid and piprost as enhancers of cytotoxicity in drug resistant and sensitive cell lines. *Cancer Res* 48:3622-3625

Tew KD, Houghton PJ, Houghton JA (1993): *Preclinical and Clinical Modulation of Anticancer Drugs.* Boca Raton: CRC Press

Tsuchida S, Sekine Y, Shineha R, Nishihira T, Sato K (1989): Elevation of the placental glutathione S-transferase form (GST-pi) in tumor tissues and the levels in sera of patients with cancer. *Cancer Res* 49:5225-5229

Tsuchida S, Maki T, Sato K (1990): Purification and characterization of glutathione transferases with an activity toward nitroglycerin from human aorta and heart. Multiplicity of the human class Mu forms. *J Biol Chem* 265:7150-7157

Tutsumi M, Sugisaki T, Makino T, Miyaga N, Nakatani K, Shiratori T, Takahashi S, Konishi Y (1987): Oncofetal expression of glutathione s-transferase placental form in human stomach carcinomas. *Jpn J Cancer Res* 78:631-633

Volm M, Mattern J, Samsel B (1992): Relationship of inherent resistance to doxorubicin, proliferative activity and expression of P-glycoprotein 170, and glutathione s-transferase-p in human lung tumors. *Cancer* 70:764-769

Wang AL, Tew KD (1985): Increased glutathione-S-transferase activity in a cell line with acquired resistance to nitrogen mustards. *Cancer Treat Rep* 69:677-682

Wang YY, Teicher BA, Shea TC, Holden SA, Rosbe KW, al AA, Henner WD (1989): Cross-resistance and glutathione-S-transferase-pi levels among four human melanoma cell lines selected for alkylating agent resistance. *Cancer Res* 49:6185-6192

Warholm M, Guthenberg C, Mannervik B, von BC, Glaumann H (1980): Identification of a new glutathione S-transferase in human liver. *Acta Chem Scand [b]* 34:607-21

Warholm M, Guthenberg C, Mannervik B (1983): Molecular and catalytic properties of glutathione transferase mu from human liver: an enzyme efficiently conjugating epoxides. *Biochemistry* 22:3610-3617

Williams D (1985): S-nitrosation and the reactions of S-nitroso compounds. *Chem Soc Rev* 14:171-196

Wolf CR, Macpherson JS, Smyth JF (1986): Evidence for the metabolism of mitozantrone by microsomal glutathione transferases and 3-methylcholanthrene-inducible glucuronosyl transferases. *Biochem Pharmacol* 35:1577-1581

Woolley PV, Tew KD (1988): *Mechanisms of Drug Resistance in Neoplastic Cells.* San Diego: Academic Press

Zhong S, Howie AF, Ketterer B, Taylor J, Hayes JD, Beckett GJ, Wathen CG, Wolf CR, Spurr NK (1991): Glutathione S-transferase mu locus: use of genotyping and phenotyping assays to assess association with lung cancer susceptibility. *Carcinogenesis* 12:1533-1537

3. PHARMACOLOGY OF DRUG TRANSPORT IN MULTIDRUG RESISTANT TUMOR CELLS

Henk J. Broxterman and Carolien H.M. Versantvoort

INTRODUCTION

In this chapter we will discuss mainly pharmacological aspects of drug transport in *intact* multidrug resistant tumor cells as opposed to studies on plasma membrane vesicles. Multidrug resistance (MDR) is defined as cross-resistance to several classes of drugs including drugs that act at different target sites. The underlying basis for MDR in *in vitro* selected resistant tumor cell lines is often a reduced intracellular accumulation of cytostatic drugs due to increased outward transport of these drugs over the cellular plasma membrane. We will discuss the pharmacological properties of MDR-related drug transport, focussed on the two human drug transporter proteins, that have been proven by transfection of full length cDNA to confer the MDR phenotype to sensitive cells. These proteins are the *MDR*1 encoded P-glycoprotein (Pgp or P170) and the *MRP* encoded multidrug resistance-associated protein (MRP or P190) (Gottesman and Pastan, 1988; Cole et al., 1992; Zaman et al., 1994). In particular, properties of these proteins will be addressed, that are derived from studies on *intact* tumor cells. Studies on purified protein or reconstituted protein into phospholipid vesicles are particularly suited for the investigation of biochemical and biophysical characteristics of drug transport.

However, information on the properties of drug transporters in their natural localization, the membrane of *intact* cells, may provide additional relevant data regarding the impact of the drug transporter proteins on the cellular pharmacology of drugs. In particular we will emphasize the energy-dependence of drug transport, transport of drugs against a concentration gradient, saturation of drug transport, competition with drug transport by "resistance modulators" and intra-cellular distribution of drugs. Finally, we will discuss the relevance of these data in relation to drug resistance of human cancer.

ATP DEPENDENCE OF DRUG TRANSPORT

In the earliest studies on multidrug resistance it was found that the plasma membrane barrier for drugs, later to be identified as the drug transporter Pgp, was ATP-dependent (Carlsen et al., 1977). This characteristic is now widely believed to be an essential property of all transmembrane transport mediated by proteins belonging to the ATP-binding cassette (ABC) transporter superfamily. ABC transporters utilize the energy of ATP hydrolysis to pump substrates across the membrane against a concentration gradient (Higgins, 1992). Therefore, the transport of drugs by a pump such as Pgp will be at the expense of cellular energy. In fact we have estimated that a highly Pgp overexpressing tumor cell line (10^5-10^6 Pgp molecules per cell) may expend as much as 10% of its energy turnover to get rid of a substrate like the MDR modulator verapamil (Broxterman et al., 1989). This was one of the first pieces of evidence that modulators of cytostatic drug transport themselves might be pumped out by Pgp. Since Pgp needs ATP to pump out drugs from the cell, the question what the K_m for ATP of the drug transport activity is, has relevance for its *in vivo* action. Table 1 shows several reference values for the apparent K_m for ATP of *in vitro* Pgp ATPase activities and in addition "K_m" values, at which the daunorubicin pump rate by Pgp (Feller et al., 1994) or MRP (Versantvoort et al., 1994) was half-maximally inhibited. Since human solid tumors are generally considered to have low and heterogeneous ATP levels (<0.5 - 3 mM), compared to the levels in cell culture (> 5mM) (Vaupel et al., 1989), these data may well be physiologically relevant. Based on these results it has to be considered that *in vivo* drug pumping by Pgp or MRP may be limited by cytosolic ATP concentrations. It would also imply the possibility to modulate MDR by using inhibitors of glycolysis, which is the main energy-producing pathway in many tumors (Broxterman and Pinedo, 1991). Little is known yet with respect to the stoichiometry of drug pumping.

Table 1. ATP dependence of various Pgp and MRP activities.

K_m for ATP (mM)	activity	material	reference
$K_m = 0.94$ $K_m = 0.51$	ATPase ATPase	Pgp in detergent Pgp in phospholipid	Shapiro
$K_m = 1.4$	ATPase	Pgp plasma membrane	Al-Shawi
$K_m = 0.5$	ATPase	Pgp plasma membrane	Sarkadi
$K_m \approx 1.5$[a]	V_{pump}[b]	Pgp in intact cells	Feller
$K_m \approx 1.5$[a]	V_{pump}[b]	MRP in intact cells	Versant-voort

[a] Apparent K_m in intact cells (Pgp in KB8-5 and MRP in GLC$_4$/ADR cells) is based on the assumption of homogeneous ATP distribution over the whole cell volume. The experimental uncertainty is larger than for plasma membrane studies. [b] V_{pump} is the daunorubicin efflux rate by Pgp or MRP, calculated according to Versantvoort et al., 1994.

Shapiro and Ling (1994) estimated that their purified Pgp had an ATPase activity that could account for about 2 molecules of daunorubicin exported per sec per Pgp molecule. Based on data on ATP consumption in Pgp-overexpressing cells and the assumption of 2 ATP hydrolysed per verapamil molecule transported, we calculated a transport rate of 100 molecules verapamil per sec per Pgp molecule. (Broxterman and Pinedo, 1991).These data seem to suggest that maximal verapamil turnover by Pgp is much higher than maximal daunorubicin turnover (Broxterman et al., 1989). However, since pump rates for verapamil have not been measured directly and all calculations are based on major assumptions, these figures have to be regarded only as a frame of thinking and further experimentation.

DRUG TRANSPORT AGAINST A CONCENTRATION GRADIENT

Apart from ATP-dependence of transport, another characteristic that has to be proven in order to classify drug transport as an active process, is transport against a concentration gradient (Higgins, 1992). For Pgp this has been an unresolved issue for a long time, since mostly drug transport activity is measured by drug efflux from

preloaded cells into drug-free medium *in vitro*. Recently, two studies
have shown evidence for transport against a concentration gradient of
colchicine in Pgp-containing secretory vesicles (Ruetz and Gros, 1994)
and of vinblastine in inside-out plasma membrane vesicles (Schlemmer
and Sirotnak, 1994). In our laboratory we have provided evidence for
daunorubicin transport against a concentration gradient in *intact* Pgp-
as well as MRP-overexpressing cells. This was done by measuring the
dynamic response of daunorubicin influx and efflux from cells exposed
to a short pulse of verapamil in a daunorubicin-containing medium
(Lankelma et al., 1990). A second method made use of the selective
permeabilization of plasma membranes by a low concentration of
digitonin (Versantvoort et al., 1992). If after loading the cells with
daunorubicin until steady state was reached a concentration gradient of
daunorubicin over the plasma membrane is present, caused by active
efflux, then upon permeabilization of the plasma membrane, extra
daunorubicin will flow into the cells and rapidly bind to its DNA
target until equilibrium is reached (Fig. 1). In sensitive cells no
change will occur, because intra- and extracellular free daunorubicin
concentrations are equal. These experiments have provided evidence
for active drug efflux by Pgp and MRP (Zaman et al., 1994;
Versantvoort et al., 1992).

In addition it should be mentioned that the intracellular (cytosolic)
pH in Pgp as well as MRP overexpressing cells and MRP transfectants
was not different from the sensitive parent cells when measured under
the same conditions as used for drug accumulation studies, that is with
fetal calf serum present. This excludes a significant contribution of a
pH gradient to the observed daunorubicin transport, also concluded
recently for rhodamine 123 transport (Altenberg et al., 1993).

Moreover, Ruetz and Gros (1994) recently showed evidence that
Pgp-mediated vinblastine transport was independent of proton or
electrochemical gradients over the membrane. In sum, these data
support the model that Pgp and MRP are ATP-dependent drug transporters, actively reducing the intracellular drug concentration.

Figure 1. A model showing the effect of digitonin on daunorubicin (DNR) uptake in sensitive and MDR tumor cells. In MDR cells by active efflux the cytosolic DNR concentration is lower than the outside concentration, causing a concentration gradient, which is abolished by digitonin.

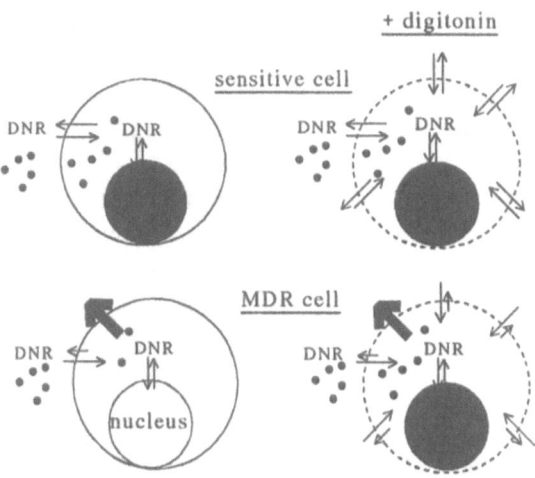

SATURATION OF DRUG TRANSPORT

A property of protein-mediated drug transport is that one should be able to demonstrate saturation of drug transport. Such saturation of drug transport has generally been very difficult to show for Pgp-mediated drug transport (Hammond et al., 1989) using *intact* cells. However, recently several papers have provided evidence for saturation of Pgp-mediated drug transport. Hunter et al. (1993) studying vinblastine transport through polarized human intestinal adenocarcinoma cells found a V_{max} for its polarized transport, described to Pgp, since it was inhibited by the anti-Pgp antibody MRK-16. Horio et al. (1990) reported a K_m of 1 µM for vinblastine pumping by Pgp. Spoelstra et al. (1992) in a kinetic study have shown saturation of daunorubicin transport in a number of Pgp-expressing tumor cell lines. In the highly Pgp-expressing cell line 2780[AD] saturation of daunorubicin transport could not be found, probably by the inability to reach sufficiently high intracellular concentrations of substrate at the high pump rate in these cells.

Versantvoort et al. (1994) have shown saturation of daunorubicin transport in the MRP-overexpressing cell line GLC$_4$/ADR from which an apparent K$_m$ of 1.4 µM for active daunorubicin transport was derived. These experiments showed that the used drug concentration may be important in determining the apparent cellular accumulation defect (see Fig. 2). For daunorubicin concentrations ([DNR]$_o$) higher than 2 µM the accumulation in the GLC$_4$/ADR cells is no longer linear with its concentration because saturation of the active transport. In addition, the accumulation in sensitive cells becomes alinear, probably because of saturation of DNA binding sites. The net effect is an apparently smaller accumulation defect at higher drug concentrations. Now that more kinetic studies are being pursued (Dordal et al., 1992; Pereira et al., 1994; Stein et al., 1994), kinetic constants for the active transport of an increasing number of drugs will become available in the near future.

Figure 2. Saturation of daunorubicin transport in GLC4/ADR cells. Steady-state accumulation of daunorubicin in GLC4 and GLC4/ADR cells. Reprinted from Biochem Pharmacol, CHM Versantvoort et al. (1994) in press, with kind permission from Elsevier Science Ltd, the Boulevard, Langford Lane, Kidlington 0X5 1GB, UK.

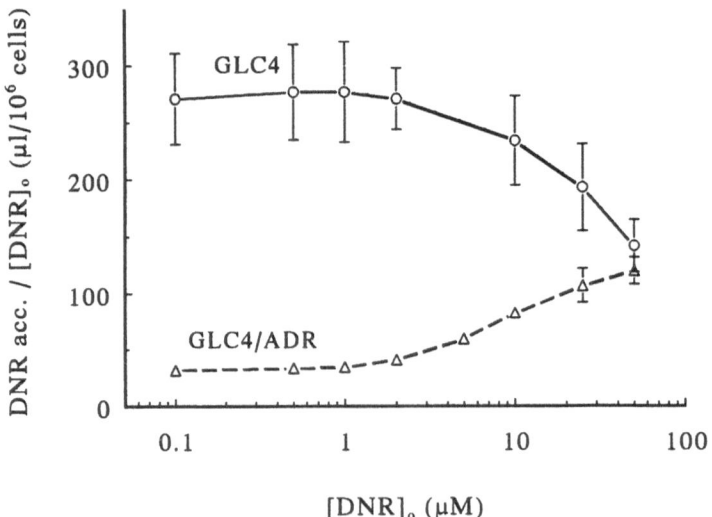

COMPETITION FOR TRANSPORT BY REVERSAL AGENTS

An important part of clinical research into MDR focusses on the potential of "reversal agents" or "resistance modulators" to improve chemotherapy with MDR drugs. Reversal agents are relatively non-cytotoxic agents that inhibit the transport of anticancer agents by Pgp or MRP. Hereby these agents increase the cytosolic and consequently target site concentration of anticancer drug in the MDR cell. A large number of drugs and chemicals have been identified as reversal agents for Pgp-mediated resistance (Ford and Hait, 1990). In general, these compounds have some, but less potent activity as modulators of MRP-mediated drug transport (Cole et al., 1989). The first class of compounds shown to selectively inhibit MRP-mediated daunorubicin transport probably by competition with daunorubicin are the (iso)flavonoids, such as genistein (Versantvoort et al., 1993; 1994). The effect of buthionine sulfoximine (BSO) on daunorubicin accumulation in the MRP-overexpressing HL60/AR cells suggests a role of glutathione in anthracycline transport (Lutzky et al., 1989). The effect of flavonoids or BSO on active transport of other cytostatic drugs is not yet known.

A theoretically, but potentially also important question in clinical practice is whether reversal agents for Pgp-mediated resistance are transported themselves by Pgp out of the cell and whether they act competitively or non-competitively with the cytostatic drugs. In plasma membrane studies, evidence for competitive and non-competitive interactions has been reported for the combination of cyclosporins with vinca alkaloids (Tamai and Safa, 1990) and azidopine with vinblastine or cyclosporin A (Tamai and Safa, 1991) respectively. Using *intact* cells, non-competitive behaviour has been observed for the effect of verapamil on 4'-o-tetrahydropyranyladriamycin (Pereira et al., 1994) and daunorubicin (Spoelstra et al., 1994).

As far as the active transport of the two most studied reversal agents, verapamil and cyclosporin A is concerned, there seems to be general consent between studies that verapamil is transported by Pgp (Cano-Gauchi and Riordan, 1987; Broxterman and Pinedo , 1991). While transport data for cyclosporins also indicate the presence of Pgp-mediated cyclosporin transport (Saeki et al., 1993; Naito et al, 1993), the absence of effect of cyclosporins on the Pgp-ATPase activity (Rao and Scarborough, 1994) and cellular energy metabolism (Broxterman et al., 1990) seems to point at mechanistic differences between the interaction of verapamil and cyclosporin with Pgp. Mutant Pgps are now used to establish whether drugs and reversal agents bind to the same or other sites on the Pgp molecule (Kajiji et al., 1994). Mutant Pgps might exist that are affected by verapamil but not by cyclosporins (Ma and Melera, 1994; Dietel et al., 1994). Analysis of cooperativity of Pgp-mediated daunorubicin transport suggested a model in which Pgp pumps two molecules of daunorubicin per cycle (Guiral et al, 1994). No evidence of cooperativity was found for verapamil-induced stimulation of Pgp-ATPase activity (Garrigos et al., 1993). Moreover the Pgp-ATPase (and drug transport?) activity may be differently influenced by phosphorylation by different protein kinase isoforms (Sachs et al., 1994). These studies show that there is still much to learn about the mechanisms of interaction of individual drugs and reversal agents with Pgp, while for MRP virtually nothing is known yet. It is hoped that more quantitative knowledge of the kinetics of drug transport will lead to more rational and refined application of reversal agents in the clinic.

INTRACELLULAR DISTRIBUTION OF ANTHRACYCLINES

A frequently observed aspect of MDR in tumor cell lines is that the distribution of drugs, mainly studied for anthracyclines, in subcellular compartments seems to be changed compared to that in the drug sensitive cell lines. This aspect will be discussed extensively in Chapter   of this volume. However, it has to be mentioned here that the most frequently reported change in drug distribution, a decrease in the nuclear to cytoplasmic ratio (N/C ratio) of anthracycline fluorescence, occurs both in Pgp and MRP related MDR cell lines, including cell lines with a low resistance factor (Gervasoni et al., 1991; Schuurhuis et al., 1991). Moreover, the contribution of this factor to the resistance compared to the contribution of the drug accumulation defect might be relatively greater in cell lines with a low resistance factor (Schuurhuis et al., 1993b). Although there are many papers formulating hypotheses that this phenomenon might contribute to drug resistance, mainly by means of a putative sequestration of drugs away from their target sites (Marquardt and Center, 1992; Lutzky et al., 1989), the mechanistic cause for the apparently different drug distribution in MDR cells is still unknown. An important observation in this respect might be the finding by Wood et al. (1994), that there was no apparent "redistribution" of daunorubicin in Pgp-expressing cells when measured with [³H]- daunorubicin, while it was observable with fluorescence microscopy. However, in a quantitative study comparing the quenched (i.e. mainly DNA bound) with the unquenched fraction of daunorubicin in Pgp and wild-type cells, it was confirmed that in Pgp-expressing cells, relatively more daunorubicin was present in the cytoplasm (Lankelma et al, 1991). In spite of the lack of mechanistic information, differences in doxorubicin fluorescence N/C ratio may have diagnostic value for prediction of chemotherapy failure in certain diseases, such as acute myeloid leukemia (Schuurhuis et al., 1993a).

CONCLUSIONS

Two drug transporter proteins, Pgp and MRP are known to cause MDR in tumor cell lines. Also, these proteins are known to be expressed to a variable extent in many human tumors. The important question to be addressed is, what the contribution of these proteins to clinical resistance to chemotherapy is. Therefore, essentially one would like to know the impact of these drug transporters on the intracellular drug concentration at their target sites. An *in vivo* method for functional Pgp imaging using an organotechnetium complex as recently proposed (Piwnica-Worms et al.,1993) would be a step forward. Refined, more sensitive techniques to determine *ex vivo* tumor cell drug concentrations to probe specifically various drug transporters will have to be developed. Finally, guided by an increased knowledge on the interaction of drugs with their transport proteins and on cellular pharmacokinetics of cytostatic drugs in MDR tumor cells, hopefully more selective reversal agents will be developed and applied in the clinic.

REFERENCES

Al-Shawi MK, Senior AE (1993): Characterization of the adenosine triphosphatase activity of chinese hamster P-glycoprotein. *J Biol Chem* 268: 4197-4206

Altenberg GA, Young G, Horton JK, Glass D, Belli JA, Reuss L (1993):
       Changes in intra- or extracellular pH do not mediate P-glycoprotein-
       dependent multidrug resistance. *Proc Natl Acad Sci USA* 90: 9735-
       9738
Broxterman HJ, Pinedo HM (1991): Energy metabolism in multidrug
       resistant tumor cells: a review. *J Cell Pharmacol* 2: 239-247
Broxterman HJ, Pinedo HM, Kuiper CM, Schuurhuis GJ, Lankelma J
       (1989): Glycolysis in P-glycoprotein overexpressing human tumor
       cell lines. *FEBS Lett* 247: 405-410
Broxterman HJ, Pinedo HM, Schuurhuis GJ, Lankelma J (1990):
       Cyclosporin A and verapamil have different effects on energy
       metabolism in multidrug-resistant tumour cells. *Br J Cancer* 62: 85-
       88
Cano-Gauchi DF, Riordan JR (1987): Action of calcium antagonists on
       multidrug resistant cells. *Biochem Pharmacol* 36: 2115-2123
Cole SPC, Bhardwaj G, Gerlach JH, Mackie JE, Grant CE, Almquist KC,
       Stewart AJ, Kurz EU, Duncan AMV, Deeley RG (1992):
       Overexpression of a transporter gene in a multidrug-resistant human
       lung cancer cell line. *Science* 258: 1650-1654
Cole SPC, Downes HF, Slovak ML (1989): Effect of calcium antagonists
       on the chemosensitivity of two multidrug-resistant tumour cell lines
       which do not overexpress P-glycoprotein. *Br J Cancer* 59: 42-46
Carlsen SA, Till JE, Ling V (1977): Modulation of drug permeability in
       chinese hamster ovary cells. *Biochem Biophys Acta* 467: 238-250
Dietel M, Herzig I, Reymann A, Brandt I, Schaefer B, Bunge A,
       Heidebrecht HJ, Seidel A (1994): Secondary combined resistance to
       the multidrug-resistance-reversing activity of cyclosporin A in the
       cell line F4-6RADR-CsA. *J Cancer Res Clin Oncol* 120: 263-271
Dordal MS, Winter JN, Atkinson AJ (1992): Kinetic analysis of P-glyco-
       protein mediated doxorubicin efflux. *J Pharmacol Exp Ther* 263:
       762-766
Feller N, Versantvoort CHM, Boven E, Lankelma J, Pinedo HM,
       Broxterman HJ (1994): ATP dependence and activity of drug
       transporters in vivo and in intact tumor cells. *Proc Am Assoc Cancer
       Res* 35: 349
Ford JM, Hait WN (1990): Pharmacology of drugs that alter multidrug
       resistance in cancer. *Pharmacol Rev* 42: 155-199
Garrigos M, Belehradek J, Mir LM, Orlowski S (1993): Absence of
       cooperativity for MgATP and verapamil effects on the ATPase
       activity of P-glycoprotein containing membrane vesicles. *Biochem
       Biophys Res Comm* 196: 1034-1041

Gervasoni JE, Fields SZ, Krishna S, Baker MA, Rosado M, Thuraisamy
        K, Hindenburg AA, Taub RN (1991): Subcellular distribution of
        dauno-rubicin in P-glycoprotein-positive and -negative drug-resistant
        cell lines using laser-assisted confocal microscopy. *Cancer Res* 51:
        4955-4963
Gottesman MM, Pastan I (1988): The multidrug-transporter, a double-
        edged sword. *J Biol Chem* 263: 12163-12166
Guiral M, Viratelle O, Westerhoff HV, Lankelma J (1994): Cooperative
        P-glycoprotein mediated daunorubicin transport into DNA-loaded
        plasma membrane vesicles. *FEBS Lett* 346: 141-145
Hammond JR, Johnstone RM, Gros P (1989): Enhanced efflux of [^{3}H]
        vinblastine from chinese hamster ovary cells transfected with a full-
        length complementary DNA clone for the *mdr*1 gene. *Cancer Res* 49:
        3867-3871
Higgins CF (1992): ABC transporters: from microorganims to man. *Annu
        Rev Cell Biol* 8: 67-113
Horio M, Pastan I, Gottesman MM, Handler JS (1990): Transepithelial
        transport of vinblastine by kidney-derived cell lines. Application of
        new kinetic model to estimate in situ K_m of the pump. *Biochem
        Biophys Acta* 1027: 116-122
Hunter J, Jepson MA, Tsuruo T, Simmons NL, Hirst BH (1993):
        Functional expression of P-glycoprotein in apical membranes of
        human intestinal Caco-2 cells. *J Biol Chem* 268: 14991-14997
Kajiji S, Dreslin JA, Grizzuti K, Gros P (1994): Structurally distinct
        modulators show specific patterns of reversal against P-glycoproteins
        bearing unique mutations at serine[939/941]. *Biochemistry* 33: 5041-5048
Lankelma J, Spoelstra E, Dekker H, Broxterman HJ (1990): Evidence for
        daunomycin efflux from multidrug-resistant 2780[AD] human ovarian
        carcinoma cells against a concentration gradient. *Biochim Biophys
        Acta* 1055: 217-222
Lankelma J, Mülder HS, van Mourik F, Wong Fong Sang HW,
        Kraayenhof R, van Grondelle R (1991): Cellular daunomycin
        fluorescence in multidrug resistant 2780[AD] cells and its relation to
        cellular drug localisation. *Biochim Biophys Acta* 1093: 147-152
Lutzky J, Astor MB, Taub RN, Baker MA, Bhalla K, Gervasoni JE,
        Rosado M, Stewart V, Krishna S, Hindenburg AA (1989): Role of
        glutathione and dependent enzymes in anthracycline-resistant
        HL60/AR cells. *Cancer Res* 49: 4120-4125
Ma JF, Melera PW (1994): Expression of a mutant pgp1 confers a
        multidrug resistance phenotype insensitive to cyclosporin A reversal.
        Proc Am Assoc Cancer Res 35: 358

Marquardt D, Center MS (1992): Drug transport mechanisms in HL60
    cells isolated for resistance to adriamycin: evidence for nuclear drug
    accumulation and redistribution in resistant cells. *Cancer Res* 52:
    3157-3163

Naito M, Tsuge H, Kuroko C, Koyama T, Tomida A, Tatsuta T, Heike Y,
    Tsuruo T (1993): Enhancement of cellular accumulation of
    cyclosporine by anti-P-glycoprotein monoclonal antibody MRK-16
    and synergistic modulation of multidrug resistance. *J Natl Cancer
    Inst* 85: 311-316

Pereira E, Borrel MN, Fiallo M, Garnier-Suillerot A (1994): Non
    -competitive inhibition of P-glycoprotein-associated efflux of THP-
    adriamycin by verapamil in living K562 leukemia cells. *Biochim
    Biophys Acta* 1225: 209-216

Piwnica-Worms D, Chiu ML, Budding M, Kronauge JF, Kramer RA,
    Croop JM (1993): Functional imaging of multidrug-resistant P-
    glycoprotein with an organotechnetium complex. *Cancer Res* 53:
    977-984

Rao US, Scarborough GA (1994): Direct demonstration of high affinity
    interactions of immunosuppressant drugs with the drug binding site
    of the human P-glycoprotein. *Mol Pharmacol* 45: 773-776

Ruetz S, Gros P (1994): Functional expression of P-glycoproteins in
    secretory vesicles. *J Biol Chem* 269: 12277-12284

Sachs CW, Blobe GC, Rao us, Fabbro D, Scarborough GA, Hannum YA,
    Fine RL (1994): Phosphorylation of P-glycoprotein by protein kinase
    C isoenzymes ß$_I$ and ß$_{II}$ inhibits drug-stimulated ATPase activity *in
    vitro*. *Proc Am Assoc Cancer Res* 35: 352

Saeki T, Ueda K, Tanigawara Y, Hori R, Komano T (1993): Human P-
    glycoprotein transports cyclosporin A and FK506. *J Biol Chem* 268:
    6077-6080

Sarkadi B, Price EM, Boucher RC, Germann UA, Scarborough GA
    (1992): Expression of the human multidrug resistance cDNA in insect
    cells generates a high activity drug-stimulated membrane ATPase. *J
    Biol Chem* 267: 4854-4858

Schlemmer SR, Sirotnak FM (1994): Evidence for active transport of
    vinblastine mediated by P-glycoprotein in inside-out plasma
    membrane vesicles derived from murine erythroleukemia cells over-
    expressing MDR-3. *Proc Am Assoc Cancer Res* 35: 431

Schuurhuis G, Broxterman HJ, de Lange JHM, Pinedo HM, van
    Heijningen THM, Kuiper CM, Scheffer GL, Scheper RJ, van Kalken
    CK, Baak JPA, Lankelma J (1991): Early multidrug resistance,
    defined by changes in intracellular doxorubicin distribution,
    independent of P-glycoprotein. *Br J Cancer* 64: 857-861

Schuurhuis GJ, Broxterman HJ, Ossenkoppele GJ, Baak JPA, Lankelma J, Eekman JK, Pinedo HM (1993a): Functional detection of MDR phenotype in acute myeloid leukemia. Correlation with clinical response. *Exp Hematol* 21: 1079

Schuurhuis GJ, van Heijningen THM, Cervantes A, Pinedo HM, de Lange JHM, Keizer HG, Broxterman HJ, Baak JPA, Lankelma J. (1993b) Changes in subcellular doxorubicin distribution and cellular accumulation alone can largely account for doxorubicin resistance in SW-1573 lung cancer and MCF-7 breast cancer multidrug resistant tumour cells. *Br J Cancer* 68: 898-908

Shapiro AB and Ling V (1994): ATPase activity of purified and reconstituted P-glycoprotein from Chinese hamster ovary cells. *J Biol Chem.* 269: 3745-3754

Spoelstra EC, Westerhoff HV, Dekker H, Lankelma J (1992): Kinetics of daunorubicin transport by P-glycoprotein of intact cancer cells. *Eur J Biochem* 207: 567-579

Spoelstra EC, Westerhoff HV, Pinedo HM, Dekker H, Lankelma J (1994): the multidrug-resistance-reverser verapamil interferes with cellular P-glycoprotein mediated pumping of daunorubicin as a non-competing substrate. *Eur J Biochem* 221: 363-373

Stein WD, Cardarelli C, Pastan I, Gottesman MM (1994): Kinetic evidence suggesting that the multidrug transporter differentially handles influx and efflux of its substrates. *Mol Pharmacol* 45: 763-772

Tamai I, Safa AR (1990): Competitive interaction of cyclosporins with the Vinca-alkaloid binding site of P-glycoprotein in multidrug-resistant cells. *J Biol Chem* 265: 16509-16513

Tamai I, Safa AR (1991): Azidopine noncompetitively interacts with vinblastine and cyclosprin A binding to P-glycoprotein in multidrug resistant cells. *J Biol Chem* 266: 16796-16800

Vaupel P, Kallinowski F, Okunieff P (1989): Blood flow, oxygen and nutrient supply, and metabolic microenvironment of human tumors: a review. *Cancer Res* 49: 6449-6465

Versantvoort CHM, Broxterman HJ, Feller N, Dekker H, Kuiper CM, Lankelma J (1992): Probing daunorubicin accumulation defects in non-P-glycoprotein expressing multidrug resistant cell lines using digitonin. *Int J Cancer* 50: 906-911

Versantvoort CHM, Broxterman HJ, Lankelma J, Feller N, Pinedo HM (1994): Competitive inhibition by genistein and ATP dependence of daunorubicin transport in intact MRP overexpressing human small cell lung cancer cells. *Biochem Pharmacol* in press

Versantvoort CHM, Schuurhuis GJ, Pinedo HM, Eekman CA, Kuiper CM, Lankelma J, Broxterman HJ (1993); Genistein modulates the decreased drug accumulation in non-P-glycoprotein mediated multidrug resistant tumour cells. *Br J Cancer* 68:939-946

Wood DJT, Rumsby MG, Warr JR (1994): Subcellular redistribution of [^{3}H] daunomycin by multidrug resistant KB cells. *Proc Am Assoc Cancer Res* 35: 355

Zaman GJR, Flens MJ, van Leusden MR, de Haas M, Mülder HS, Lankelma J, Pinedo HM, Scheper RJ, Baas F, Broxterman HJ, Borst P (1994): The human multidrug resistance-associated protein (MRP) is a plasma membrane drug efflux pump. *Proc Natl Acad Sci USA* in press

4. THE MULTIDRUG RESISTANCE-ASSOCIATED PROTEIN - MRP

Dominic Fan, Diane R. Bielenberg, Yun-Fang Wang, Robert Radinsky, and Pedro J. Beltran

INTRODUCTION

The development of the multidrug resistant (MDR) phenotype in cancer cells is the major obstacle to successful chemotherapy. Elucidation of the mechanisms that determine inherent resistance or chemotherapy-induced resistance of human tumors to many of the anticancer agents currently used in the clinic, is of great interest to researchers and great importance to patients. The MDR phenotype has classically been associated with the overexpression of the transmembrane energy-dependent P-glycoprotein transporter coded for by the *mdr1* gene (Kartner et al. 1983; Pastan and Gottesman 1987; Bradley et al. 1988; Endicott and Ling 1989; Biedler 1994). However, the frequent findings of certain cancer cell lines possessing an MDR phenotype but lacking the overexpression of P-glycoprotein, prompted scientists to search for other potential molecules which could be responsible for an increased resistance to structurally unrelated chemotherapeutic drugs (McGrath and Center 1987; Cole et al. 1989; Haber et al. 1989; Baas et al. 1990; Coley et al. 1991; Versantvoort et al. 1992; Jachez and Loor 1993; Hill and Hosking 1994).

NON-P-GLYCOPROTEIN MEDIATED MDR: NEW PROTEINS

A novel 96-kDa membrane protein has been characterized in human breast cancer MCF-7/AdrVp subline that did not overexpress

P-glycoprotein. This protein has been correlated with drug resistance to doxorubicin and found at high levels in clinical samples obtained from patients refractory to doxorubicin (Chen et al. 1990). Similarly, a 42- and 85-kDa membrane proteins were identified by a polyclonal antibody directed against the putative ATP binding domain of P-glycoprotein in MCF/MX cells selected by mitoxantrone. These cells were cross-resistant to doxorubicin and etoposide but without P-glycoprotein overexpression (Nakagawa et al. 1992). More recently, a 110-kDa ATP-dependent cytoplasmic transporter protein has been identified in many non-P-glycoprotein mediated MDR tumor cell lines and normal cells and tissues by the use of a p110-specific monoclonal antibody LRP-56 (Scheper et al. 1993). The involvement of this LRP-reacting protein in the energy-dependent drug transport process remains to be elucidated. While searching for such alternative molecules, many investigators analyzed the HL60 human leukemia cell line and its drug-selected resistant variants. HL60 cells resistant to vincristine have been found to have elevated levels of three highly phosphorylated surface membrane proteins, P210, P180, and P150 (McGrath and Center 1988). All three proteins contributed to MDR in these cells by means of reduced accumulation of drug. P210 and P180 were determined to be structurally related proteins that reacted with the C219 P-glycoprotein monoclonal antibody. However, P150 was distinct because it was also present in the sensitive and revertant HL60 cells, and did not react with C219. Presumably, phosphorylation of the P150 in sensitive cells could convert this protein to a form active in drug resistance (McGrath and Center 1988). On the other hand, HL60 cells selected for resistance to doxorubicin exhibited MDR but did not contain detectable levels of P-glycoprotein (McGrath and Center 1987). Comparison of membrane proteins between the HL60 and HL60/ADR cell lines, using antibodies raised against synthetic peptides derived from P-glycoprotein, revealed in the HL60/ADR cells the presence of a 190-kDa ATP-binding protein that was primarily localized in the endoplasmic reticulum. This protein was not detectable in the membranes of parental cells and could easily bind 8-azido[alpha-^{32}P] ATP (Marquardt et al. 1990).

MRP: THE MOLECULAR ASPECTS

In order to further characterize this unique 190-kDa protein, investigators resolved to studying gene expression in various cell systems. Many cell lines derived from lung cancers manifest atypical MDR phenotypes

Table 1. Non-P-glycoprotein MDR Cell Lines with MRP Overexpression

Cells	Types	Resistance by	Ref
H69AR	SCLC	ADR-selection	Cole et al. 1992
			Slovak et al. 1993
HL60/ADR	Leukemia	ADR-selection	McGrath et al. 1989
			Marquardt et al. 1990
COR-L23/R	Large cell LC	ADR-selection	Barrand et al. 1993
			Barrand et al. 1994
GLC4/ADR	SCLC	ADR-selection	Zaman et al. 1993
			Kuiper et al. 1994
HT1080/DR4	Fibrosarcoma	ADR-selection	Slovak et al. 1993
MCF7/VP	Breast ca.	VP-16-selection	Schneider et al. 1994
MOR/R	Adenocar. LC	ADR-selection	Barrand et al. 1993
			Barrand et al. 1994
SW-1573-S1-R	NSCLC	ADR-selection	Zaman et al. 1993
U937 U-A's	Leukemia	ADR-selection	Slapak et al. 1994
UMCC-1/VP	Breast ca.	VP-16-selection	Doyle et al. 1994
HeLa T2, T5	Cervical ca.	*mrp* transfection	Grant et al. 1994
NIH/3T3 clones	Mu fibroblasts	*mrp* transfection	Kruh et al. 1994

without P-glycoprotein overexpression (Cole et al. 1989; Baas et al. 1990; Eijdems et al. 1992; Barrand et al. 1993). The small cell lung cancer line NCI-H69 and its resistant variant NCI-H69AR were used to construct a randomly primed H69AR cDNA library and screened by differential hybridization with total cDNA prepared from H69 and H69AR mRNA (Cole et al. 1992). One of the 2.8-kb cDNA clones had a strong differential signal hybridized with a single class of mRNA of approximately 7.8 to 8.2 kb that was overexpressed 100 to 200 fold in the resistant cells. A single open reading frame of 1531 amino acids was defined (Cole and Deeley 1993), encoding a protein designated as multidrug resistance-associated protein (MRP). The gene coding for this message was named MRP gene. Southern blot analysis indicated that the overexpression of MRP transcripts was directly associated with gene amplification (Cole et al. 1992).

CYTOGENETIC EVIDENCE

Karyotypic composition analysis of the parental and resistant cell lines showed some significant differences. Both parental and resistant cell lines contained a morphologically normal chromosome 16, one der(16), and the same variability in the number of double minutes. However, the NCI-H69AR cell line also displayed a new der(16) that exhibited structural alterations involving band 16p13.1 (Slovak et al. 1993). This finding was consequential since Cole and colleagues had previously mapped the MRP gene to band 16p13.1 by radioisotopic chromosomal *in situ* hybridization (Cole et al. 1992). In addition, the NCI-H69AR resistant cells had two large hsr-bearing marker chromosomes. In order to demonstrate that these cytogenetic changes were relevant for MRP expression,a partial revertant of the NCI-H69AR line was also analyzed. The NCI-H69PR revertant line contained approximately one-twentieth of the 7.8 to 8.2 kb mRNA and no longer possessed the hsr-bearing chromosomal markers and the double minutes containing the chromosome 16 material, proving the importance of these alterations for MRP overexpression (Cole et al. 1992).

CELL BIOLOGY OF MRP

Similar overexpression of the 190-kDa plasma membrane protein have been found in many MDR cell lines to include the human MCF7/VP breast cancer and the human small cell UMCC-1/VP, large cell COR-L23/R and adenocarcinoma MOR/R lung cancer (Table 1), as well as human tissues (Table 2), and the protein is likely to be the encoded product of the MRP gene (Barrand et al. 1993; Barrand et al. 1994; Doyle et al. 1994; Schneider et al. 1994b). These studies provided evidence for a unique molecular determinant for non-P-glycoprotein MDR phenotypes. In an effort to determine if the p190 novel protein that produced an MDR phenotype in the HL60/ADR cells may be related to the MRP gene first identified in the H69AR cells (Cole et al. 1992), antisera were prepared by using three synthetic peptides derived from the deduced sequence of the H69AR MRP protein (Krishnamachary and Center 1993). By immunoblot analysis, all antisera reacted with a 190 kDa protein in the membranes of resistant but not sensitive HL60 cells. Antiserum ASPKE, prepared against amino acids sequence of 246-260

Table 2. MRP Expression in Normal Human Tissues

Tissues	Relative MRP mRNA Levels
Muscle	5+
Lung	4+
Spleen	3+
Testis	3+
Bladder	3+
Thyroid	3+
Adrenal gland	2+
Gall bladder	2+
Stomach	+
Duodenum	+
Colon	+
Kidney	+
Heart	±
Placenta	±
Pancreas	±
Ovary	±
Brain	±
Liver	±

Expression of MRP in various normal human tissues are assigned by the relative mRNA levels visualized by RNase protection assays. Ref. Zaman et al. 1993.

(KEDTSEQVVPVLVKN) and did not cross-react with P-glycoprotein, localized p190 mainly in the endoplasmic reticulum with lower levels also found in the plasma membrane fraction, consistent with previous findings (Marquardt et al. 1990). By blocking the N-linked carbohydrate addition of the NCI-H69 AR cells with tunicamycin, a 165-kDa reduced glycosylated form of p190 was generated in the endoplasmic reticulum membranes (Krishnamachary and Center 1993). Alignment-parameter analysis of the MRP gene performed by Cole and colleagues (Cole et al. 1992) revealed that the MRP protein is a member of the adenosine triphosphate (ATP)-binding cassette (ABC) superfamily of transport systems (Hyde et al. 1990) that are consistently being clustered into two major subgroups.   One such cluster includes the human MRP (Hum/MRP), the leishmania P-glycoprotein-related molecule (Lei/PgpA), and the cystic fibrosis transmembrane conductance regulators (CFTRs) of human (Hum/CFTR), bovine (Bov/CFTR), mouse (Mus/CFTR), and dogfish (Squ/CFTR). The other cluster includes the P-glycoproteins, the major histocompatibility complex class II-linked peptide transporters (Hum/Tap2 and Mus/Tap1), the bacterial exporters (Eco/HlyB and Pas/LktB), the heterocyst differentiation protein (Ana/HetA), the malarial parasite transporter (Pfa/Mdr1), and the yeast mating factor exporter (Ysc/Ste6). Therefore, MRP is only distantly related to P-glycoprotein (14% homology confined to the predicted ATP-binding domain) (Grant et al. 1994) and other members of the ABC transporters superfamily. The analysis suggests that MRP may be more closely related to the Leishmania P-glycoprotein-related molecule Lei/pgpA, and to the human cystic fibrosis transmembrane conductance regulator CFTR with similarity in the C-terminal regions containing signatures of the nucleotide-binding folds (NBFs) (Cole et al. 1992).

TRANSFECTION OF THE MRP GENE

It has become evident that MRP may play an important role in non-P-glycoprotein mediated drug resistance. However, the possibility that MRP does not confer MDR but its overexpression is simply a result of coamplification with the gene that actually mediates drug resistance, has not been ruled out. In order to address this issue, Grant and colleagues transfected HeLa cells with an pRc/CMV-MRP expression vector (Grant et al. 1994). Some of those transfected clones that exhibited an MDR phenotype also displayed a 20- to 80-fold higher mRNA levels than parental cells and were accompanied by more than 10-fold increase in the level of MRP protein and a 15-fold increase in drug resistance. These cells were cross-resistant to vincristine and VP-16 but not to cisplatin. Molecular analysis of the transfected cells revealed that cellular mRNA transcripts for topoisomerase IIα and IIß, annexin II, and P-glycoprotein levels were not different from the parental cells. Similarly, using a λpCEV27 phagemid DNA library prepared from the polyadenylated RNA of the doxorubicin-resistant HL60R cells, Kruh and colleagues transfected the NIH/3T3 fibroblasts with the drug resistant DNA. The transfer of an expression cDNA library material to these cells conferred a MRP-mediated MDR phenotype to doxorubicin, vinblastine, and VP16 in several of the transfectants (Kruh et al. 1994).

These observations strongly suggest that MRP overexpression may be sufficient in conferring an MDR phenotype in cancer cells similar to that mediated by P-glycoprotein overexpression (Grant et al. 1994).

OTHER CONSIDERATIONS

It must be noted that MRP is not responsible for every non-P-glycoprotein mediated MDR phenotype, and that in many cases other factors might be involved in conferring resistance (Zwelling et al. 1990; Fan et al. 1992; de la Torre et al. 1993; Hamaguchi et al. 1993; Scheper et al. 1993; Fan et al. 1994; Moore et al. 1994; Schneider et al. 1994a; Takeda et al. 1994). Zaman and colleagues used a RNAse protection assay to examine MRP expression in several non-P-glycoprotein mediated MDR cell lines derived from GLC4, a small cell lung cancer, and from SW 1573, a non-small cell lung cancer. The results showed that none of the ten cell lines derived from SW 1573 overexpressed MRP and that only one of the cell lines derived from GLC4 displayed a 25-fold increase in MRP mRNA and gene copy number (Zaman et al. 1993). In another study, it was shown that MRP overexpression was highest in the human leukemia U937 cells selected with a shorter exposure time in lower, more clinically relevant concentrations of doxorubicin. However, there was no evidence for MRP gene amplification. When the same cell line was exposed to higher concentrations of doxorubicin or for longer periods of time, MRP overexpression started to decline and the cells progressively overexpressed P-glycoprotein (Slapak et al. 1994). These data imply that pharmacologic and physiologic considerations are important for modeling MDR and might explain the lack of correlation between P-glycoprotein overexpression and clinical drug resistance manifested by certain cancers.

Studies from our laboratory analyzing if host-tumor interactions modulate MRP or mdr1 gene expression suggest that mdr1 but not MRP can be upmodulated by host environment. We determined the levels of the ~ 7.8-kb MRP and ~ 4.3-kb mdr1 mRNA transcripts by nothern blot analysis of the KM12SM human colon carcinoma cells growing in tissue culturte, as subcutaneous and spleen tumors, as cecal tumor and liver metastases in athymic nude mice, and as cultures derived from those tumors. When compared to the original KM12SM cells in culture, mRNA analyses demonstrated an reduced expression of the 7.8-kb MRP specific transcript under all conditions (Fig. 1). In contrast, expression

Figure 1. Northern blot analyses of MRP and *mdr*1 expression in the KM12SM human colon carcinoma cells growing ectopically (skin and spleen), orthotopically (cecum and liver), or *in vitro*. Lanes A, KM12SM human colon carcinoma cells growing *in vitro*; B, subcutaneous tumor; C, subcutaneous tumor cells recultured *in vitro* for 4 days; D, spleen tumor; E, spleen tumor cells recultured *in vitro* for 4 days; F, cecal tumor; G, cecal tumor cells recultured *in vitro* for 7 days; H, liver metastases; I, liver metastases recultured *in vitro* for 4 days. Poly (A)+ mRNA (5 µg/lane) was used in all cases. The probes used were a 1-kb Eco RI restriction endonuclease cDNA fragment from the 3' end of the MRP 10.1 clone (Cole et al., 1992), a 1.38-kb Eco RI fragment from clone pHDR5A corresponding to the human P-glycoprotein 1 (*mdr*1) cDNA (Galski et al., 1989), and a 1.3-kb Pst I gene fragment corresponding to rat glyceraldehyde-3-phosphate dehydrogenase (GAPDH) (Fort et al., 1985).

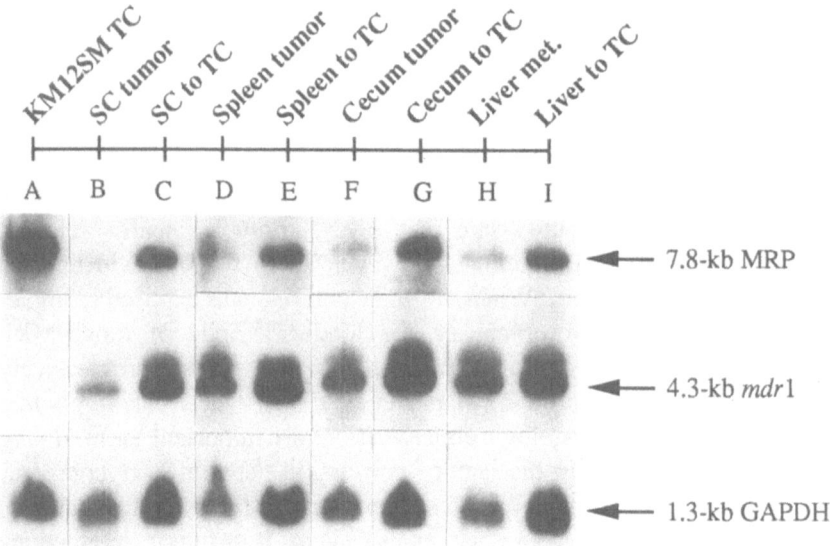

of the 4.3-kb *mdr*1-specific transcript was upmodulated in KM12SM cells grown as tumors in the athymic nude mice and as transient cultures of the same tumors. Subcutaneous and spleen tumors expressed lower levels of the *mdr*1 transcript when compared with cecal or liver tumors (Fig. 1). These findings demonstrate that the organ environment can differentiallymodulate the expression of the *mdr*1 and MRP genes in the KM12SM human colon carcinoma cells.

Other observations from studies on MRP-related MDR phenotypes suggested that although MRP alone may be sufficient in causing drug resistance in cancer cells, it may also function as a factor of collateral MDR. In the case of the human small cell H69AR, large cell COR-L23/R, and adenocarcinoma MOR/R lung cancer cell lines, MRP gene amplification parallels with the levels of its mRNA, MRP protein and *in vitro* drug resistance, indicating that MRP could be solely accountable for the resistant phenotype (Cole et al. 1992; Barrand et al. 1993; Barrand et al. 1994).On the other hand, in the P-glycoprotein-negative human fibrosarcoma cell line HT1080/DR4, a 200-fold increase in drug resistance has been found, but only a 14-fold increase in the MRP mRNA and a 5-fold amplification in the MRP gene. Although one should not align scales of molecular parameters to quantify gradation of pharmacological responses, these observations nevertheless point to the possibility that other factors might also play a collateral role in the development of non-P-glycoprotein mediated MDR phenotypes (Mirski and Cole 1989; Slovak et al. 1993).

PERSPECTIVE

MRP is found in many cancer cell lines as well as normal tissues, and is considered as a transporter which could function in a putative P-glycoprotein-like fashion to alter intracellular accumulation and/or distribution of drugs. While the importance of MRP in experimental drug resistance is becoming more obvious, the actual mechanism for MRP-mediated drug resistance is still not understood. However, the MRP-overexpressing drug resistant human small cell lung cancer line H69AR has been found to have an inwardly rectifying K^+ channel current and an increased volume-regulated Cl^- anion current (Jirsch et al. 1993). Although MRP expression in some clinical hematological (Burger et al. 1994; Abbaszadegan et al. 1994) (Broxterman et al. 1994) and lung (Rubio et al. 1994; Savaraj et al. 1994) cancers appeared to be detectable but ubiquitous, higher levels of MRP have been noted in some acute lymphoblastic leukemia (ALL) relapses and chronic myeloid leukemia (CML) samples (Beck et al. 1994). Furthermore, it has been found that acute myeloid leukemia (AML) patients with an inversion in chromosome 16 could result in deletion of MRP and a relatively favorable prognosis (Kuss et al. 1994). Therefore, even the possible role for MRP to play in clinical drug resistance is not certain, its significance should not be underestimated.

REFERENCES

Abbaszadegan MR, Futscher BW, Domann F, List A, Dalton WS (1994): Analysis of MRP expression in drug resistant cell lines and clinical specimens. *Proc Amer Assoc Cancer Res* 35:207

Baas F, Jongsma APM, Broxterman HJ, Arceci RJ, Housman D, Scheffer GL, Riethorst A, van Groenigen M, Nieuwint AWM, Joenje H (1990): Non-P-glycoprotein mediated mechanism for multidrug resistance precedes P-glycoprotein expression during *in vitro* selection for doxorubicin resistance in a human lung cancer cell line. *Cancer Res* 50:5392-5398

Barrand MA, Heppell-Parton AC, Wright KA, Rabbitts PH, Twentyman PR (1994): A 190-kilodalton protein overexpressed in non-P-glycoprotein-containing multidrug-resistant cells and its relationship to the MRP gene. *J Natl Cancer Inst* 86:110-117

Barrand MA, Rhodes T, Center MS, Twentyman PR (1993): Chemosensitisation and drug accumulation effects of cyclosporin A, PSC-833 and verapamil in human MDR large cell lung cancer cells expressing a 190k membrane protein distinct from P-glycoprotein. *Eur J Cancer* 29:408-415

Beck J, Gekeler V, Handgretinger R, Niethammer D (1994): PCR gene expression analysis of multidrug resistance associated genes in primary and relapsed state leukemias: comparison of mdr1, mrp, topoisomerase IIα, topoisomerase IIß and cyclin A mRNA levels. *Proc Amer Assoc Cancer Res* 35:337

Biedler JL (1994): Drug resistance: genotype versus phenotype--Thirty-second G. H. A. Clowes Memorial Award Lecture. *Cancer Res* 54:666-678

Bradley G, Juranka PF, Ling V (1988): Mechanism of multidrug resistance. *Biochim Biophys Acta* 948:87-128

Broxterman HJ, Kuiper CM, Schuurhuis GJ, Ossenkoppele GJ, Feller N, Scheper RJ, Lankelma J, Pinedo HM (1994): Analysis of P-glycoprotein (pgp) and non-Pgp multidrug resistance in acute myeloid leukemia. *Proc Amer Assoc Cancer Res* 35:348

Burger H, Nooter K, van Wingerden KE, Oostrum RG, Sonneveld P, Zaman GJR, Borst P, Splinter TAW, Stoter G (1994): Analysis of the expression of multidrug resistance-associated protein (MRP) in hematological malignancies. *Proc Amer Assoc Cancer Res* 35:206

Chen YN, Mickley LA, Schwartz AM, Acton EM, Hwang JL, Fojo AT (1990): Characterization of Adriamycin-resistant human breast cancer cells which display overexpression of a novel resistance-related membrane protein. *J Biol Chem* 265:10073-10080

Cole SPC, Bhardwaj G, Gerlach JH, Mackie JE, Grant CE, Almquist KC, Stewart AJ, Kurz EU, Duncan AMV, Deeley RG (1992): Overexpression of a transporter gene in a multidrug-resistant human lung cancer cell line. *Science* 258:1650-1654

Cole SPC, Deeley RG (1993): Multidrug resistance-associated protein: sequence correction. *Science* 260:879

Cole SPC, Downes HF, Slovak ML (1989): Effect of calcium antagonists on the chemosensitivity of two multidrug-resistant human tumour cell lines which do not overexpress P-glycoprotein. *Br J Cancer* 59:42-46

Coley HW, Workman P, Twentyman PR (1991): Retention of activity by selected anthracyclines in a multidrug resistant human large cell lung carcinoma line without P-glycoprotein hyperexpression. *Br J Cancer* 63:351-357

de la Torre M, Hao XY, Larsson R, Nygren P, Tsuruo T, Mannervik B, Bergh J (1993): Characterization of four doxorubicin adapted human breast cancer cell lines with respect to chemotherapeutic drug sensitivity, drug resistance associated membrane proteins and glutathione transferases. *Anticancer Res* 13:1425-1430

Doyle LA, Ross DD, Ordonez JV, Yang W, Gao Y, Tong Y, Belani CP, Gutheil JC (1994): An etoposide-resistant small cell lung cancer subline overexpresses the MRP gene. *Proc Amer Assoc Cancer Res* 35:467

Eijdems EWHM, Borst P, Jongsma APM, de Jong S, de Vries EGE, van Groenigen M, Versantvoort CHM, Nieuwint AWM, Baas F (1992): Genetic transfer of non-P-glycoprotein-mediated multidrug resistance (MDR) in somatic cell fusion: dissection of a compound MDR phenotype. *Proc Natl Acad Sci USA* 89:3498-3502

Endicott JA, Ling V (1989): The biochemistry of P-glycoprotein-mediated multidrug resistance. *Annu Rev Biochem* 58:137-171

Fan D, Beltran PJ, O'Brian CA (1994): Reversal of multidrug resistance. In: *Reversal of Multidrug Resistance in Cancer,* (ed. JA Kellen), pp. 93-125. Boca Raton: CRC Press

Fan D, Fidler IJ, Ward NE, Seid C, Earnest LE, Housey GM, O'Brian CA (1992): Stable expression of a cDNA encoding rat brain protein kinase C-beta I confers a multidrug-resistant phenotype on rat fibroblasts. *Anticancer Res* 12:661-667

Fort P, Marty L, Piechaczyk M, Sabrouty DE, Dani C, Jeanteur P, Blanchard JM (1985) Various rat adult tissues express only one major species from the glyceraldehyde-3-phosphate dehydrogenase multigene family. *Nucleic Acids Res* 13:1431-1442

Galski H, Sullivan M, Willingham MC, Chin K-V, Gottesman MM, Pastan I, Merlino GT (1989) Expression of a human multidrug resistance cDNA (*mdr*1) in the bone marrow of transgenic mice: resistance to danunomycin-induced leukopenia. *Mol Cell Biol* 9:4357-4363

Grant CE, Valdimarsson G, Hipfner DR, Almquist KC, Cole SPC, Deeley RG (1994): Overexpression of multidrug resistance-associated protein (MRP) increases resistance to natural product drugs. *Cancer Res* 54:357-361

Haber M, Norris MD, Kavallaris M, Bell DR, Davey RA, White L, Stewart BW (1989): Atypical multidrug resistance in a therapy-induced drug-resistant human leukemia cell line (LALW-2): resistance to vinca alkaloid independent of P-glycoprotein. *Cancer Res* 49:5281-5287

Hamaguchi K, Godwin AK, Yakushiji M, ODwyer PJ, Ozols RF, Hamilton TC (1993): Cross-resistance to diverse drugs is associated with primary cisplatin resistance in ovarian cancer cell lines. *Cancer Res* 53:5225-5232

Hill BT, Hosking LK (1994): Differential effectiveness of a range of novel drug-resistance modulators, relative to verapamil, in influencing vinblastine or teniposide cytotoxicity in human lymphoblastoid CCRF-CEM sublines expressing classic or atypical multidrug resistance. *Cancer Chemother Pharmacol* 33:317-24

Hyde SC, P. E, Hartshorn MJ, Mimmack MM, Gileadi U, Pearce SR, Gallagher MP, Gill DR, Hubbard RE, Higgins CF (1990): Structural model of ATP-binding proteins associated with cystic fibrosis, multidrug resistance and bacterial transport. *Nature* 346:362-365

Jachez B, Loor F (1993): Atypical multi-drug resistance (MDR): low sensitivity of a P-glycoprotein-expressing human T lymphoblastoid MDR cell line to classical P-glycoprotein-directed resistance-modulating agents. *Anticancer Drugs* 4:605-615

Jirsch J, Deeley RG, Cole SPC, Stewart AJ, Fedida D (1993): Inwardly rectifying K+ channels and volume-regulated anion channels in multidrug-resistant small cell lung cancer cells. *Cancer Res* 53:4156-4160

Kartner N, Riordan JR, Ling V (1983): Cell surface P-glycoprotein associated with multidrug resistance in mammalian cell lines. *Science* 221:1285-1288

Krishnamachary N, Center MS (1993): The MRP gene associated with a non-P-glycoprotein multidrug resistance encodes a 190-kDa membrane bound glycoprotein. *Cancer Res* 53:3658-3661

Kuss BJ, Deeley RG, Cole SPC, Willman CL, Kopecky KJ, Wolman SR, Eyre HJ, Lane SA, Nancarrow JK, Whitmore SA (1994): Deletion of gene for multidrug resistance in acute myeloid leukaemia with inversion in chromosome 16: prognostic implications. *Lancet* 343:1531-1534

Kruh GD, Chan A, Myers K, Gaughan K, Miki T, Aaronson SA (1994): Expression complementary DNA library transfer establishes *mrp* as a multidrug resistance gene. *Cancer Res* 54:1649-1652

Marquardt D, McCrone S, Center MS (1990): Mechanisms of multidrug resistance in HL60 cells: detection of resistance-associated proteins with antibodies against synthetic peptides that correspond to the deduced sequence of P-glycoprotein. *Cancer Res* 50:1426-1430

McGrath T, Center MS (1987): Adriamycin resistance in HL60 cells in the absence of detectable P-glycoprotein. *Biochem Biophys Res Commun* 145:1171-1176

McGrath T, Center MS (1988): Mechanisms of multidrug resistance in HL60 cells: evidence that a surface membrane protein distinct fromP-glycoprotein contributes to reduced cellular accumulation of drug. *Cancer Res* 48:3959-3963

Mirski SE, Cole SPC (1989): Antigens associated with multidrug resistance in H69AR, a small cell lung cancer cell line. *Cancer Res* 49:5719-5724

Moore M, Wang X, Lu YF, Wormke M, Craig A, Gerlach JH, Burghardt R, Barhoumi R, Safe S (1994): Benzo-alpha pyrene-resistant MCF-7 human breast cancer cells. A unique aryl hydrocarbon-nonresponsive clone. *J Biol Chem* 269:11751-11759

Nakagawa M, Schneider E, Dixon KH, Horton J, Kelley K, Morrow C, Cowan KH (1992): Reduced intracellular drug accumulation in the absence of P-glycoprotein (*mdr*1) overexpression in mitoxantrone-resistant human MCF-7 breast cancer cells. *Cancer Res* 52:6175-6181

Pastan I, Gottesman MM (1987): Multiple drug resistance in human cancer. *N Engl J Med* 28:1388-1393

Rubio GJ, Pinedo HM, Gazdar AF, Van Ark-Otte J, Giaccone G (1994): MRP gene assessment in human cancer, normal lung, and lung cancer cell lines. *Proc Amer Assoc Cancer Res* 35:206

Savaraj N, Wu CJ, Bao JJ, Solomon J, Donnelly E, Feun LG, Lampidis TJ, Kuo MT (1994): Multidrug resistance associated protein gene expression in small cell and non small cell lung cancer. *Proc Amer Assoc Cancer Res* 35:242

Scheper RJ, Broxterman HJ, Scheffer GL, Kaaijk P, Dalton WS, van Heijningen THM, van Kalken CK, Slovak ML, de Vries EGE, van der Valk P, Meijer CJLM, Pinedo HM (1993): Overexpression of a Mr 110,000 vesicular protein in non-P-glycoprotein-mediated multidrug resistance. *Cancer Res* 53:1475-1479

Schneider E, Horton JK, Yang CH, Nakagawa M, Cowan KH (1994a): Multidrug resistance-associated protein gene overexpression and reduced drug sensitivity of topoisomerase II in a human breast carcinoma MCF7 cell line selected for etoposide resistance. *Cancer Res* 54:152-158

Schneider E, Yamazaki H, Sinha BK, Cowan KH (1994b): Chemosensitization of drug-sensitive and resistant human breast cancer MCF-7 cells expressing the multidrug resistance-associated protein (MRP). *Proc Amer Assoc Cancer Res* 35:359

Slapak CA, Mizunuma N, Kufe DW (1994): Overexpression of the multidrug resistance-associated protein without gene amplification in doxorubicin selected U937 cells. *Proc Amer Assoc Cancer Res* 35:342

Slovak ML, Ho JP, Bhardwaj G, Kurz EU, Deeley RG, Cole SPC (1993): Localization of a novel multidrug resistance-associated gene in the HT1080/DR4 and H69AR human tumor cell lines. *Cancer Res* 53:3221-3225

Takeda Y, Nishio K, Niitani H, Saijo N (1994): Reversal of multidrug resistance by tyrosine-kinase inhibitors in a non-P-glycoprotein-mediated multidrug-resistant cell line. *Int J Cancer* 57:229-239

Versantvoort CHM, Broxterman HJ, Pinedo HM, de Vries EGE, Feller N, Kuiper CM, Lankelma J (1992): Energy-dependent processes involved in reduced drug accumulation in multidrug-resistant human lung cancer cell lines without P-glycoprotein expression. *Cancer Res* 52:17-23

Zaman GJ, Versantvoort CH, Smit JJ, Eijdems EW, de Haas M, Smith AJ, Broxterman HJ, Mulder NH, de Vries EG, Baas F, Borst P (1993): Analysis of the expression of MRP, the gene for a new putative transmembrane drug transporter, in human multidrug resistant lung cancer cell lines. *Cancer Res* 53:1747-1750

Zwelling LA, Slovak ML, Doroshow JH, Hinds M, Chan D, Parker E, Mayes J, Sie KL, Meltzer PS, Trent JM (1990): HT1080/DR4: a P-glycoprotein-negative human fibrosarcoma cell line exhibiting resistance to topoisomerase II-reactive drugs despite the presence of a drug-sensitive topoisomerase II. *J Natl Cancer Inst* 82:1553-1561

5. TOPOISOMERASES IN MULTIDRUG RESISTANCE

Teruhiro Utsugi, Cynthia E. Herzog, and Dominic Fan

INTRODUCTION

Multidrug resistance (MDR) in cancer refers to the phenomenon whereby the treatment with one chemotherapeutic drug induces pleiotropic resistance toward drugs that are unrelated to the original compound. Since the acquisition of MDR in cancer is one of the obstacles in the management of cancer, the elucidation of the MDR mechanisms and the development of therapeutics to overcome clinical MDR are major concerns in cancer chemotherapy.

Topoisomerases are important targets for certain anticancer drugs widely used in the clinic. Adriamycin (ADR), etoposide (VP-16), and teniposide (VM-26) are being used to target topoisomerase II (Tewey et al., 1984a; Ross et al., 1984). Camptothecin analogues such as CPT-11 (Kunimoto et al., 1987), which has been approved for clinical use in Japan, and Topotecan (Johnson et al., 1989), which is under clinical trial in the U.S.A., are drugs being used to target topoisomerase I. Recently, a variety of structurally unrelated agents have been found to be capable of inhibiting both topoisomerase I and II, and are being developed as chemotherapeutic agents.

At least two types of MDR can be distinguished on the basis of different mechanisms: so called "classical MDR" and "atypical MDR". The "classical MDR" phenotype is resistance to a group of structurally unrelated lipophilic drugs caused by reduced intracellular drug levels due to the expression of the membrane bound P-glycoprotein (P-gp) efflux pump. Cells selected for P-gp mediated MDR are generally resistant to vinca alkaloids, actinomycin-D, anthracyclines and epipodophyllotoxins.

Cells with "atypical MDR" have no or low levels of P-gp, instead resistance is associated with mechanisms such as an alteration of topoisomerase II (Danks et al., 1987; Beck et al., 1987; Danks et al., 1988). Resistant cells selected with the topoisomerase II inhibitor VP-16 often express cross resistance to the other topoisomerase II inhibitors such as amsacrine (*m*-AMSA) and ADR (Glisson et al., 1986), but not to vinca alkaloids. In this chapter, the role of topoisomerases in MDR, especially the mechanism of resistance to topoisomerase inhibitors and the attempts at the reversal of such resistance are discussed.

TOPOISOMERASES

All eukaryotic cells have two classes of topoisomerases which can be distinguished as type I and type II topoisomerase on the basis of their divergent physical and mechanistic properties (Wang, 1985; Osheroff, 1989). The role of type I topoisomerase is to relax DNA twist made in the process of DNA and/or RNA synthesis by altering DNA topology with the reaction passing or swiveling a single strand of DNA through a transient single-strand break made in the other strand (Wang, 1985). Type I topoisomerase is a monomeric protein having a molecular weight of 100-kDa, requires no energy-cofactor for its action, and its gene is encoded on chromosome 20q12-13.2 as an unique gene (Liu and Miller, 1981).

Type II topoisomerase alters DNA topology by passing the DNA helix through a transient double strand break made in the DNA helix *via* an ATP-dependent process (Wang, 1985). Topoisomerase II is an essential enzyme for the survival of eukaryotic cells and plays an important role in relaxing DNA twist made in the process of DNA replication and recombination. At least two isoforms of topoisomerase II exist and are distinguished by their different molecular masses. Topoisomerase IIα is a 170-kDa polypeptide and topoisomerase IIß a 180-kDa polypeptide (Drake et al., 1987; Chung et al., 1989). The apparent structure of topoisomerase IIα (Danks et al., 1993) is shown in Figure 1. The mammalian topoisomerase II can be further divided into three domains on the basis of its amino acid sequence comparison with the bacterial type II topoisomerase; DNA gyrase (Lynn et al., 1986; Wychoff et al., 1989). The amino-terminal domain of the mammalian topoisomerase II has a homology with the B-subunit of the bacterial DNA gyrase and contains the ATP binding consensus sequences. The central domain has homology with the A-subunit of DNA gyrase which contains tyrosine

Figure 1. Schematic sequences and functional sites of the human topoisomerase IIα. Motif A and motif B: ATP-binding sites. DNBS: ATP-binding dinucleotide binding sequence. DBD: DNA binding domain containing tyrosine residue at amino acid position 804 that binds covalently to DNA during strand passing cycle. gyr: bacterial gyrase. Reference: Danks et al, 1993.

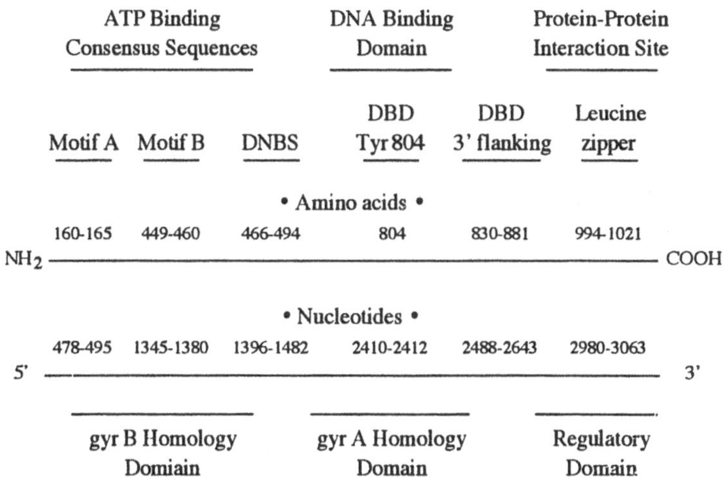

ATP Binding Consensus Sequences			DNA Binding Domain		Protein-Protein Interaction Site
Motif A	Motif B	DNBS	DBD Tyr 804	DBD 3' flanking	Leucine zipper

• Amino acids •

| 160-165 | 449-460 | 466-494 | 804 | 830-881 | 994-1021 |

NH₂ —— COOH

• Nucleotides •

| 478-495 | 1345-1380 | 1396-1482 | 2410-2412 | 2488-2643 | 2980-3063 |

5' —— 3'

| gyr B Homology Domiain | gyr A Homology Domain | Regulatory Domain |

residues that can link covalently to DNA and act as breakage and reunion points. The carboxyl-terminal domain contains a number of phosphorylation sites which are highly variable (homologues to histone H1) and lack homology with bacterial DNA gyrase. Topoisomerase IIα and topoisomerase IIß have 70% homology, and when the non-conserved carboxyl-terminal domain is excluded, homology between the two increases to 80% (Chung et al., 1989; Austin et al., 1990; Jenkins et al., 1992; Austin et al., 1993).

Since the carboxyl-terminal contains a number of sites which can be phosphorylated *in vivo* (Cardenas et al., 1992), it is postulated to play an important role in the physiological regulation of the enzyme. The differences in the carboxyl-terminal domain between topoisomerase IIα and topoisomerase IIß may contribute to their dissimilar characteristics. Although topoisomerase IIα and topoisomerase IIß are highly homologous, the encoding genes are located on distinct chromosomes; 17q21-22 for topoisomerase IIα and 3q24 for topoisomerase IIß (Tsai-Pflugfelder et al., 1988; Chung et al., 1989; Tan et al., 1992; Jenkins et al., 1992). The significance of cells having two types of topoisomerase

II and their biological roles and reactivity to chemotherapeutic drugs are not well defined.   The characteristics of topoisomerase IIα and topoisomerase IIß are summarized in Table 1.   The analysis of drug stimulated cleavage suggested that topoisomerase IIα prefers A-T rich sequences, while topoisomerase IIß prefers G-C rich sequences (Fosse et al., 1988). The cellular distribution for these enzymes are also different with topoisomerase IIα found in the nuclear matrix and topoisomerase IIß in the nucleolus (Negri et al., 1992; Zini et al., 1991).

Another   major   difference   between   topoisomerase   IIα   and topoisomerase IIβ is their expression profile during cell proliferation (Woessner et al., 1991).   The cellular amount of topoisomerase IIα increases during growth phase and falls sharply when approaching plateau phase (Drake et al., 1989; Prosperi et al., 1992). This suggests that the expression of topoisomerase IIα is intimately associated with replication and chromosomal condensation-segregation during cell growth and division.   In contrast, the expression of topoisomerase IIβ is not associated with cell proliferation, if anything the amount of topoisomerase IIβ actually increases in plateau phase (Drake et al., 1989). It has been suggested that topoisomerase IIβ may be involved in the process of DNA transcription (Prosperi et al., 1992).

Reduced levels of topoisomerase IIα are commonly found in cells resistant to VP-16, VM-26, or m-AMSA, while the expression of topoisomerase IIβ does not change (Drake et al., 1987). Topoisomerase II inhibitors show 3-8 fold greater inhibition of the catalytic activity of topoisomerase IIα than topoisomerase IIβ (Drake et al., 1989). These findings indicate that chemotherapeutic drugs may induce cytotoxicity selectively via topoisomerase IIα (Woessner at al., 1990).   Since the significance of topoisomerase IIβ in "atypical MDR" and its role on DNA metabolism are more equivocal, we will focus on topoisomerase IIα in this chapter and refer to it synonymously as topoisomerase II.

TOPOISOMERASE INHIBITORS

A number of chemotherapeutic drugs inhibit topoisomerases as their primary cellular targets. The inhibitors of topoisomerase I, topoisomerase II, and both topoisomerase I and II are listed in Table 2. These agents are structurally diverse, and one of the few shared properties of these agents is their ability to bind DNA. These agents can be divided into two groups; the DNA-intercalative agents and the non-intercalative agents (Liu, 1990).

Table 1. Characteristics of Topoisomerase II alpha and beta.

Characteristics	Topoisomerase II alpha	Topoisomerase II beta
Molecular weight	170 kDa homodimer	180 kDa homodimer
Chromosomal	17q21-22	3q24
Distribution	Nucleoplasm	Nucleolus
Affinity to DNA	A+T rich domain	G+C rich domain
Cell cycle-dependency	High: exponential phase (S/G2), peaks G2/M, decrease in G1	High: plateau-phase (G0/G1) constant throughout cell cycle
Topo II inhibitors	High sensitivity	Low sensitivity
Function	DNA synthesis ?	DNA transcription ?

Topoisomerase II Inhibitors

Topoisomerase II inhibitors include many clinically used antineoplastic agents such as ADR, VP-16, and VM-26. The group of drugs which exhibit intercalative property includes anthracyclines (e.g., ADR, daunomycin), mitoxantrone (Tewey et al., 1984a), *m*-AMSA (Nelson et al., 1984; Rowe et al., 1986), elliptecine (Tewey et al., 1984b), and amonafide (Hsiang et al., 1989). The other group of drugs which exhibits non-intercalative property includes epipodophyllotoxins (e.g., VP-16, VM-26), genestein (Yamashita et al., 1990), and quinolines (Elsea et al., 1993). The common mechanism of action for these agents is their ability to stabilize a transient covalent complex between DNA and topoisomerase II. In the presence of these agents, the binding to and cleavage of DNA by topoisomerase II can occur, however, the rejoining of DNA strands is blocked, resulting in the formation of a stable enzyme-DNA complex (cleavable complex) with double strand DNA breaks (Liu, 1989). The formation of cleavable complex is the initial step for producing tumor cells death. There is a good correlation between the antitumor activity and the ability of drugs to form cleavable complex (Liu, 1990; Pommier, 1993; Corbett and Osheroff, 1993, Elsea et al., 1993). The precise mechanisms leading to eventual cell death after formation of cleavable complex are not fully understood. However, the presence of DNA breaks is known to induce mutations during nucleic acid synthesis (Han et al., 1993), formation of chromosome abnormalities (Lonn et al., 1989; Andersson et al., 1989), and triggering of programmed cell death (apoptosis) (Roy et al., 1992; Hickman, 1992; Onishi et al., 1993).

Table 2. DNA Topoisomerase-Targeting Drugs.

Target Enzymes	Drug class	Drug name
Topo II	Intercalators	
	Anthracyclines	Adriamycin (Doxorubicin)
		Daunomycin (Daunorubicin)
	Anthracenediones	Mitoxanthrone
	Acridines	m-AMSA (amsacrine)
	Ellipticines	2-methyl-9-hydroxyellipticine
	Benzoisoquinolinediones	Amonafide
	Non-intercatators	
	Epipodophyllotoxins	VP-16 (Etoposide)
		VM-26 (Teniposide)
	Isoflavones	Genestein
	Quinolones	CP-115,953
	Dioxapiperadines	ICRF-193
	Thiobarbituric acid	Merbarone
	Hexasulfated naphthylurea	Suramin
Topo I	Intercalators	
	Indolocarbazoles	ED-110
	Bisbenzimides	Hoechst 33342
	(minor groove binder)	
	Non-intercalators	
	Camptothecins	CPT-11
		Topotecan
		9-AC
Topo I & II	Intercalators	
	Pyridobenzoindoles	RP-60475 (Intoplicine)
	Fagaronine	Fagaronine
	Actinomycins	Actinomycin D
	Saintopin	Saintopin

Abbreviations: CPT-11: 7-ethyl-10-[4-(1-piperidino)-1-piperidino]carbonyloxy camptothecin; Topotecan: 10,11-methylenedioxy-camptothecin; 9-AC: 9-amino-camptothecin; Fagaronine: 2-hydroxy-3,8,9-trimethoxy-5-methyl-benzo[c]-phenanthridine.

It must be noted that some of the topoisomerase II inhibitors, such as ICRF-193 (Tanabe et al., 1991), merbarone (Drake et al., 1989), and suramin (Bojanowski et al., 1992) are not known to induce cleavable complex formation in cancer cells. These agents instead induce cytotoxic activity by preventing topoisomerase II from binding to DNA, hence formation of cleavable complex mediated by VP-16 could be inhibited (Tanabe et al., 1991; Bojanowski et al., 1992).

Topoisomerase I Inhibitors

Camptothecin (Wall et al., 1966) is currently the best characterized topoisomerase I inhibitor (Hsiang et al., 1985). Despite its good activity in various experimental tumors models, the outcome of earlier clinical trials with camptothecin was disappointing due to severe toxicity such as bone marrow depression and hemorrhagic cystitis. In order to circumvent clinical toxicities, many derivatives of camptothecin have been developed. Among these derivatives, CPT-11 has shown good efficacy against various human cancers in clinical studies, and has recently been approved for clinical use in Japan. The cytotoxic effect of camptothecin is mediated by the formation of a stable enzyme-DNA complex with single-strand breaks. Camptothecin and many of its derivatives are not substrates for the P-gp efflux pump, hence "classical MDR" will not confer resistance to these drugs. However, Topotecan has been found to be associated with the classical MDR phenotype because of the charged amino group in the molecule that was introduced to improve solubility (Chen et al., 1991).

Other topoisomerase I inhibitors include the derivatives of indolcarbazoles (Yoshinari et al., 1993) and a minor groove binder Hoechst 33342 (Chen et al., 1993). Extensive efforts are being invested in the development of indolcarbazoles derivatives because they show promise as a new series of agents capable of targeting topoisomerase I.

Dual Topoisomerase I and II Inhibitors

Recently, a new class of agents targeting both topoisomerase I and topoisomerase II has been reported. Among them, RP-60475 (intoplicine) is the first agent to enter clinical trials with dose-limiting hepatotoxicity (Poddevin et al., 1993). RP-60475 is a strong DNA intercalator and induces cleavable complexes with both topoisomerase I and topoisomerase II. Although it does not exhibit cross-resistance with camptothecin- or m-AMSA-resistant cell lines, it exhibits cross-resistance with P-gp-mediated MDR cells. The other dual inhibitors of topoisomerase I and topoisomerase II include the antibiotic saintopin (Yamashita et al., 1991) and the plant alkaloid fagaronine (Larsen et al., 1993). Actinomycin D has also been found to inhibit both topoisomerase I (Trask and Muller, 1988) and topoisomerase II (Tewey et al., 1984a).

RESISTANT MECHANISMS AGAINST TOPOISOMERASE
INHIBITORS

The development, mechanism, and reversal of resistance to anticancer
drug are multifaceted (Fan et al, 1994). For example, resistance to the
folate analogue methotrexate can be caused by either decreased uptake of
the drug (Schuetz et al., 1988) or increased dehydrofolate reductase,
which is the cellular target for methotrexate, due to amplification of the
gene (Alf et al., 1978). It is possible for the cells to become resistant to
topoisomerase II reactive drugs by reducing drug uptake as seen with P-
gp mediated MDR. However, gene amplification would increase
topoisomerase II levels and further the formation of cleavable complexes
and cells death. Studies employing various tumor cell lines resistant to
topoisomerase inhibitors correlates their resistance with a reduced
expression of the enzymes or expression of a mutated form of enzyme.

Resistance to Topoisomerase II Inhibitors

The atypical MDR phenotype refers to drug resistance exhibited by
cancer cells selected by one topoisomerase II inhibitor and having cross-
resistance toward other topoisomerase II inhibitors. Some of the
characteristics of cells that are resistant to topoisomerase II inhibitors are
listed in Table 3. Since VP-16 and ADR are substrates of the P-gp efflux
pump, several of the cell lines selected with these drugs became MDR
due to P-gp overexpression. For example, H69/V9, P388/MTT, and
P388/DOX cells exhibit both P-gp overexpression and topoisomerase II
alternation (Kunikane et al., 1993; Kamath et al., 1992). However, the
majority of topoisomerase II inhibitor-resistant cell lines have MDR
mediated by the alteration of topoisomerase II alone. These resistant cells
can be divided into two groups; those exhibiting reduced expression of
topoisomerase II or those exhibiting topoisomerase II gene mutations.

   In the case of the altered-expression of topoisomerase II, the cells are
frequently found to have lower levels of the topoisomerase II mRNA as
well as reduced activity of the enzyme (e.g., KB/VP-2, KB/VM-4)
(Matsuo et al., 1990; Takano et al., 1991). Reduced topoisomerase
II levels can occur as a result of genomic alterations (Deffie et al., 1989;
Tan et al., 1989). In these cells, the synthesis of the enzyme is reduced
secondary to decreased transcription of the topoisomerase II gene. The
reduced level of the enzyme lessens the formation of the cleavable
complexes produced by topoisomerase II inhibitors and therefore

Table 3. Characteristics of Resistant Cell Lines to DNA Topoisomerase II Inhibitors.

Cell lines	Selecting Drugs	Resistance rate*	P-gp mdr1	Accumulation	Topoisomerase II activity	mRNA	protein	Distribution	Mutation	Molecular weight	References
P-gp MDR Type:											
H69/VP	VP-16		↑	↓		+/-	+/-				Kunikane et al,1993
P388/MTT	MTX		↑			→	→				Kamath et al, 1992
P388/DOX	DOX		↑				→				
Altered Expression Type:											
KB/VP-2	VP-16	50		+/-	↓	→					Takano et al,1991
KB/VM-4	VM-26	100		↓	↓	→					Matsuo et al,1990
Mutation Type:											
Vpm^R-5	VM-26								Arg^493 → Gln (G^1478 → A)		Chan et al,1993
CEM/VM-1	VM-26	50	--	↓					Agr^449 → Gln (G^1346 → A)		Danks et al,1988
CEM/VM-1-5	VM-26	140	--	↓					Agr^449 → Gln (G^1346 → A)		Bugg et al,1991
HL-60/AMSA	mAMSA	50-100		+/-			+/-		Arg^486 → Lys (G^1457 → A)		Hinds et al,1991
KBM-3/AMSA	mAMSA	200		+/-			+/-		Arg^486 → Lys (G^1457 → A) Lys^479 → Glu (A^1435 → G) Lys^519 → Stop codon (A^1555 → T)		Lee et al,1992
CEM/VP-1	VP-16	16							Lys^797 → Asn (G^2391 → T)		Patel and Fisher,1993
V-511	VP-16								Asp^851 → Gly (A^2552 → G)		Hashimoto et al,1994
Altered Distribution Type:											
H209/V6	VP-16	22	--	+/-	+/-	IIα:↓ IIβ:+/-	IIα:↓ IIβ:+/-	IIα: nucleus → cytoplasm IIβ: +/-		IIα: 170K→160K IIβ: +/-	Feldhoff et al,1994
HL-60/MX-2	MTX	35	--	+/-	IIα:↓	IIα:↓	IIα:↓ IIβ:↓	IIα: nucleus & cytoplasm IIβ: +/-		IIα: 170K+160K IIβ: +/-	Harker et al,1994

Abbreviations: P-gp, P-glycoprotein; VP-16, etoposide; VM-26, teniposide; DOX, Doxorubicin; mAMSA, amsacrine; MTX, mitoxantrone; +/-, no change; --, not expressed. *Resistance rate, fold increase relative to the agent used for selecting resistant line.

Table 4. Characteristics of Resistant Cell Lines to DNA Topoisomerase I Inhibitors.

Cell lines	Drugs	Resistance rate*	P-gp mdr1	Accumu-lation	Topoisomerase I activity	mRNA	protein	HyperMe-thylation	Mutation	Topoisomerase II activity	References
PC-7/CPT	CPT-11	8.8	--	+/-	↓	↓	↓				Kanazawa et al.,1990
HT-29/CPT	CPT	6.9			+/-		↓			↑	Sugimoto et al.,1990b
St-4/CPT	CPT	8.8					↓				Sugimoto et al.,1990a
P388/CPT	CPT-11	45	--		↓	↓	↓	Yes			Sugimoto et al.,1990a; Tan et al.,1989;
P388/CPT	CPT	8	--				↓			↑	Eng et al.,1990
CPT-K5	CPT	300		+/-	+/-		↓		Asp^533 -> Gly (A^1598 -> G)		Andoh et al.,1987; Tamura et al.,1990

Abbreviations: CPT, camptothecin; P-gp, P-glycoprotein; --, not expressed; +/-, not changed   *Resistance rate, fold increase relative to camptothecin (CPT) against parental cells.

Table 5. Resistant Cell Lines to Dual Inhibitor of DNA Topoisomerase I and II: RP-60475.

Cell lines	Resistance rate against RP60475	CPT	VP-16	P-gp mdr1	Accumu-lation	Topoisomerase I Activity	mRNA level	Topoisomerase II Activity	mRNA level
P388RP19	34	0.6	29	↑	↓	+/-	↓	↓	↓
P388RP20	46	1.2	50	↑	↓	+/-	↑		↓
P388RPc2	10	>35	10	--		+/-	+/-	↓	↓

Abbreviations: RP-60475, intoplicine; CPT, camptothecin; VP-16, etoposide; P-gp, P-glycoprotein; --, not expressed; +/-, not changed. Reference: Muriaux et al., 1993.

manifests a resistance phenotype. It is believed that hypermethylation of the topoisomerase II gene and/or reduction of transcriptional activity of the topoisomerase II gene may be involved in downregulation of topoisomerase gene transcription.

In the case of mutations of topoisomerase II, the enzyme extracted from resistant cell lines forms fewer cleavable complexes and has a higher dependency for ATP. The mutation sites of these resistance cell lines (Vpm[R]-5, CEM/VM-1, CEM/VM-1-5, HL-60/AMSA, KBM-3/AMSA) were localized within the ATP-binding domain of topoisomerase IIα (Chan et al., 1993; Bugg et al., 1991; Hinds et al., 1991; Lee et al., 1992). The mutations in this region may reduce the affinity between the enzyme and ATP, or ATPase activity. Other cell lines (CEM/VP-1, V-511) have mutations in the DNA binding domain containing tyrosine 804 (Patel and Fisher, 1993; Hashimoto et al, 1994). In those cell lines, the point mutation lies close to the catalytic tyrosine 804 residue of the protein and may induce conformational change of the DNA binding site and interfere with drug-induced trapping of the cleavable complex. These results suggest that the mutations in the topoisomerase II gene may generate drug-resistant enzymes.

Recently, topoisomerase II-resistant cells (H209/V6, HL-60/MX2) (Feldhoff et al., 1994; Harker et al., 1994) have been found to have altered cellular distribution of the enzyme. A 3'-terminal deletion in the 6.1kb topoisomerase IIα mRNA produces a 4.8kb mRNA transcript in the human small cell lung cancer line H209/V6 selected by VP-16 (Feldhoff et al., 1994). Although the deleted fragment does not contain sequences affecting enzyme activity, it contains the nuclear localization signal for topoisomerase IIα. As a result of such modification, the resistant cells have a 160-kDa topoisomerase IIα found only in the cytoplasm, whereas the parental cells profiled a 170-kDa topoisomerase IIα mainly in the nucleus (Feldhoff et al., 1994). Therefore, an altered distribution of topoisomerase IIα due to a loss of the mRNA nuclear localization signal may mediate resistance against topoisomerase II inhibitors.

Resistance to Topoisomerase I Inhibitors

Table 4 summarizes the characteristics of cells resistant to topoisomerase I inhibitors. These cell lines have no cross resistance to other drugs, including topoisomerase II inhibitors. Like cells resistant to topoisomerase II inhibitors, camptothecin-resistant cells can be divided into two types; those cells with decreased topoisomerase I levels and those cells with mutations in topoisomerase I gene. The reduction of cellular topoisomerase I expression in resistant cell lines such as PC-7/CPT, HT-29/CPT, St-4/CPT, P388/CPT (Kanazawa et al., 1990; Sugimoto et al., 1990a; Sugimoto 1990b; Tan et al., 1989, Eng et al., 1990) has been postulated to correlate with the reduced levels of topoisomerase I mRNA by hypermethylation of the topoisomerase I gene (Eng et al., 1990). Such expressional modification usually produces 10-50-fold resistance to topoisomerase I inhibitors. On the other hand, a 300-fold resistance to camptothecin has been shown in the CPT-K5 cell line (Andoh et al., 1987; Tamura et al., 1990), as a result of a point mutation. Camptothecin inhibits the rejoining of single strand breaks made by topoisomerase I. The point mutation (A^{1598} -> G) is located in the highly conservative region responsible for the rejoining of single strand breaks in DNA (Tamura et al., 1990). This mutation is believed to produce a drug-resistant enzyme.

Resistance to Topoisomerase I and II Inhibitors

There is little known about cancer cell resistance to agent targeting both topoisomerase I and II. Three cell lines selected with RP-60475 are the only resistant model currently available (Muriaux et al., 1993). The characteristics of these cell lines are summarized in Table 5. Cell lines P388RP19 and P388RP20 developed complex resistant profiles with reduced mRNA levels of both topoisomerase I and II, and overexpression of the P-gp efflux pump. However, the other cell line P388RPc2 exhibited only a reduction of topoisomerase II mRNA and activity. The common trait among these cell lines has been alteration of the enzyme expression, however, the levels of enzyme are not proportional to the resistant rate against CPT and VP-16. It remains to be determined whether mutations play a role in such topoisomerase I/II-resistant phenotypes, and the significance of multiple alterations of topoisomerase I, topoisomerase II, and P-pg.

Resistance Related to bcl-2

Bcl-2 is being extensively investigated for its role in drug resistant phenotypes. *bcl-2* is a protooncogene localized at the chromosomal breakpoint of the t(14;18) found in human follicular lymphoma (Tsujimoto et al., 1985) and has the oncogenic function of blocking programmed cell death (apoptosis). It encodes a 25-kDa protein localized in the inner mitochondrial membrane (Hockenbery et al., 1990). Little is known of the mechanism by which *bcl2* protein inhibits apoptosis triggered by various stimuli. Deregulated *bcl-2* has been shown to extend the survival of certain hematopoietic and neuronal cell lines following growth factor deprivation (Nunez et al., 1990; Garcia et al. 1992; Allsopp et al., 1993), or cells irradiated with x-ray (Wyllie et al., 1980). It has also been noted that *bcl-2* inhibits apoptosis induced by various anticancer drugs, including topoisomerase inhibitors (Miyashita and Reed, 1992; Miyashita and Reed, 1993; Fisher et al, 1993). B*cl-2* transfected human non-small cell lung cancer line SBC-3/bcl2 developed resistance to camptothecin and ADR (Ohmori et al., 1993). Murine B cell clones transfected with *bcl-2* were resistant to VP-16. However, the overexpression of *bcl-2* did not affect the formation and disappearance of DNA strand breaks by VP-16 which is the initial step leading to topoisomerase inhibitor-mediated cell death (Kamesaki et al., 1993). This finding suggests that *bcl-2* protein may interfere with late events related to cell death subsequent to cleavable complex formation.

EXPRESSION OF TOPOISOMERASES IN CANCER

The sensitivity of cells to the topoisomerase-targeting drugs, with few exceptions, is directly proportional to enzyme levels in the nucleus (Davies et al., 1988; Daffie et al., 1989; Bjornsti et al., 1989; Madden and Champoux, 1992). The levels of topoisomerase II varies with DNA replication traversing the cell cycle (maximum at G_2-M phase) (Heck and Earnshaw 1986; Chow and Ross, 1987; Hech et al., 1989). Topoisomerase II inhibitors generally induce cytotoxicity in rapidly proliferating tumor cells (Sullivan et al., 1986; Fry et al., 1991; Webb et al., 1991), likely due to higher levels of topoisomerase II in the fast growing cells compared to quiescent cells. In contrast, topoisomerase I levels does not change significantly throughout cell cycle (Heck et al., 1989). However, some tumors have been found to have elevated levels of topoisomerase I relative to normal tissues, and expressed selective sensitivity to topoisomerase I inhibitors. Table 6 summarizes the expression of topoisomerases in several cancers. Tumors of the colorectum, prostate, ovary, and malignant lymphoma, but not of the kidney, contained higher levels of topoisomerase I compared to their normal tissue counterparts (van der Zee et al., 1991; Giovanella et al 1989; Husain et al., 1994). It has been shown that the levels of topoisomerase II are elevated in some tumors such as breast cancers,

Table 6. Expression of Topoisomerases in Cancer.

Topoisomerase I		Topoisomerase II	
High	Low	High	Low
Colon ca.	Renal ca.	Breast ca.	Gastric ca.
Prostate ca.	Gastric ca.	Ovarian ca.	Chronic lympho-
Ovarian ca.		Malignant lymphoma	cytic leukemia
Malignant lymphoma		Colon ca.	

References: Potmesil et al., 1988; Giovanella et al., 1989; van der Zee et al., 1991; Holden et al., 1992; Hirabayashi et al., 1992; Husain et al., 1994.

ovarian cancers, malignant lymphoma, but not in gastric cancers or chronic lymphocytic leukemia (Potmesil et al., 1988; van der Zee et al., 1991; Holden et al., 1992; Hirabayashi et al., 1992).

The different expression profiles of topoisomerases in cancers may reflect the degrees of sensitivity to topoisomerase inhibitors. Topoisomerase I and topoisomerase II inhibitors are expected to produce selective activity in tumors having elevated levels of the respective topoisomerase. Table 7 shows the clinical efficacy of CPT-11, ADR, and VP-16 in various tumors. The results indicate that the topoisomerase I inhibitor CPT-11 is relatively more active against colorectal tumors and malignant lymphoma which express elevated levels of topoisomerase I, however, a similar degree of responses were seen in ovarian and gastric cancer which reportedly had respectively high and normal topoisomerase I levels. The topoisomerase II inhibitor ADR is relatively more active against breast cancer and malignant lymphomas that express elevatedlevels of topoisomerase II, but again the degree of responses seen in gastric and colon cancers are inverse to what would be expected from reports of topoisomerase II levels in these tumors. Notably, normal tissues with high expression of topoisomerase II such as thymus and bone marrow manifested clinical toxicities when treated with ADR or VP-16 (Holden et al., 1990). No attempt has been made to correlate the response of individual tumors to their levels of topoisomerase I or topoisomerase II. These results suggest that monitoring of topoisomerase levels in cancer may be a useful tool for predicting the responsiveness

Table 7. Clinical Responses (% CR+PR) to Topo I & Topo II Inhibitors.

Cancer Type	CPT-11 (%)	ADR (%)	VP-16 (%)
Malignant lymphoma	39	33	41
Small cell lung ca.	37	27	38
Non-small cell lung ca.	34	13	11
Breast ca.	18	50	
Gastric ca.	23	30	
Colon ca.	33	15	
Pancreas ca.	11		
Ovarian ca.	24		
Cervical ca.	24		
Renal ca.	0		
Osteosarcoma		26	
Acute leukemia			25

Abbreviations: ADR, adriamycin; VP-16, etoposide.
References: Negoro et al., 1991; Takeuchi et al., 1991; Ogawa and Taguchi, 1992; Furue, 1994; Ogawa et al., 1972; Yokoyama et al., 1974; Schmoll, 1982; Konno et al., 1986; Kimura et al., 1986.

and selective efficacy of topoisomerase-targeted drugs. However, other factors will probably also impact on clinical responses to topoisomerase-reactive drugs.

REVERSAL OF RESISTANCE TO TOPOISOMERASE INHIBITORS

As reviewed above, the resistance of cancer cell to topoisomerase I inhibitors is generally due to a reduction of cellular topoisomerase I levels. Conversely, some of these resistant cells (HT-29/CPT, P388/CPT) increased their expression of topoisomerase II (Tan et al., 1989; Sugimotoet al., 1990b). Similar compensatory overexpression of topoisomerase I has been observed in cells resistant to topoisomerase II inhibitors due to reduced topoisomerase II levels (Tan et al., 1989). Thus, topoisomerases I and II may be functionally complementary to each other. As one of the approaches to overcome clinical resistance against topoisomerase inhibitors, the development of effective compounds capable of targeting both topoisomerases I and II will bear obvious importance. Alternatively, combination therapy employing inhibitors for both topoisomerases may be feasible in suppressing responsive tumors and also preventing development of resistance to topoisomerase inhibitors.

Combinations of inhibitors to topoisomerase I and II have been tested. When human leukemia cell lines were treated in vitro with combinations of camptothecin, topotecan, VP-16, m-AMSA, or daunomycin, mutual interference with cytotoxicity was observed between inhibitors of the two enzyme types (Kaufmann, 1991). However, when topoisomerase I inhibitors and topoisomerase II inhibitor were sequentially used to treat cultured tumor cells, enhanced cytotoxic effects could be obtained (Bertrand et al., 1992). Moreover, pretreatmentwith topoisomerase I inhibitor CPT-11 significantly enhanced the cytotoxicity of the topoisomerase II inhibitor ADR against human tumor xenografts in nude mice (Kim et al., 1992). It was postulated that the elevation of topoisomerase II expression by CPT-11 pretreatment potentiated the effects of subsequent ADR therapy. These results indicate that proper scheduling may be one of the most critical factors for combination therapy with topoisomerase I and topoisomerase II inhibitors.

PERSPECTIVES

As topoisomerases are enzymes intimately associated with DNA replication and cell growth and development, their place and importance in cancer biology and therapeutics is inevitable and indisputable. Although it is becoming more obvious that the mechanisms of resistance to topoisomerase inhibitors are largely based on topoisomerase alterations such as reduction of enzyme levels, the precise mechanisms of resistance are not fully understood. Much remained to be done to identify a distinct variant in cancer cells that may be responsive to selective inhibitor of the enzymes. Resistant cell lines with different characteristics will serve as models for future investigations pertinent to the development of effective topoisomerase inhibitors. We look forward to prospective clinical studies employing monitoring of topoisomerases as well as other relevant MDR profiles, logical scheduling, and diligent clinical management. We also look forward to the development of dual topoisomerase I/II inhibitors with improved therapeutic index and broadened antitumor spectrum.

REFERENCES

Allsopp TE, Wyatt S, Paterson HF, Davies AM (1993): The proto-oncogene *bcl-2* can selectively rescue neurotrophic factor-dependent neurons from apoptosis. *Cell* 73:295-307

Alt FW, Kellems RE, Bertino JR, Schimke RT (1978): Selective multiplication of dihydrofolate in methotrexate-resistant variants of cultured murine cells. *J Biol Chem* 253:1357-1370

Andersson HC, Kihlman BA (1989): The production of chromosomal alterations in human lymphocytes by drugs known to interfere with the activity of DNA topoisomerase II. I. m-AMSA. *Carcinogenesis* 10:123-130

Andoh T, Ishii K, Suzuki Y, Ikegami Y, Kusunoki Y, Takemoto Y, Okada K (1987): Characterization of a mammalian mutant with a camptothecin-resistant DNA topoisomerase I. *Proc Natl Acad Sci USA* 84:5565-5569

Austin CA, Fisher LH (1990): Isolation and characterization of a human cDNA clone encoding a novel DNA topoisomerase II homologue from HeLa cells. *FABS Lett* 266:115-117

Austin CA, Sng JH, Petel S, Fisher LM (1993): Novel HeLa topoisomerase II is the II-beta isoform: Complete coding sequence and homology with other type II topoisomerases. *Biochim Biophys Acta* 1172:283-291

Beck WT, Cirtain MC, Danks MK, Felsted RL, Safa AR, Wolverton JS, Suttle DP, Trent JM (1987): Pharmacological, molecular, and cytogenetic analysis of "atypical" multidrug-resistant human leukemic cells. *Cancer Res* 47:5455-5460

Bertrand R, O'Connor PM, Kerrigan D, Pommier Y (1992): Sequential administration of camptothecin and etoposide circumvents the antagonistic cytotoxicity of simultaneous drug administration in slowly growing human colon carcinoma HT-29 cells. *Eur J Cancer* 28A:743-748

Bjornsti M-A, Benedetti P, Viglianti GA, Wang JC (1989): Expression of human DNA topoisomerase I in yeast cells lacking yeast DNA topoisomerase I: Restoration of sensitivity of the cells to the antitumor drug camptothecin. *Cancer Res* 49:6318-6323

Bojanowski K, Lelievre S, Markovits J, Couprie J, Jacquemin-Sablon A, Larsen AK (1992): Suramin is an inhibitor of DNA topoisomerase II in vitro and in Chinese hamster fibrosarcoma cells. *Proc Nalt Acad Sci USA* 89:3025-3029

Bugg BY, Danks MK, Beck WT, Suttle DP (1991): Expression of a mutant DNA topoisomerase II in CCRF-CEM human leukemia cells selected for resistance to teniposide. *Proc Nalt Acad Sci USA* 88:7654-7658

Cardenas ME, Dang Q, Glover CVC, Gasser SM (1992): Casein kinase II phosphorylates the eukaryote-specific C-terminal domain of topoisomerase II in vivo. *EMBO* J 11:1785-1796

Chan VT-W, Ng S, Eder JP, Schnipper LE (1993): Molecular cloning and identification of a point mutation in the topoisomerase II cDNA from an etoposide-resistant Chinese hamster ovary cell line. *J Biol Chem* 268:2160-2165

Chen AY, Yu C, Potmesil M, Wall ME, Wani MC, Liu LF (1991): Camptothecin overcomes MDR1-mediated resistance in human KB carcinoma cells. *Cancer Res* 51:6039-6044

Chen AY, Yu C, Bodley A, Peng LF, Liu LF (1993): A new mammalian DNA topoisomerase I poison Hoechst 33342: Cytotoxicity and drug resistance in human cell cultures. *Cancer Res* 53:1332-1337

Chow K-C, Ross WE (1987): Topoisomerase II-specific drug sensitivity in relation to cell cycle progression. *Mol Cell Biol* 7:3119-3123

Chung TDY, Drake FH, Tan KB, Per SR, Crooke ST, Mirabelli CK (1989): Characterization and immunological identification of cDNA clones encoding two human DNA topoisomerase II isozymes. *Proc Natl Acd Sci USA* 86: 9431-9435

Corbett AH, Osheroff N (1993): When good enzymes go bad: Conversion of topoisomerase II to a cellular toxin by antitumor drugs. *Chem Res Toxicol* 6:585-597

Danks MK, Yalowich JC, Beck WT (1987): Atypical multiple drug resistance in a human leukemic cell line selected for resistance to teniposide (VM-26). *Cancer Res* 47:1297-1301

Danks MK, Schmidt CA, Cirtain MC, Suttle DP, Beck WT (1988): Altered catalytic activity of and DNA cleavage by DNA topoisomerase II from human leukemia cells selected for resistance to VM26. *Biochemistry* 27:8861-8869

Danks MK, Warmouth MR, Friche E, Granzen B, Bugg BY, Harker WG, Zwelling LA, Futscher BW, Suttle DP, Beck WT (1993): Single-strand conformational polymorphism analysis of the Mr 170.000 isozyme of DNA topoisomerase II in human tumor cells. *Cancer Res* 53:1373-1379

Davies SM, Robson CN, Davies SL, Hickson ID (1988): Nuclear topoisomerase II levels correlate with the sensitivity of mammalian cells to intercalating agents and epipodophyllotoxins. *J Biol Chem* 263:17724-17729

Deffie AM, Batra JK, Goldenberg GJ (1989): Direct correlation between DNA topoisomerase II activity and cytotoxicity in Adriamycin-sensitive and -resistant P388 leukemia cell lines. *Cancer Res* 49:58-62

DeVore RF, Corbett AH, Osheroff N (1992): Phosphorylation of topoisomerase II by casein kinase II and protein kinase C: Effects on enzyme-mediated DNA cleavage/religation and sensitivity to the antineoplastic drugs etoposide and 4'-(9-acridinylamino)-methane-sulfon-m-aniside. *Cancer Res* 52:2156-2161

Drake FH, Zimmerman JP, McCabe FL, Bartus HF, Per SR, Sullivan DM, Ross WE, Mattern MR, Johnson RK, Crooke ST, Mirabelli CK (1987): Purification of topoisomerase II from amsacrine-resistant P388 leukemia cells: Evidence for two forms of the enzyme. *J Biol Chem* 262:16739-16747

Drake FH, Hofman GA, Bartus HF, Mattern MR, Crooke ST, Mirabelli CK (1989): Biochemical and pharmacological properties of p170 and p180 forms of topoisomerase II. *Biochemistry* 28:8154-8160

Elsea SH, McGuirk PR, Gootz TD, Moynihan M, Osheroff N (1993): Drug features that contribute to the activity of quinolones against mammalian topoisomerase II and cultured cells: Correlation between enhancement of enzyme-mediated DNA cleavage in vitro and cytotoxic potential. *Antimicrob Agents Chemother* 37:2179-2186

Eng WK, McCabe FL, Tan KB, Mattern MR, Hofmann GA, Woessner RD, Hertzberg RP, Johnson RK (1990): Development of a stable camptothecin-resistant subline of P388 leukemia with reduced topoisomerase I content. *Mol. Pharmacol* 38:471-480

Fan D, Beltran PJ, OBrian CA (1994): Reversal of multidrug resistance. In: *Reversal of Multidrug Resistance in Cancer,* (ed. JA Kellen), pp. 93-125. Boca Raton: CRC Press

Feldhoff PW, Mirski SEL, Cole SPC, Sullivan DM (1994): Altered subcellular distribution of topoisomerase IIα in a drug-resistant human small cell lung cancer cell line. *Cancer Res* 54:756-762

Fisher TC, Milner AE, Gregory CD, Jackman AL, Aherne GW, Hartley JA, Dive C, Hickman JA (1993): *bcl-2* modulation of apoptosis induced by anticancer drugs: Resistance to thymidylate stress is independent to classical resistance pathways. *Cancer Res* 53:3321-3326

Fosse P, Paoletti C, Saucier J-M (1988): Pattern of recognition of DNA by mammalian DNA topoisomerase II. *Biochem Biophys Res Commun* 151:1233-1240

Fry AM, Chresta CM, Davies SM, Walker MC, Harris AL, Hartley JA, Masters JRW, Hichson ID (1991): Relationship between topoisomerase II level and chemosensitivity in human tumor cell lines. *Cancer Res* 51:6592-6595

Furue H (1994): Irinotecan hydrochloride (CPT-11). *Jpn J Cancer Chemother* 21:709-717

Garcia I, Martinou I, Tsujimoto Y, Martinou J-C (1992): Prevention of programmed cell death of sympathetic neurons by the *bcl-2* proto-oncogene. *Science* 258:302-304

Giovanella BC, Stehlin JS, Wall ME, Wani MC, Nicholas AW, Liu LF, Silber R, Potmesil M (1989): DNA topoisomerase I-targeted chemotherapy of human colon cancer in xenografts. *Science* 246:1046-1048

Glisson B, Gupta R, Hodges P, Ross W (1986): Cross-resistance to intercalating agents in an epipodophyllotoxin-resistant chinese hamster ovary cell line: Evidence for a common intracellular target. *Cancer Res* 46:1939-1942

Han Y-H, Austin MJF, Pommier Y, Povirk LF (1993): Small deletion and insertion mutations induced by the topoisomerase II inhibitor teniposide in CHO cells and comparison with sites of drug-stimulated DNA cleavage in vitro. *J Mol Biol* 229:52-66

Harker WG, Slade DL, Holguin MH, Feldhoff PW, Sullivan DM (1994): Mitoxantrone-resistant HL-60 leukemia cells contain an altered topoisomerase II alpha gene, mRNA and subcellular protein distribution. *Proc Am Assoc Cancer Res* 35:2707

Hashimoto S, Chatterjee S, Danks KM, Beck WT (1994): Point mutation in the vicinity of the DNA binding domain of topoisomerase II gene is associated with the development of resistance to VP-16. *Proc Am Assoc Cancer Res* 35:2720

Hech MMS, Hittelman WN, Earnshaw WC (1989): In vivo phosphorylation of the 170-kDa form of eukaryotic DNA topoisomerase II: Cell cycle analysis. *J Biol Chem* 264:15161-15164

Heck MMS, Earnshaw (1986): Topoisomerase II: Specific marker for cell proliferation. *J Cell Biol* 103:2569-2581

Hickman JA (1992): Apoptosis induced by anticancer drugs. *Cancer Metastasis Rev* 11:121-139

Hinds M, Disseroth K, Mayes J, Altschuler E, Jansen R, Ledley FD, Zwelling LA (1991): Identification of a point mutation in the topoisomerase II gene from a human leukemia cell line containing an amsacrine-resistant form of topoisomerase II. *Cancer Res* 51:4729-4731

Hirabayashi N, Kim R, Nishiyama M, Aogi K, Saeki S, Toge T, Okada K (1992): Tissue expression of topoisomerase I and II in digestive tract cancers and adjacent normal tissues. *Pro Am Assoc Cancer Res* 33:2603

Hockenbery D, Nunez G, Milliman C, Schreiber RD, Korsmeyer SJ (1990): Bcl-2 is an inner mitochondrial membrane protein that blocks programmed cell death. *Nature* 348:334-336

Holden JA, Rolfson DH, Wittwer CT (1990): Human DNA topoisomerase II: Evaluation of enzyme activity in normal and neoplastic tissues. *Biochemistry* 29:2127-2134

Holden JA, Rolfson DH, Wittwer CT (1992): The distribution of immunoreactive topoisomerase II protein in human tissue and neoplasms. *Oncol Res* 4:157-166

Hsiang Y-H, Hertzberg R, Hecht S, Liu LF (1985): Camptothecin induces protein-linked DNA breaks via mammalian DNA topoisomerase I. *J Biol Chem* 260:14873-14878

Hsiang Y-H, Jiang JB, Liu LF (1989): Topoisomerase II-mediated DNA cleavage by amonafide and its structural analogs. *Mol Pharmacol* 36:371-376

Husain I, Mohler JL, Seigler HF, Besterman JM (1994): Elevation of topoisomerase messenger RNA, protein, and catalytic activity in human tumor: Demonstration of tumor-type specificity and implications for cancer chemotherapy. *Cancer Res* 54:539-546

Jenkins JR, Ayton P, Jones T, Davies SL, Simmons DL, Harris AL, Sheer D, Hickson ID (1992): Isolation of cDNA clones encoding the β isozyme of human DNA topoisomerase II and localization of the gene to chromosome 3p24. *Nucleic Acids Res* 20:5587-5592

Johnson RK, McCabe FL, Faucette LF, Hertzberg RP, Kingsbury WD, Boehm JC, Caranfa MJ, Holden KG (1989): SK&F10864, a water-soluble analog of camptothecin with broad-spectrum activity in preclinical tumor models. *Proc Am Assoc Cancer Res* 30:623

Kamath N, Grabowski D, Ford J, Kerrigan D, Pommier Y, Ganapathi R (1992): Overexpression of P-glycoprotein and alterations in topoisomerase II in P388 mouse leukemia cells selected in vivo for resistance to mitoxantrone. *Biochem Pharmacol* 44:937-945

Kamesaki S, Kamesaki H, Jorgensen TJ, Tanizawa A, Pommier Y, Cossman J (1993): *bcl-2* protein inhibits etoposide-induced apoptosis through its effects on events subsequent to topoisomerase II-induced DNA strand breaks and their repair. *Cancer Res* 53:4251-4256

Kanzawa F, Sugimoto Y, Minato K, Kasahara K, Bungo M, Nakagawa K, Fujiwara Y, Liu LF, Saijo N (1990): Establishment of a camptothecin analogue (CPT-11)-resistant cell line of human non-small cell lung cancer: Characterization and mechanism of resistance. *Cancer Res* 50:5919-5924

Kaufmann SH (1991): Antagonism between camptothecin and topoisomerase II-directed chemotherapeutic agents in a human leukemia cell line. *Cancer Res* 51:1129-1136

Kim R, Hirabayashi N, Nishiyama M, Jinushi K, Toge T, Okada K (1992): Experimental studies on biochemical modulation targeting topoisomerase I and II in human tumor xenografts in nude mice. *Int J Cancer* 50:760-766

Kimura K, Yamada K, Yoshida T (1986): Phase II study of NK171 (etoposide) on malignant lymphomas and acute leukemia. *Jpn J Cancer Chemother* 13:496-501

Konno K, Nagahama F, Nakai Y, Nakabayashi T, Hiraga Y, Takebe K, Tamura M, Oizumi K, Sato M, Ito T, Hayashi I (1986): A phase II study of intravenous VP-16-213 in small cell and non-small cell carcinoma of the lung. *Jpn J Cancer Chemother* 13:931-937

Kunikane H, Ohta S, Kubota N, Takeda Y, Nishino K, Saijo N, Krisham A (1990): Relationship between amount of P-glycoprotein and cellular adriamycin retention in lung cancer cell lines. *Proc Am Assoc Cancer Res* 34:1836

Kunimoto T, Nitta K, Tanaka T, Uehara N, Baba H, Takeuchi M, Yokokura T, Sawada S, Miyasaka T, Mutai M (1987): Antitumor activity of 7-Ethyl-10-[4-(1-piperidino)-1-piperidino]carbonyloxy-c amptothecin, a novel water-soluble derivative of camptothecin, against murine tumors. *Cancer Res* 47:5944-5947

Larsen AK, Grondard L, Couprie J, Desoize B, Comoe L, Jardillier J-C, Riou J-F. (1993): The antileukemic alkaloid fagaronine is an inhibitor of DNA topoisomerase I and II. *Biochem Pharmcol* 46:1403-1412

Lee M-S, Wang JC, Beran M (1992): Two independent amsacrine-resistant leukemia cell lines share an identical point mutation in the 170 kDa form of human topoisomerase II. *J Mol Biol* 223:837-843

Liu LF, Miller KG (1981): Eukaryotic DNA topoisomerases: Two forms of type I DNA topoisomerases from HeLa cell nuclei. *Proc Natl Acad Sci USA* 78:3487-3491

Liu LF (1989): DNA topoisomerase poisons as antitumor drugs. *Annu Rev Biochem* 58:351-375

Liu LF (1990): Anticancer drugs that convert DNA topoisomerases into DNA damaging agents. In: *DNA Topology and Its Biological Effects,* (ed. NR Cozzarelli and JC Wang), pp. 371-389. Cold Spring Harbor: Cold Spring Harbor Laboratory Press

Lonn U, Lonn S, Nylen U, Winbald G (1989): Altered formation of DNA in human cells treated with inhibitors of DNA topoisomerase II (etoposide and teniposide). *Cancer Res* 49:6202-6207

Lynn R, Giaever G, Swanberg SL, Wang JC (1986): Tandem regions of yeast DNA topoisomerase II share homology with different subunits of bacterial gyrase. *Science* 233:647-649

Madden KR, Champoux JJ (1992): Overexpression of human topoisomerase I in baby hamster kidney cells: Hypersensitivity of clonal isolates to camptothecin. *Cancer Res* 52:525-532

Matsuo K, Kohno K, Takano H, Sato S, Kiue A, Kuwano M (1990): Reduction of drug accumulation and DNA topoisomerase II activity in acquired teniposide-resistant human cancer KB cell lines. *Cancer Res* 50:5819-5824

Miyashita T, Reed JC (1992): *bcl-2* gene transfer increases relative resistance of S49.1 and WEHI7.2 lymphoid cells to cell death and DNA fragmentation induced by glucocorticoids and multiple chemotherapeutic drugs. *Cancer Res* 52:5407-5411

Miyashita T, Reed JC (1993): *Bcl-2* oncoprotein blocks chemotherapy-induced apoptosis in a human leukemia cell line. *Blood* 81:151-157

Muriaux D, Lavelle F, Riou JF (1993): Establishment of murine cell lines resistant to the topoisomerase I and II inhibitor intoplicine. *Proc Am Assoc Cancer Res* 34:2542

Negoro S, Fukuoka M, Niitani H, Suzuki A, Nakabayashi T, Kimura M, Motomiya M, Kurita Y, Hasegawa K, Kuriyama T, Nishiwaki Y, Ogawa M, Nakao I, Saijyo N, Obo K, Furue H, Aryiyoshi Y, Shimokawa K, Furuse K, Nakajima S, Irie K, Kimura I, Ogura T, Fujii M, Hara N, Hara Y, Nakano S, Araki J, Miyata Y, Taguchi T (1991): A phase II study of CPT-11, a camptothecin derivative, in patients with primary lung cancer. *Jpn J Cancer Chemother* 18:1013-1019

Nelson EM, Tewey KM, Liu LF (1984): Mechanism of antitumor drug action: Poisoning of mammalian DNA topoisomerase II by 4'-(9-acridinylamino)methanesulfon-m-anisidide. *Proc Nalt Acad Sci USA* 81:1361-1365

Nergi C, Chiesa R, Cerino A, Bestagno M, Sala C, Zini N, Naraldi AM, Ricotti GCBA (1992): Monoclonal antibodies to human DNA topoisomerase I and the two isoforms of DNA topoisomerase II: 170- and 180-kDa isozymes. *Exp Cell Res* 200:452-459

Nunez G, London L, Hockenbery D, Alexander M, McKearn JP, Korsmeyer SJ (1990): Deregulated *bcl-2* gene expression selectively prolongs survival of growth factor-deprived hemopoietic cell lines. *J Immunol* 144:3602-3610

Ogawa M, Kurita S, Nishimura J, Kamei Y, Ariyoshi Y, Murakami M, Oyama A, Sugiura T, Kato R, Ohta K, Nakamura A (1972): Clinical trial with adriamycin, a new antibiotic, in treatment of malignant neoplasms. *Jpn J Cancer Clin* 18:806-812

Ogawa M, Taguchi T (1992): Clinical studies with CPT-11: The Japanese experience. *Ann Oncol* 3:118

Ohmori T, Podack ER, Nishio K, Takahashi M, Miyahara Y, Takeda Y, Kubota N, Funayama Y, Ogasawara H, Ohira T, Saijo N (1993): Apoptosis of lung cancer cells caused by some anti-cancer agents (MMC, CPT-11, ADR) is inhibited by *bcl-2*. *Biochem Biophys Res Commun* 15:30-36

Onishi Y, Azuma Y, Sato Y, Mizuno Y, Tadakuma T, Kizaki H (1993): Topoisomerase inhibitors induce apoptosis in thymocytes. *Biochim Biophys Acta* 1175:147-154

Osheroff N (1989): Biochemical basis for the interactions of type I and type II topoisomerases with DNA. *Pharmacol Ther* 41:223-241

Patel S, Fisher LM (1993): Novel skeleton and genetic characterization of an etoposide-resistant human leukemic CCRF-CEM cell line. *Br J Cancer* 67:456-463

Poddevin B, Riou J-F, Lavelle F, Pommier Y (1993): Dual topoisomerase I and II inhibition by intoplicine (RP-60475), a new antitumor agent in early clinical trials. *Mol Pharmacol* 44:767-774

Pommier Y (1993): DNA topoisomerase I and II in cancer chemotherapy: Update and perspectives. *Cancer Chemother Pharmacol* 32:103-108

Potmesil M, Hsiang Y-H, Liu LF, Bank B, Grossberg H, Kirschenbaum S, Forlenzar TJ, Penziner A, Kanganis D, Knowles D, Traganos F, Silber R (1988): Resistance of human leukemic and normal lymphocytes to drug-induced DNA cleavage and low levels of DNA topoisomerase II. *Cancer Res* 48:3537-3543

Prosperi E, Sala E, Negri C, Oliani C, Supino R, Ricotti G BCA, Bottiroli G (1992): Topoisomerase II a and β in human tumor cells grown in vitro and in vivo. *Anticancer Res* 12:2093-2100

Ross W, Rowe T, Glisson B, Yalowich J, Liu LF (1984): Role of topoisomerase II in mediating epipodophyllotoxin-induced DNA cleavage. *Cancer Res* 44:5857-5860

Rowe TC, Chen GC, Hsiang Y, Liu LF (1986): DNA damage by antitumor acridines mediated by mammalian DNA topoisomerase II. *Cancer Res* 46:2021-2026

Roy C, Brown DL, Little JE, Valentine BK, Walker PR. Sikorska M, LeBlanc J. Chaly N (1992): The topoisomerase II inhibitor teniposide (VM-26) induces apoptosis in unstimulated mature murine lymphocytes. *Exp Cell Res* 200:416-424

Schmoll H (1982): Review of etoposide single-agent activity. *Cancer Treat Rev* 9:21-30

Schuetz JD, Matherly LH, Westin EH, Goldman ID (1988): Evidence for a functional defect in the translocation of the methotrexate transport carrier in a methotrexate-resistant murine L1210 leukemia cell line. *J Biol Chem* 263:9840-9847

Sugimoto Y, Tsukahara S, Oh-hara T, Isoe T, Tsuruo T (1990a): Decreased expression of DNA topoisomerase I in camptothecin-resistant tumor cell lines as determined by a monoclonal antibody. *Cancer Res* 50:6925-6930

Sugimoto Y, Tsukahara S, Oh-hara T, Liu LF, Tsuruo T (1990b): Elevated expression of DNA topoisomerase II in camptothecin-resistant human tumor cell lines. *Cancer Res* 50:7962-7965

Sullivan DM, Glisson BS, Hodges PK, Smallwood-Kentro S, Ross WE (1986): Proliferation dependence of topoisomerase II mediated Drug action. *Biochemistry* 25:2248-2256

Takano H, Kohono K, Ono M, Uchida Y, Kuwano M (1991): Increased phosphorylation of DNA topoisomerase II in etoposide-resistant mutants of human cancer KB cells. *Cancer Res* 51:3951-3957

Takeuchi S, Dobashi K, Fujimoto S, Tanaka K, Suzuki M, Terashima Y, Hasumi K, Akiya K, Negishi Y, Tamaya T, Tanizawa O, Sugawa T, Umesaki N, Sekiba K, Aono T, Nakano H, Noda K, Shiota M, Yakushiji M, Sugiyama T, Hashimoto M, Yajima A, Takamizawa H, Sonoda T, Takeda Y, Tomoda Y, Ohta M, Ozaki M, Hirabayashi K, Hiura M, Hatae M, Nishigaki K, Taguchi T (1991): A late phase II study of CPT-11 in gynecologic cancers. *Jpn J Cancer Chemother* 18:1681-1689

Tamura H, Kohchi C, Yamada R, Ikeda T, Koiwai O, Patterson E, Keene J, Okada K, Kjeldsen E, Nishikawa K, Andoh T (1990): Molecular cloning of a cDNA of a camptothecin-resistant human DNA topoisomerase I and identification of mutation sites. *Nucleic Acids Res* 19:69-75

Tan KB, Mattern MR, Eng W-K, McCabe FL, Johnson RK (1989): Nonproductive rearrangement of DNA topoisomerase I and II genes: Correlation with resistance to topoisomerase inhibitors. *J Natl Cancer Inst* 81:1732-1735

Tan KB, Dorman TE, Falls KM, Chung TDY, Mirabelli CK, Crooke ST, Mao J (1992): Topoisomerase IIα and topoisomerase IIβ genes: Characterization and mapping to human chromosomes 17 and 3, respectively. *Cancer Res* 52:231-234

Tanabe K, Ikegami Y, Ishida R, Andoh T (1991): Inhibition of topoisomerase II by antitumor agents Bis(2,6-dioxopiperazine) derivatives. *Cancer Res* 51:4903-4908

Tewey KM, Rowe TC, Yang L, Halligan BD, Liu LF (1984a): Adriamycin-induced DNA damage mediated by mammalian DNA topoisomerase II. *Science* 226:466-468

Tewey KM, Chen GL, Nelson EM, Liu LF (1984b): Intercalative antitumor drugs interfere with the breakage-reunion reaction of mammalian DNA topoisomerase II. *J Biol Chem* 259:9182-9187

Trask DK, Muller MT (1988): Stabilization of type I topoisomerase-DNA covalent complexes by actinomycin D. *Proc Natl Acd Sci USA* 85:1417-1421

Tsai-Pflugfelder M, Liu LF, Liu AA, Tewey KM, Whang-Peng J, Knutsen T, Huebner K, Kroce CM, Wang JC. (1988): Cloning and sequencing of cDNA encoding human DNA topoisomerase II and localization of the gene to chromosome region 17q21-22. *Proc Natl Acad Sci USA* 85:7177-7181

Tsujimoto Y, Gorham J, Cossman J, Jaffe E, Croce CM (1985): The t(14;18) chromosome translocations involved in B-cell neoplasms result from mistakes in VDJ joining. *Science* 229:1390-1393

van der Zee AGJ, Hollema H, de Jong S, Boonstra H, Gouw A, Willemse PHB, Zijlstra JG, de Vries EGE (1991): P-glycoprotein expression and DNA topoisomerase I and II activity in benign tumor of the ovary and in malignant tumor of the ovary, before and after platinum/cyclophosphamide chemotherapy. *Cancer Res* 51:5915-5920

Wang JC (1985): DNA topoisomerases. *Annu Rev Biochem* 54:665-697

Wall ME, Wani MC, Cooke CE, Palmer KH, McPhail AT, Slim GA (1966): The isolation and structure of camptothecin, a novel alkaloidal leukemia and tumor inhibitor from Camptotheca acuminata. *J Am Chem Soc* 88:3888-3890

Webb CD, Latham MD, Lock RB, Sullivan DM (1991): Attenuated topoisomerase II content directly correlates with a low level of drug resistance in a chinese hamster ovary cell line. *Cancer Res* 51:6543-6549

Woessner RD, Chung TDY, Hofman GA, Mattern MR, Mirabelli CK, Drake FH, Johnson RK (1990): Differences between normal and ras-transfected NIH-3T3 cells in expression of the 170kD and the 180kD forms of topoisomerase II. *Cancer Res* 50:2901-2908

Woessner RD, Mattern MR, Mirabelli CK, Johnson RK, Drake FH (1991): Proliferation- and cell cycle-dependent differences in expression of the 170 kilodalton and 180 kilodalton forms of topoisomerase II in NIH-3T3 cells. *Cell Growth Differ* 2:209-214

Wyckoff E, Natalie D, Nolan JM, Lee M, Hsieh T-S (1989): Structure of the Drosophila DNA topoisomerase II gene: Nucleotide sequence and homology . *J Mol Biol* 205:1-13

Wyllie AH, Kerr JFR, Currie AR (1980): Cell death: The significance of apoptosis. *Int Rev Cytol* 68:251-305

Yamashita Y, Kawada S, Nakano H (1990): Induction of mammalian topoisomerase II dependent DNA cleavage by non-intercalative flavonoids, genestein and orobol. *Biochem Pharmacol* 39:737-744

Yamashita Y, Kawada S, Fujii N, Nakano H (1991): Induction of mammalian DNA topoisomerase I and II mediated DNA cleavage by saintopin, a new antitumor agent from fungus. *Biochemistry* 30:5838-5845

Yokoyama M, Himori T, Ujiie S, Saito T (1974): Treatment of malignant neoplasms with Adriamycin. *Jpn J Cancer Clin* 20:536-544

Yoshinari T, Yamada A, Uemura D, Nomura K, Arakawa H, Kojiri K, Yoshida E, Suda H, Okura A (1993): Induction of topoisomerase I-mediated DNA cleavage by a new indolocarbazole, ED-110. *Cancer Res* 53:490-494

Zini N, Martelli AM, Sabatelli P, Santi S, Negri C, Ricotti GSBA, Naraldi AM (1992): The 180-kDa isoform of topoisomerase II is located in the nucleolus and belongs to the structural elements of the nuclear remnant. *Exp Cell Res* 200:460-466

6. GENOTOXICITY OF TOPOISOMERASE II INHIBITORS: CONSEQUENCES FOR CHEMOTHERAPY

Frank Gieseler

A primary step in the unveiling of cellular reistance is the understanding of the determinats of cellular sensitivity to chemotherapeutic drugs. In this chapter, the factors which are necessary for cellular sensitivity in the treatment with topoisomerase II (topo II) inhibiting drugs are elucidated and reasons for cellular resistance resulting in therapeutic failure are discussed.

TWO-STEP MODEL OF DRUG INDUCED CELL DEATH

Topoisomerases are the enzymes which control the three-dimensional organization of the DNA. Several distinctive steps in their action cycle have been defined. Topo II inhibiting drugs are substances from several chemical classes which inhibit topoisomerases in different ways. A block of the enzymes' activity-cycle by these drugs results in the accumulation of intermediate products which must be removed by the cell. Additionally, the physiological function of the inhibited enzymes is lost. The consequences for the cell depend upon the concentration of the drug, the genotoxicity resulting from inhibition of the topoisomerase action, as well as upon the cellular status (e.g. quiescent, proliferative, differentiated, etc.). The cellular effects of topo II inhibitors highly depend upon the concentration in which they are used:

At ultra-low drug concentrations (10 - 100 fold below the lethal dose) the effect of the drug depends upon its mode of action (e.g. DNA intercalation site, inhibition of DNA binding of topo II, inhibition of isoenzymes, etc.) and results in specific cellular reactions such as inhibition or induction of cellular differentiation or proliferation. At these concentrations, the cells are still able to compensate for the functional loss of the enzymes.

At therapeutic drug concentrations, the outcome depends highly upon the reaction of the cell to the molecular effects of drug treatment. In most cases, the cells do not die immediately, but after the initiation of a frustrated rescue attempt. In the treatment of sensitive cells with lethal doses of topo II inhibiting drugs, two steps can be distinguished. With a few exceptions, which will be discussed later, the drugs stabilize a topo II-DNA complex at different stages of the enzymes' action-cycle after the induction of DNA strand breaks by the enzyme. Obviously, this genotoxicity is a prerequisite for the initiation of cellular reactions which depend upon the expression of specific genes, such as p53, c-myc or bcl2 and on the effect of growth factors.

At high drug concentrations, all cells can be killed by topo II inhibitors *in vitro*. When using such high does, cell death correlates to the amount of DNA damage. Also, one must take in consideration that a number of topo II inhibiting drugs, especially the DNA intercalators, have additional intracellular effects which are clearly dose dependent.

The cellular response after treatment with topo II inhibitors are especially critical in the doses which are used in therapy. If the DNA damage can be repaired which also requires enough intact topoisomerase to remodulate DNA, the cell survives and is "resistant to the drug. The primary effects, the events from the administration of the drugs to the induction of DNA strand breaks, have been studied in detail, whereas the secondary part, the recognition of the strand breaks by the cell and the induction of a cellular reaction which finally results in cell death, are still far from being completely unveiled. Cellular resistance might occur either through events which decrease genotoxicity (e.g. lower drug concentration, lower DNA binding, resistant topo II) or throught events which modulate the cellular reaction (e.g. mutant or low expression of p53, deregulated c-myc, overexpression of bcl2, growth factors).

BIOCHEMISTRY OF THE TOPOISOMERASE-ACTION

Controlling the three dimensional DNA structure is essential for every cell. This is not only true for cell division with chromosome formation (Uemura et al., 1987), but also for gene transcription regulation since DNA-polymerases favor a certain degree of torsional stress in the DNA

(Tsao et al., 1989). In these areas gene transcription is more likely to occur and *vice versa*, the synthesis of topoisomerases is influenced by the degree of DNA - relaxation (Menzel and Gellert, 1983).

Topoisomerases are a family of isoenzymes. Up to date, we know of three different genes, the one encoding for topo I is located on chromosome 20, whereas the encoding gene for topo II alpha is located at chromosome 17 and located on chromosome 3 is the one for topo II beta (Tan et al., 1992). These genes encode for three different proteins that are additionally heavily posttranscriptionally modified. Ribosylation and phosphorylation, both with consequences for the enzymes' activity and their drug sensitivity have been described (Heck et al., 1989; Schroder et al., 1989; Takano et al., 1991; Gasser et al., 1992; Samuels and Shimizu, 1992). This might explain why we find several distinct topoisomerase - activities in intact cells.

The way of processing DNA is obviously very similar for topo I and II isoenzymes. We are able to differentiate at least six different steps which are important for the understanding of differences in the mode of action of inhibiting cytostatic drugs (Osheroff, 1986):
• loose (non-covalent) binding of the enzyme to the DNA
• tight (covalent) binding
• DNA cleavage
• DNA strand passage
• DNA religation
• enzyme turn over.

As it is extremely difficult to examine DNA - processing enzymes *in vivo*, it is still not known how these enzymes actually function in intact human cells and several divergent models exist (Gieseler et al., 1993). The principle difference between topo I and topo II is not their way of action *in vitro*, but probably their intranuclear localisation. In contrast to topo I, topo II is a major component of the nuclear matrix (NM) (Earnshaw et al., 1985). The DNA is organised in "loops" which are fixed to the NM at the "matrix attached regions" (MAR) (Tsutsui et al., 1988). Localized at the footpoints of these loops, topo II is able to control the torsional stress of the attached DNA-loop (Laemmli and Gasser, 1987). This is true at least for topo II alpha, its expression is tightly associated with proliferation and this isoenzyme also seems to be the main target of cytostatic drugs inhibiting topo II.

Topo II beta is considered to be localized in the nucleolus of the cells (Jensen et al., 1991). Its functional role seems to be more associated with cellular differentiation than with proliferation (Zwelling et al., 1988;

Gieseler et al., 1990; Gieseler et al., 1991), which is supported by the fact that topo II alpha is found in all eucaryotes, whereas topo II beta is found only in vertebrates (Tan et al., 1992). Nevertheless, the cellular function of both isoenzymes can only be understood in the context of all DNA - binding proteins. In other words, purified topo does not necessarily act in the same way as it does in its physiological environment. This perception is important for the interpretation of *in vitro* experiments when drawing conclusions for therapy.

INDUCTION OF GENOTOXICITY BY TOPO II INHIBITORS

The first step in the successful treatment with topo II inhibiting drugs is the induction of DNA strand-breaks. In order to interact with topo II and induce genotoxicity, topo II inhibiting drugs must cross the outer cell membrane, the cytoplasma, enter the nucleus and bind to the DNA (Fig. 1). For daunorubicin and idarubicin, two of the most important anthracyclines, and idarubicinol, the active derivation of idarubicin, the drug-concentrations inside the cells, inside the nucleus and the amount bound to the DNA has been determined. Several sensitive and resistant cell lines as well as blood lymphocytes (pbl) from healthy volunteers have been examined (Gieseler et al., 1993; Gieseler et al., 1994).

In all cells examined, we wound a several thousand fold accumulation of daunorubicin, idarubicin and idarubicinol in the cytoplasm and nucleus. 30-60% of the drugs are found in the nucleus, resulting in a 200 to 300 fold difference of concentration between nucleus and extracellular fluids. The nuclear/cytoplasmatic ratio did not correlated with resistance of the cells. Within 10 minutes daunorubicin, idarubicin and idarubicinol cross the outer cell membrane, the cytoplasma and arrive in the nucleus. Nevertheless, the time required to reach their highest DNA binding-rate is between 20 and 45 minutes depending on cell type and drugs (Gieseler et al., 1994).

In order to determine the DNA binding rates of anthracyclines *in vitro* and *in vivo*, we assessed the quenching of the fluorescent AT-binder Hoechst 33342 which has been shown to correlate directly with the amount of DNA bound anthracyclines (Schroder et al., 1989).

All drugs were able to quench 100% of the Hoechst dye fluorescence *in vitro*. *In vivo*, on the other hand, there are differences in the quenching capabilities of the various drugs. Idarubicin and it's derivative idarubicinol were capable of quenching 91.5% of the Hoechst

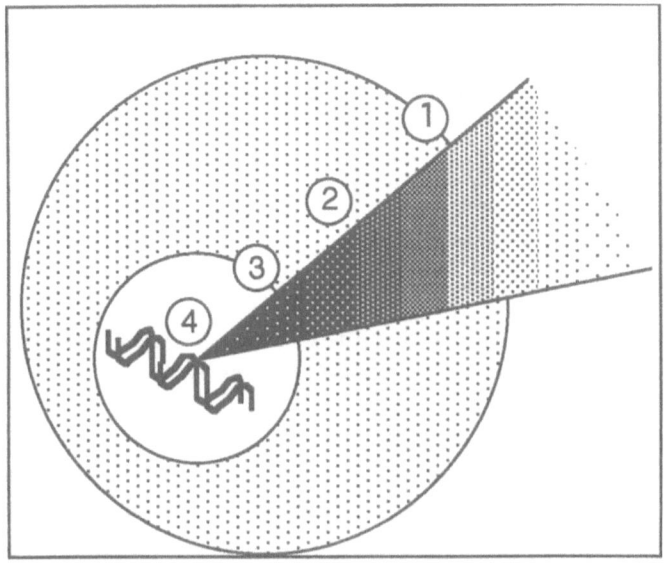

Figure 1. Intracellular pharmacokinetic of topo II targeting drugs (1, cell membrane; 2, cytoplasma; 3, nuclear membrane; 4, DNA).

dye, while daunorubicin only managed to quench 76% under the same conditions. The amount of DNA binding is of exceptional importance for the induction of genotoxicity in the treatment with anthracyclines. There is a direct correlation between cell death and the quantity of DNA-bound drugs, and it seems to be a valid tool to determine cellular sensitivity to anthracyclines (Gieseler et al., 1993; Gieseler et al., 1994).

CELLULAR EFFECTS OF TOPOISOMERASE INHIBITORS AT ULTRA-LOW CONCENTRATIONS

Another hint at the importance of genotoxicity for the cellular effects of topoisomerase inhibiting drugs comes from the following experiments. There is accumulating evidence that both type I and type II topoisomerases play a key role in cellular differentiation. The activity of topo I increased rapidly after treatment of HL-60 cells with phorbol myristate acetate (PMA); reaching its maximum increase (150% of control activity) at 3 h post-treatment and remained elevated for at least

Table 1. Differentiation inducing capacity of topo II inhibiting drugs.

induction[0]	drug*	mode of action
no (0-8%)	novobiocin, coumermycin	ATP site binder
low (18-22%)	mAMSA, anthracyclines	DNA-intercalator
high (26-53%)	epipodophyllotoxines	non-intercalator

*optimal concentration of induction 10-100 times below lethal concentration
[0]number of differentiated cells in percent from all living cells

24 h, whereas the decrease in topo II activity occurs at a later time, concomitantly with the loss of proliferative potential in differentiating HL-60 cells (Gorsky, 1989). Topoisomerase inhibitors, given in appropriate concentrations, are cytotoxic for hematopoetic cells; sub in sub-lethal doses several inhibitors are able to induce cellular differentiation. HL-60 cells have been induced to metamyelocytes, banded and segmented neutrophils by 10-hydroxy-camptothecin, a potent topo I inhibitor (Ling et al., 1991) as well as VP-16, a potent topo II inhibitor (Nakaya et al., 1991). Cells resistant to higher doses of these inhibitors could not be induced and analogues of these substances which do not inhibit topoisomerases had no inducing capacity. The addition of mAMSA, also a potent topo II inhibitor, to the medium in the concentration of 15 ng/ml had not effect on the growth of undifferentiated HL-60 cells, but the induction of differentiation by DNSO (1% vol/vol) was blocked effectively in the presence of mAMSA: the cells remained NBT-negative with a viability of more than 80% when simultaneously incubated with 1% DMSO and 15 ng/ml of mAMSA (Gieseler et al., 1991). It has been previously described that mAMSA also inhibits phorbol-ester induced differentiation of HL-60 cells (Sahyoun et al., 1986).

According to their differentiation inducing capacity, Topo II inhibiting drugs can be divided into three different classes:

For the induction of differentiation in hematopoietic cells, a complex alteration of gene transcription is necessary. It seems that the DNA-binding affinity of the drugs in relation to their protein- (topo II-) binding capacity is important for their potency to induce differentiation.

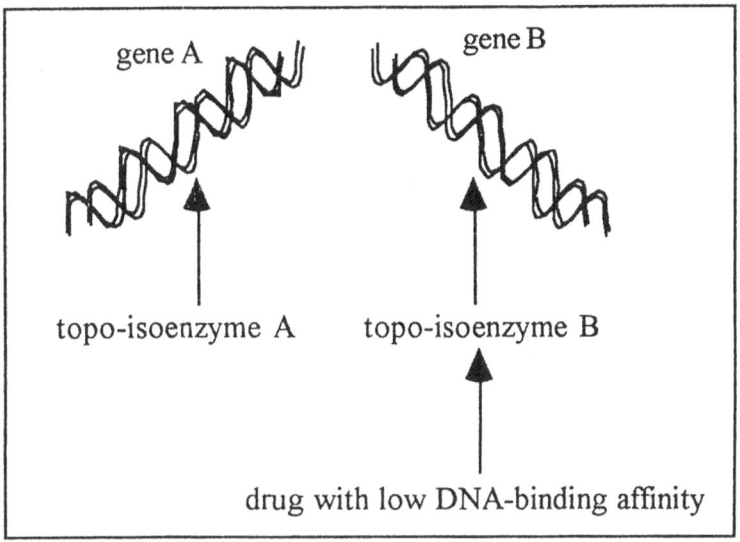

Figure.2. Model of the alteration of DNA-processing by the inhibition of topo II isoenzymes

A model for gene transcription alteration through topo II inhibition shown in figure 2: In contrast to anthracyclines, which have a high DNA-binding affinity, podophyllotoxines in ultra-low concentrations inhibit specific topo II sub-fractions which are lost for their physiological role of DNA processing. This results in the alteration of gene transcription in certain DNA areas, thus inducing cellular differentiation.

CELLULAR EFFECTS OF TOPOISOMERASE INHIBITORS IN THERAPEUTICAL CONCENTRATIONS

In the clinical situation, the concentration of cytostatic drugs must be high enough to result in the desired cytotoxicity but low enough to avoid severe side effects. In these concentration ranges, the drugs inhibit the action-cycles of topo II at different stages (Figure 3). Aclarubicin inhibits the DNA-binding of topo-II, whereas daunorubicin and doxorubicin stabilize the cleavable complex (CC) before DNA strand-passage (CC1). The podophyllotoxines inhibit both CC1 and CC2 and amsidyl stabilized CC2, resulting in inhibition of the religation step of the enzyme (Sorensen et al., 1992); Robinson et al., 1993). These findings

Figure 3. Inhibition of the topo II action-cycle by different cytostatic drugs

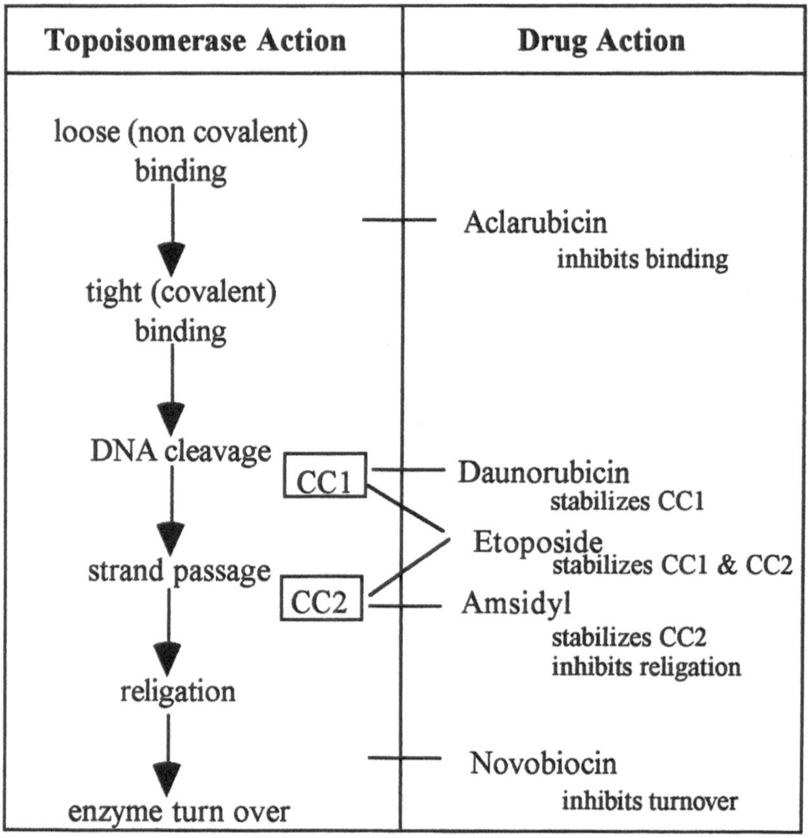

Topoisomerase Action	Drug Action

loose (non covalent) binding ↓ tight (covalent) binding ↓ DNA cleavage ↓ strand passage ↓ religation ↓ enzyme turn over	Aclarubicin
	  inhibits binding
	
	Daunorubicin
	  stabilizes CC1
	Etoposide
	  stabilizes CC1 & CC2
	Amsidyl
	  stabilizes CC2
	  inhibits religation
	
	Novobiocin
	  inhibits turnover

CC (cleavable complex)

are not only of theoretical interest, but have consequences for cellular sensitivity or resistance. Specific combinations, such as aclarubicin and daunorubicin, or aclarubicin and etoposide are not reasonable, in fact, cytotoxicity is inhibited (Jensen et al., 1990; Jensen et al., 1991). Also, sensitivity to aclarubicin is not necessarily associated with sensitivity to anthracyclines: In 1992 we published the characterization of a celline with altered topo II activity and multidrug resistance to daunorubicin, doxorubicin and idarubicin. These cells were highly sensitive to aclarubicine which underlines the relevance of the specific molecular action of these drugs for combination therapies (Erttmann et al., 1992).

CELLULAR EFFECTS OF TOPOISOMERASE II INHIBITORS AT HIGH CONCENTRATIONS

Especially the DNA-intercalaters, such as anthracyclines, amsidyl and mitoxantrone, have a number of additional cellular effects which must be taken into account at higher concentrations. Due to their high lipophilicity, they have direct membrane toxicity. Free oxygen radicals are also formed, which might play an important role in cardiotoxicity, as heart cells have reduced repair capacities because the peroxide reducing capacity of myocardial cells rests solely on their glutathion/glutathion peroxidase cycle (Dorshow et al., 1980; Dorshow et al., 1990). Additionally, the mitochondrial oxygen chain is inhibited. These effects are clearly dose dependent and play an increasing role at higher drug concentrations, they also certainly contribute to side effects. Whether they are important for cellular sensitivity at clinically relevant drug concentrations is still unclear.

CELLULAR RESISTANCE ACCORDING TO THE TWO-STEP MODEL OF CELL DEATH

The intracellular events which result in cell death in the treatment with topo II inhibiting drugs can be separated in two major steps:
• the primary events from the cellular uptake of the drugs, intracellular pharmacokinetic, binding to the DNA and inhibition of topo II, resulting in genotoxicity
• the secondary events which are the reaction of the cell, from the recognition of DNA damage, activation of repair mechanisms with the topo II is inhibited, resulting in apoptotic cell death.

Although genotoxicity is a prerequisite for the secondary events, there might be a considerable time lapse between both steps. The occurance of cellular resistance can be due to alterations which inhibit genotoxicity or those which modulate the cellular reaction. Molecular alterations resulting in decreased genotoxicity (step 1 - mechanisms) have been described for all sub-cellular levels such as membrane transport (Deffie et al., 1988; Ling, 1992), "trapping" of the drugs in intracytoplasmatic vesicules (Dietel et al., 1990) or increased detoxification, e.g. via the glutathion pathway. Additionally, the target protein topoisomerase II can be altered in several different ways such as gene mutations (Hinds et al, 1991), mRNA expression (Towatari et al., 199), mRNA splicing (Davies et al., 1993), lower activitiy (Davies et al., 1988; Erttmann et al., 1992;

Gieseler et al., 1992), altered expression of isoenzymes (Drake et al., 1989), posttranscriptional modifications (Kroll and Rowe, 1991) or resistant isoenzymes (Boege et al., 1993). The cellular reaction on the other hand, depends upon the status of the cell (e.g. proliferating, quiescent, differentiated). Step 2 - mechanisms include mutations or lower expression of p53 (its function is necessary in recognizing DNA damage) (Lowe et al., 1993), deregulated c-myc which might enhance apoptosis under certain conditions (Evan et al., 1992), higher expression of bcl2 (Kamesaki et al., 1993) and high concentrations of growth factors in cells with the necessary receptors (Loten et al., 1991).

The development of strategies to avoid or circumvent cellular resistance in therapy demands the exploration of the specific events which resulted in resistance. Step 1 - mechanisms, recognized by insufficient DNA damage after treatment, coult be avoided by the use of particular drug - combinations with the required drug concentrations. Step 2 - mechanisms, defined by the lack of apoptosis after appropriate DNA damage, might be affected by the alteration of cellular control mechanisms through interleukines, cytokines or growth factors.

REFERENCES

Boege F, Kjeldsen E, Gieseler F, Alsner J and Biersack H (1993): A drug-resistant variant of topoisomerase II alpha in human HL-60 cells exhibits alterations in catalytic pH optimum, DNA binding and sub-nuclear distribution. *Eur J Biochem* 218:757-584

Davies SL, Jenkins JR and Hickson ID (1993): Human cells express two differently spliced forms of topoisomerase beta mRNA. *Nucl Acid Res* 21:3719-3723

Davies SM, Robson CN, Davies SL and Hickson ID (1988): Nuclear topoisomerase II levels correlate with the sensitivity of mammalian cells to interclyting agents and epipodophyllotoxins. *J Biol Chem* 263:17724-17729

Deffie A, Alam T, Seneviratne C, Beenken S, Betra J and Shea S (1988): Multifactorial resistance to adriamycin: relationship of DNA repair, glutathion transferase activity, drug efflux, and p-glycoprotein in cloned cell lines of adriamycin-sensitive and -resistant p288 leukemia. *Cancer Res* 48:3595-3597

Dietel M, Arps H, Lage H and Niendorf A (1990): Membrane Vesicle formation due to Acquired Mitoxantrone Resistance in Human Gastric Carcinoma Cell Line EPG85-257. *Cancer Res* 50:6100-6106

Dorshow JH, Akman SFFC and Esworthy S (1990): Role of gluthatione - glutathione peroxidase cycle in cytotoxicity of anticancer quinones. *Pharmacol Ther* 47:359-370

Dorshow JH, Locker GY and Meaers CE (1980): Enzymatic defenses in the mouse heart against reactive oxygen metabolites: alteratnions produced by doxorubicin. *J Clin Invest* 65:128-135

Drake FH, Hofmann GA, Bartus HF, Mattern MR, Crooke ST and Mirabelli CK (1989): Biochemical and pharmacological properties of p170 and p180 forms of topoisomerase II. *Biochem* 28:8154-8160

Earnshaw WC, Halligen B, Cooke CA, Heck MM and Liu LF (1985): Topoisomerase II is a structural component of mitotic chromosome scaffolds. *J Cell Biol* 100:1706-1715

Erttmann R, Boetefür A, Erttmann KD, Gieseler F, Looft G, Münchmeyer M, Reymann A and Winkler K (1992): Conserved cytotoxic activity of aclacinomycin A in multifactorial multidrug resistance. *Haematol and Blood Transfusion* 34:49-55

Evan GI, Wyllie AH, Gibert CS, Littlewood TD, Land H, Brooks M, Waters CM, Penn LZ and Hancock DC (1992): Induction of apoptosis in fibroblasts by c-myc protein. *Cell* 69:119-122

Gasser SM, Walter R, Dang Q and Cardenas ME (1992): Topoisomerase II: its functions and phosphorylation. *Ant Van Leeuwenhoek* 62:15-24

Gieseler F, Biersack H, Brieden T, Manderscheid J and Nübler V (1994): Cytotoxicity of anthracyclines: correlation with cellular uptake, intracellular distribution and DNA-binding. *Ann Haematolg* 68:(accepted)

Gieseler F, Boege F, Biersack H, Spohn B, Clark M and Wilms K (1991): Nuclear topoisomerase II activity changes during HL-60 cell differentiation: alterations of drug sensitivity and pH-dependency. *Leukemia and Lymphoma* 5:273-279

Gieseler F, Boege F and Clark M (1990): Alteration of topoisomerase II action is a possible mechanism of HL-60 cell differentiation. *Environ Health Persp* 88:183-185

Gieseler F, Boege F, Erttmann R, Tony HP, Spohn B and Clark M (1992): Characterization of human leukemic HL-60 sublines as a model for primary and secondary resistance against cytostatics. *Haematol and Blood Transfusion* 34:44-48

Gieseler F, Boege F, Ruf B, Meyer P and Wilms K (1994): Molecular pathways of topoisomerase II regulation and consequences for chemotherapy. In Hiddemann W. et al.: *Leukemia IV*, Berlin, Springer Verlag

Gorsky LD, Cross SM and Morin MJ (1989): Rapid increase in the activity of DNA topoisomerase I, but not topoisomerase II, in HL-60 promyelocytic leukemia cells treated with a phorbol diester. *Cancer Commun* 1:83-92

Heck MM, Hittelman WN and Earnshaw WC (1989): *In vivo* phosphorylation of the 170-kDa form of eukaryotic DNA topoisomerase II. Cell cycle analysis. *J Biol Chem* 264:15161-15164

Hinds M, Deisseroth K, Mayes J, Altschuler E, Jansen R, Ledley F and Zwelling LA (1991): Identification of a Point Mutation in the Topoisomerase II Gene from a Human Leukemia Cell Line Containing an Amsacrine-resistant Form of Topoisomerase II. *Cancer* 51:4729-4731

Jensen PB, Jensen PS et al. (1991): Antagonistic effect of aclarubicin on daunorubicin-induced cytotoxicity in human small cell lung cancer cells: relationship to DNA integrity and topoisomerase II. *Cancer Res* 51:5093-5099

Jensen PB, Sorensen BS, Demant EJ, Sehested M, Jensen PS, Vindelov L and Hansen HH (1990): Antagonistic effect of aclarubicin on the cytotoxicity of etoposide and 4'-(9-acridinylamino)methanesulfon-m-anasidide in human small cell lung cancer cell lines and on topoisomerase II-mediated DNA cleavage. *Cancer Res* 50:3311-3316

Kamesaki S, Kamesaki H, Jorgensen TJ, Tanizawa A, Pommier Y and Cossman J (1993): bcl-2 Protein inhibits etoposide-induced apoptosis through its effects on events subsequent to topoisomerase II-induced DNA strand breaks and their repair. *Cancer Res* 53:4251-4256

Kroll DJ and Rowe TC (1991): Phosphorylation of DNA topoisomearse II in a human tumor cell line. *J Biol Chem* 266:7957-7961

Laemmli UK and Gasser SM (1987): A glimpse at chromosomal order. *Trends in Genetics* 3:72-77

Ling V (1992): P-glycoprotein and Resistance to Anticancer Drugs. *Cancer* 69:2603-2609

Ling YH, Tseng MT and Nelson JA (1991): Differentiation induction of human promyelocytic leukemia cells by 10-hydroxycamptothecin, a DNA topoisomerase I inhibitor. *Differentiation* 46:135-141

Lotem J, Cragoe EJ and Sachs L (1991): Rescue from programmed cell death in leukemic and normal myeloid cells. *Blood* 78:953-956

Lowe SW, Ruley HE, Jacks T and Housman DE (1993): p53-dependent apoptosis modulates the cytotoxicity of anticancer agents. *Cell* 74:957-967

Menzel R and Gellert M (1983): Regulation of the genes for E. coli DNA gyrase: homeostatic control of DNA supercoiling. *Cell* 34:105-113

Nakaya K, Chou S, Kaneko M and Makamura Y (1991): Topoisomerase inhibitors have potent differentiation-inducing activity for human and mouse myeloid leukemia cells. *Jpn J Cancer Res* 82:184-191

Osheroff N (1986): Eukaryotic topoisomerase II. *J Biol Chem* 261:9944-9950

Robinson MJ, Corbett AH and Osheroff N (1993): Effects of topoisomearse II-targeted drugs on enzyme-mediated DNA cleavage and ATP hydrolysis: evidence for distinct drug interaction domains on topoisomerase II. *Biochemistry* 32:3638-3643

Sahyoun N, Wolf M, Besterman J, Hsieh T, Sander M, LeVine H, Chang KJ and Cuatrecases P (1986): Protein kinase C phosphorylates topoisomerase II: topoisomerase activition and its possible role in phorbol ester-induced differentiation of HL-60 cells. *Proc Natl Acad Sci USA* 83:1603-1607

Samuels DS and Shimizu N (1992): DNA topoisomerase I phosphorylation in murine fibroblasts treated with 12-O-tetradecanoylphorbol-13-acetate and *in vitro* by protein kinase. *J Biol Chem* 267:11156-11162

Schroder HC, Steffen R, Wenger R, Ugarkovic D and Muller WE (1989): Age-dependent increase of DNA topoisomerase II activity in quail oviduct; modulation of the nuclear matrix-associated enzyme activity by protein phosphorylation and polyADP-ribosylation. *Mutat Res* 219:283-294

Sorensen BS, Sinding J, Andersen AH, Alsner J, Jensen PB and Westergaard O (1992): Mode of action of topoisomerase II-targeting agents at a specific DNA sequence. Uncoupling the DNA binding, cleavage and religation events. *J Mol Biol* 228:778-786

Takano H, Kohno K, Ono M, Uchida Y and Kuwano M (1991): Increased Phosphorylation of DNA Topoisomerase II in Etoposide-resistant Mutants of Human Cancer KB Cells. *Cancer Res* 51:3951-3157

Tan KB, Dorman TE, Falls KM, Chung TDY, Mirabelli CK, Crooke ST and Mao J (1992): Topoisomerase IIα and Topoisomerase IIß Genes: Characterization and Mapping to Human Chromosomes 17 and 3, Respectively. *Cancer Res* 52:231-234

Towatari M, Ito Y, Morishita Y and Saito H (1990): Enhanced expression of DNA topoisomerase II by recombinant human granulocyte colony-stimulating factor in human leukemia cells. *Cancer Res* 50:7198-7202

Tsao Y, Wu H and Liu LF (1989): Transcription-driven supercoiling of DNA: direct biochemical evidence from *in vitro* studies. *Cell* 56:111-118

Tsutsui K, Tsutsui K and Muller MT (1988): The nuclear scaffold exhibits DNA-binding sites selective for supercoiled DNA. *J Biol Chem* 263:7235-7241

Uemura T, Ohkura H, Adachi Y, Morino K, Shiozaki K and Yanagida M (1987): DNA topoisomerase II is requires for condensation and separation of mitotic chromosomes in S. pombe. *Cell* 50:917-925

Zwelling LA, Chan D, Hinds M, Mayes J, Silberman LE and Blick M (1988): Effect of phorbol ester treatment on drug-induced, topoisomerase II-mediated DNA cleavage in human leukemia cells. *Cancer Res* 48:6625-6633

7. A DISTINCTIVE MULTIPLE DRUG RESISTANCE PHENOTYPE EXPRESSED BY TUMOR CELLS FOLLOWING EXPOSURE TO X-IRRADIATION

Bridget T. Hill

Resistance to drug therapy is considered one of the main reasons for treatment failures. Laboratory-based mechanistic studies aim to elucidate the biochemical/biological bases for resistance to the varied classes of antitumor drugs in current clinical usage, so as to design rationale ways of either overcoming or circumventing any expression of drug resistance, preventing its development or interfering with the mechanisms themselves. Clinical resistance to chemotherapy is encountered not only following treatment with single agents or after multiple drugs, but also has been identified in subgroups of patients with solid tumors who have received prior radiotherapy (cf. review by Hill, 1991). Indeed, our early investigative studies of the treatment of head and neck cancer highlighted the fact that patients whose tumors had been irradiated not only had reduced response rates to subsequent combination chemotherapy, but also had significantly reduced survival figures (Hill et al., 1984). In view of the major role of radiotherapy in cancer management we considered it importance to determine the molecular basis for this expression of drug resistance by tumor cells following their exposure to X-irradiation and in particular to establish whether any novel or distinctive mechanisms operated, different from those more generally studied and known to result from drug selection or exposure.

DEVELOPMENT OF AN IN VITRO MODEL SYSTEM

In the early 1980's my group initiated a series of laboratory-based studies to investigate this drug resistance phenotype. Our plan was first to develop a suitable experimental model system and so we asked the question : Does exposure of tumor cells in vitro to a series of fractions of X-irradiation result in any expression of drug resistance by the surviving population?

Initially, using a murine lymphoblastoid leukemic cell line (L5178Y), tumor cells were exposed in vitro to ten intermittent fractions of 2Gy (a dose which reduced cell survival by approximately 90%), allowing the cell population to recover back to logarithmic growth between each X-ray fraction. The surviving tumor cell population, designated L5178Y/DXR, proved significantly resistant to vincristine and to etoposide (see Figure 1), as judged by clonogenic cell survival assays (Bellamy and Hill, 1984). More recently, similar experiments were initiated with Chinese hamster ovary (CHO) cells (Hill et al., 1990). A larger acute dose of X-irradiation of 9Gy (a dose which reduced cell survival by 99%) was selected for each fraction. The resultant surviving tumor cell population was designated CHO/DXR10 and, as shown in Figure 1, these cells also proved significantly resistant to etoposide and to vincristine. These studies provided the first evidence that exposure of tumor cells in vitro to fractionated X-irradiation resulted in the surviving population expressing resistance to certain clinically-useful antitumor drugs.

CHARACTERISATION OF IRRADIATED CHO SUBLINES

It soon became apparent that the pattern of cross resistance of these irradiated sublines did not correspond precisely with that originally identified and subsequently defined as the pleiotropic or multidrug-resistance phenotype, as reviewed recently (Hill, 1993). This finding therefore appeared to support our initial contention that exposure to X-irradiation might select for or induce a distinctive drug resistance profile.

Patterns of Resistance Expressed

In the X-irradiated sublines resistance was expressed only to certain antitumor drugs and, specifically, no evidence of resistance to the anthracyclines was noted (see Table 1). Extending our studies using the

Figure 1. Survival, assessed by colony formation, of logarithmically-growing L5178Y murine leukemic or CHO cells following a 24-hour exposure to a range of etoposide or vincristine concentrations.. Values are the mean ± SE of 2-3 experiments in which duplicate cultures were drug-treated (Bellamy and Hill, 1984; Hill et al., 1990).

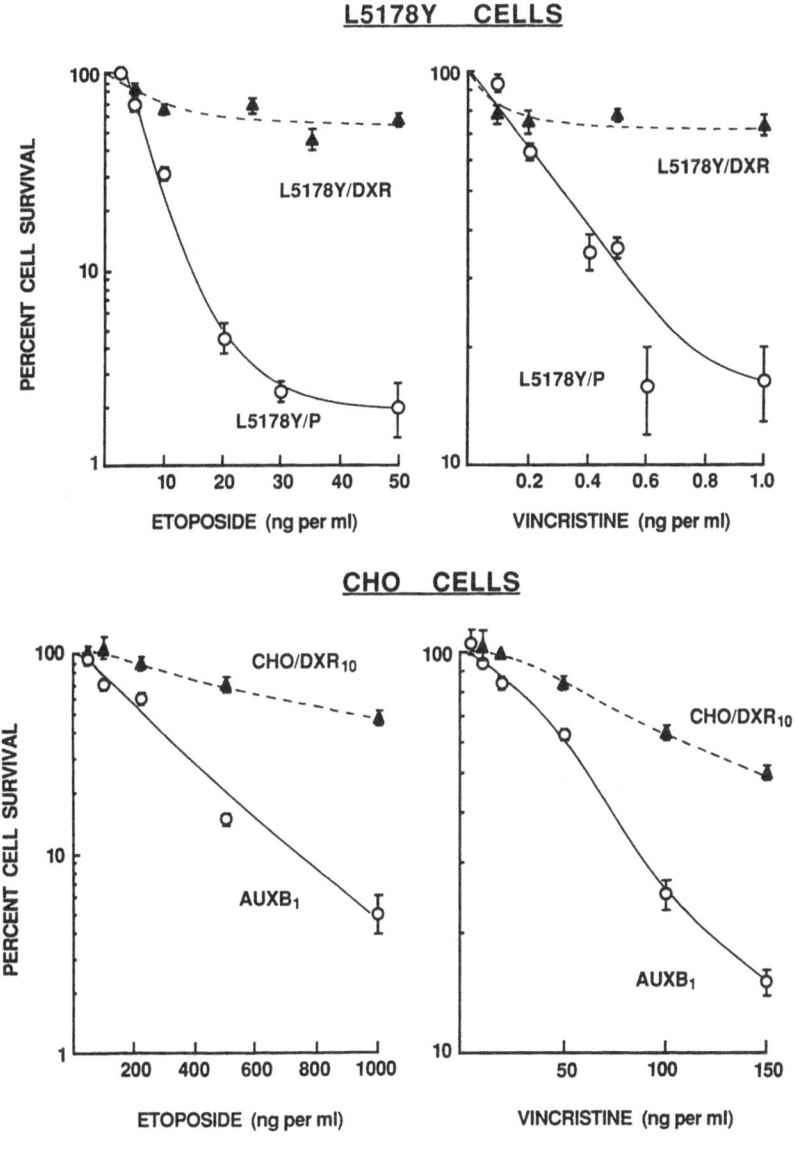

Table 1. In vitro sensitivities of Chinese hamster ovary cell lines to various antitumour agents (Hill et al., 1990; McClean et al., 1993a)

Agents tested	AuxB1 (IC_{50} µg per ml)	Resistance Index[b] DXR-10I	DXR-10II
Cisplatin	0.200	1.0	1.0
Colchicine	0.020	2.5	2.5
Daunorubicin	0.030	1.2	0.9
Doxorubicn	0.019	1.1	1.3
Etoposide	0.057	2.3	1.7
Gramacidin C	0.003	3.0	3.2
Mitoxantrone	0.052	1.3	1.4
Navelbine	0.005	3.0	3.0
Taxol	0.950	3.4	2.8
Taxotere	0.018	1.0	1.2
Vinblastine	0.008	3.5	3.8
Vincristine	0.008	6.7	8.0
X-rays[c] Do	2.26 ± 0.11	2.08 ± 0.04	2.06 ± 0.09
n	1.27 ± 0.16	1.47 ± 0.06	1.49 ± 0.26

[a] Survival curves for 24 hour exposures to each drug were obtained with the use of a minimum of these drug concentrations and four estimations per point from which IC50 values were calculated.

[b] Resistance index is the ratio obtained by dividing the IC50 values of the subline by the IC50 values of parental AuxB1 cells.

[c] Values represent the mean ± and n is the extrapolation number.

CHO cells, two independently-selected X-irradiated sublines were established from the parental AuxB1 cells and designated CHO/DXR-10I and DXR-10II. Their drug sensitivity profiles were established and their resistance indices calculated by comparing IC50 values (concentrations required to reduce cell survival by 50%). The results listed in Table 1 illustrate their resistance to colchicine, to all three Vinca alkaloids tested and to taxol, etoposide and gramicidin D in both the DXR-10 sublines. Unexpectedly, these irradiated cells showed no cross resistance to taxotere, although we have now shown that certain drug-selected multidrug-resistant sublines also failed to show any cross resistance to taxotere (Hill et al., 1994b). A lack of significant cross resistance was also noted in these DXR-10 sublines to cisplatin and to doxorubicin, daunorubicin and mitoxantrone. A finding that also requires emphasis was that these irradiated sublines showed no resistance to subsequent acute X-ray exposure i.e. this procedure did not select for or induce radioresistance. Furthermore, the differing drug responses could not be explained by any significant alterations in fundamental growth characteristics between the irradiated sublines and their parental cells. Data in Table 1 also serve to illustrate the consistency of the pattern of resistance expressed and indeed the levels of resistance identified in these two independently-derived DXR-10 sublines.

The levels of resistance expressed by these irradiated sublines are relatively modest but, as suggested earlier (Hill, 1991; Hill, 1993), might be considered more clinically relevant than many other currently used experimental model systems where resistance levels of several 100- or even 1000-fold are frequently described. The next question we therefore considered was: Are the mechanisms associated with the expression of these modest levels of drug resistance as a result of exposure to X-irradiation comparable with those identified in drug-selected resistant tumor cells?

Vinca Alkaloid Resistance Mechanisms Expressed

Resistance to Vinca alkaloids has been associated with reduced drug accumulation, increased drug efflux and overexpression of P-glycoprotein, together with sensitivity to reversal of resistance by verapamil. All of these characteristics have been identified in the CHO/DXR-10I and DXR-10II sublines (Hill et al., 1990; McClean et al., 1993a). Indeed, our data provided the first demonstration that P-glycoprotein overexpression could result from exposure of tumor cells to X-irradiation in vitro. These findings were of definite interest in view of the possible extrapolation of these methodologies used to characterise resistance mechanisms to human tumor biopsy material in studies aimed at detecting the emergence/expression of clinical resistance. Additionally, we were able to add support to our original report of a lack of cross resistance to the anthracyclines in the irradiated drug resistant sublines since

14C-doxorubicin uptake was neither diminished, relative to parental cells, nor influenced by verapamil addition and the pattern of nuclear/cytoplasmic fluorescence of doxorubicin remained predominantly nuclear (McClean et al., 1993a).

P-Glycoprotein Overexpression

Overexpression of P-glycoprotein was first identified in the CHO/DXR-10 cells by Western blot analysis using the C219 monoclonal antibody (Hill et al., 1990). Subsequent use of the C494 antibody served to confirm this and to delineate overexpression to the class I P-glycoprotein (McClean et al., 1993a). In these DXR-10 cell lines karyotypic alterations were also identified, with the most consistent ones involving the long arm of chromosome 1 (McClean et al., 1993a), which is the region to which P-glycoprotein had been localised (Trent et al., 1985).

P-glycoprotein overexpression in multidrug-resistant tumor cell lines has generally been associated with a concomitant overexpression of P-glycoprotein mRNA, sometimes accompanied in cell lines expressing high levels of resistance by gene amplification (cf. review by Hill, 1993). Southern blot analysis of the DXR-10I and DXR-10II cells provided no evidence of gene amplification (Hill et al., 1990), a finding which might be explained by their relatively modest levels of resistance. However, Northern blot analysis also failed to reveal any P-glycoprotein mRNA overexpression, even when probes for each of the three P-glycoprotein gene family members were used (Hill et al., 1990). This observation therefore suggested that overexpression of P-glycoprotein resulting from exposure to X-irradiation might be differently regulated from that identified following drug-selection of drug resistant tumor cells.

These data lead us next to consider the question: What mechanism is responsible in these irradiated cells for the overexpression of P-glycoprotein without any associated increase in P-glycoprotein mRNA?

It has been shown that expression of P-glycoprotein can be regulated by a number of diverse mechanisms, including gene amplification and transcriptional activation, as well as at the level of translation or post-translationally, as reviewed recently (Hill et al., 1990). Our observation that P-glycoprotein overexpression in these irradiated sublines was not matched by a concomitant elevation of mRNA implied that either translational or post-translational modifications of P-glycoprotein were involved in this overexpression of the protein following X-ray treatment. To investigate this aspect we examined the turnover rates of P-glycoprotein in drug-selected resistant CHO sublines, which overexpressed P-glycoprotein at both the protein and mRNA levels, and compared these with the turnover rates in our X-irradiated DXR-10 cells. Two colchicine-selected resistant sublines were examined, the highly-resistant (145-fold) 'classical' CHRC5 multidrug-resistant line (Riordan et al., 1985) and a line expressing a more modest 7-fold level of resistance (CHRA3), selected in a single step from the parental AuxB1 cells (Ling and Thompson, 1974). Stability of P-glycoprotein was estimated by following the loss of 35S-labelled-P-glycoprotein from cells with time, by quantitative immunoprecipitation and subsequent analysis on SDS-PAGE gels. Using either the C219 or the C494 monoclonal antibody, we demonstrated that while the half-life of P-glycoprotein was of the order of 10-17 hours in drug-selected CHO cells, irrespective of their levels of drug resistance, P-glycoprotein in the irradiated CHO/DXR-10II cells had a half life of > 40 hours (McClean and Hill, 1993). Overall these results provided one of the first examples of the regulation of P-glycoprotein by a post-translational increased stability.

Although the means by which X-irradiation causes the increased expression of P-glycoprotein remain to be established, the finding that irradiation of cells can alter stability of a protein has a precedent. UV irradiation of non-transformed 3T3 mouse cells resulted in an accumulation of normal p53, the tumor suppressor gene, which was found to be mediated by a post-translational stabilisation (Maltzman and Czyzyk, 1984). It is, of course, also possible that the rates of synthesis or degradation of P-glycoprotein may be altered in these irradiated cells. However, because of the low level of P-glycoprotein expression in the wild-type AuxB1 cells, existing techniques are not sufficiently sensitive to permit a quantitative examination of these possibilities.

This demonstration of P-glycoprotein regulation at the level of post-translational stability provides a basis therefore for the overexpression of P-glycoprotein in irradiated tumor cells in the absence of any elevation in P-glycoprotein mRNA. This finding raised the possibility that increased protein stabilisation may represent a new and novel mechanism for regulating drug resistance.

Dominant Expression of this Distinctive Multiple Drug Resistant Phenotype

Having identified this apparently distinctive multiple drug resistant phenotype in CHO cell lines following fractionated X-irradiation pretreatments, coupled with the fact that little appeared to be known about the specific effects of X-irradiation on surviving cells and their gene regulation, our next investigations centred on determining whether this distinctive phenotype was expressed dominantly or recessively. Intraspecies hybrids were constructed and by clonogenic assay they proved resistant to colchicine (2-fold) and to vincristine (5- to 7-fold), but not to doxorubicin. Furthermore these hybrids overexpressed P-glycoprotein, as judged by Western immunoblotting using the C219 monoclonal antibody and their vincristine resistance was sensitive, at least in part, to reversal by verapamil (McClean et al., 1992). These data were consistent with our hypothesis that this distinctive phenotype is a consequence of the dominant genetic alteration from exposure of the CHO cells to X-irradiation.

Single X-Ray Dose Selection of this Distinctive Multiple Drug Resistant Phenotype

In all these experimental studies we had used sublines which had been derived following exposure to multiple fractions of X-irradiation. The next consideration therefore was: Is this distinctive resistance phenotype a consequence of repeated stress/recovery processes or a direct result of the radiation itself?

We have now shown that exposure of the AuxB1 parental CHO cells to a single 30Gy X-ray dose similarly resulted in the survivors, designated DXR-30, expressing resistance to vincristine and to etoposide and overexpressing P-glycoprotein (McClean et al., 1993b). In agreement with data obtained on cells which received repeated X-ray exposures, in these DXR-30 cells P-glycoprotein overexpression occurred in the absence of any significant elevation of P-glycoprotein mRNA. However, the reduced ability to accumulate rhodamine 123, identified in these DXR-30 sublines and the ability of verapamil to reverse this accumulation defect implied that the P-glycoprotein which was overexpressed was functional. These results therefore indicated that a series of X-ray exposures was not necessary for expression of this distinctive multiple drug resistance phenotype, suggesting that this resulted not from a general 'stress-type' response, but rather more specifically from the radiation exposure itself, with both single-dose and repeated X-irradiation selecting for similar genetic mutants.

Influence of Further Drug- or X-Ray-Selection on the Drug Resistance Phenotype Expressed

In our original report (Hill et al., 1990), we showed that when AuxB1 cells were exposed to 20 as opposed to 10 fractions of X-rays, resistance to vincristine and to etoposide did not increase concomitantly and P-glycoprotein expression was not further enhanced.   These findings suggested that the level of resistance had reached an upper threshold in these irradiated DXR-10 cells.   This situation appeared to contrast with the more general observation in drug-selected multidrug-resistant tumor cells of increased resistance to drugs and associated elevations in P-glycoprotein and P-glycoprotein mRNA with increasing selection pressure (Shen et al., 1986; Bradley et al., 1989).

   We have now demonstrated that in these irradiated DXR-10 cells the apparent plateau in drug resistance can be overcome by drug selection although not by further X-ray selection (McClean and Hill, 1994).   When CHO/DXR-10 cells received ten pulsed 24-hour exposures to vincristine (100 ng per ml; a concentration which reduced cell survival by approximately 90%) they became more resistant to vincristine and their expression of P-glycoprotein increased.   Furthermore, the increased ability of these DXR-10 cells to efflux rhodamine 123 confirmed that there was an increase in functional P-glycoprotein expression. Additionally, certain features of the phenotype associated with the DXR-10II cells were altered as a result of their further drug selection. The subline designated DXR-10/VCR-10 proved resistant to doxorubicin, suggesting that the P-glycoprotein specificity of these cells was similar to that of other drug-selected cells (Shen et al., 1986; Bradley et al., 1989), rather than showing the distinctive drug resistance profile of the irradiated DXR-10 cells.   This development of doxorubicin resistance in these DXR-10/VCR-10 cells implied that the drug resistance phenotype that was induced in these cells following drug selection was modified from that shown following exposure to X-irradiation. One possible explanation for this was that the P-glycoprotein that was overexpressed following X-irradiation, although recognised by both C219 and C494 monoclonal antibodies (McClean and Hill, 1993a), differed from the P-glycoprotein that was overexpressed following drug selection and exhibited an altered substrate recognition profile. Although the mechanism by which P-glycoprotein can recognise and transport such a large group of structurally-unrelated substances remains to be elucidated, recent evidence suggests that membrane-associated domains participate in substrate recognition and binding. Functional analyses of chimeric and mutant P-glycoproteins have highlighted transmembrane domains as important determinants of substrate interactions (Dhir and Gros, 1992). Several reports now indicate that hamster, murine and human P-glycoproteins bearing mutations, which may result from only single amino acid substitutions, within or near transmembrane domains expressed drug resistance phenotypes distinct from that of their respective wild-types (cf. review by Hill, 1993). However, it can be predicted that the frequency of point mutations following a 9Gy dose of X-rays would be approximately 10-5 per cell (Thacker, 1992). Therefore, because of the manner in which the DXR-10 cells were derived, with the AuxB1 cells receiving doses of X-rays resulting in only a two log cell kill per fraction, and the fact that the surviving population was not cloned, it is unlikely that single amino acid mutations resulted in P-glycoprotein overexpression throughout the DXR-10 cell population. Nevertheless, it is possible that any alteration in P-glycoprotein, whether it involved qualitative changes in glycosylation or phosphorylation, or even in subcellular distribution, might modulate the ability of P-glycoprotein to ransport doxorubicin. Whilst elevated expression of P-glycoprotein in the CHO/DXR-10 cells was associated with a post-translational increase in P-glycoprotein stability rather than with any elevation of P-glycoprotein mRNA (McClean and Hill, 1993), comparative densitometry of Northern blots revealed that P-glycoprotein expression in the DXR-10/VCR-10 cells was associated with a 6-fold increase in P-glycoprotein mRNA, implicating transcriptional regulation. Furthermore, the half-life of P-glycoprotein in these DXR-10/VCR-10 cells was found to be approximately 20 hours (McClean et al., 1994), which, as discussed above, was similar to that of the drug-selected CHO sublines studied, rather than the much longer time identified for the DXR-10II cells from whom this subline was derived (McClean and Hill, 1993). It was also interesting to note that the P-glycoprotein expressed in cells showing some resistance to doxorubicin had a half-life of 12-20 hours, while the DXR-10 cells, in which P-glycoprotein had been demonstrated to have an extended half-life, did not show any doxorubicin resistance. While this observation could be fortuitous, it is also possible that a relationship may exist between factors that regulate P-glycoprotein stability and the drug resistance profile expressed. These data therefore appear to confirm that regulation of P-glycoprotein expression differs in drug resistant cells which have been selected with X-rays only, as opposed to those selected with cytotoxic drugs alone or with drugs following after X-ray selection.

This finding that further drug-selection of X-irradiated sublines proved additive to the expression of multiple drug resistance resulting from the initial X-ray exposure, represents a novel observation. It would appear that this subsequent drug selection resulted in an additional 'classical' multiple drug resistance-like phenotype (including elevations in P-glycoprotein mRNA, reduced P-glycoprotein half-life and the expression of resistance to doxorubicin) rather than merely enhancing expression of the specific and distinctive phenotype identified following fractionated X-irradiation treatment. These observations, if confirmed in similarly-derived human tumor sublines, may have some relevance in designing clinical combined modality therapies.

X-Ray-Selection for Drug Resistance in the Presence of Verapamil

Since ionizing radiation is considered to induce multiple biological effects, we were also interested in establishing a model system useful for identifying other resistance mechanisms which might be operating in these DXR-10 sublines. Therefore we attempted to use conditions which selected against P-glycoprotein-associated mechanisms, namely irradiation in the presence of the resistance modulator, verapamil. This principle had been adopted in earlier studies using human tumor cell lines and selecting for doxorubicin resistance in the presence of verapamil (Chen et al., 1990; Dalton, 1990; Futscher et al., 1992). When AuxB1 parental CHO cells were exposed to fractionated X-irradiation in the presence of verapamil, expression of P-glycoprotein in the surviving cells, designated VRP/DXR-10, was not significantly altered and P-glycoprotein mRNA levels were actually reduced (Hill and McClean, 1994), consistent with earlier reports (Chen et al., 1990; Futscher et al., 1992). Nevertheless VRP/DXR-10 cells showed resistance to vincristine and to etoposide. This seemed to indicate that alternative non-P-glycoprotein-related mechanisms of resistance were operating in these cells. Significantly, as shown earlier with the DXR-10 cells, these VRP/DXR-10 cells showed no cross resistance to doxorubicin, so strengthening the link between X-ray-selected multiple drug resistance and doxorubicin sensitivity. Although the resistance mechanisms expressed by these VRP/DXR-10 cells remain to be elucidated, these preliminary studies suggested that the resistance expressed to vincristine and to etoposide was independent, at least in part, of P-glycoprotein. This observation, if confirmed, would again appear of potential clinical relevance.

Table 2. In vitro sensitivities of human tumor sublines, established after exposure to fractionated x-irradiation, to various antitumor drugs.

Cell Line	Origin	Total X-ray Dosage	Subline Established	Order of Drug Resistance:[a] VCR[b]	VP-16[b]	DOX[b]
HN-1	scc tongue	50 Gy	HN-1/DXR-11[c]	3	4	1
MCF-7	ca breast	60 Gy	MCF-7/DXR-10[d]	4	2	1
JA-T	ca ovary	50Gy	JA-T/DXR-10[e]	3	2	1
SKOV3	ca ovary	50Gy	SKOV3/DXR-10[e]	2	2	1
SuSa	testicular teratoma	30Gy	SuSa/DXR-10[f]	2	3	1

[a] Derived from a comparison of IC_{50} values obtained using clonogenic cell survival assays and 24-hour drug exposures.
[b] VCR-vincristine, VP-16-etoposide; DOX-doxorubin.
[c] Lock and Hill, 1988; [d] Whelan and Hill, 1993; [e] Dempke et al., 1992; [f] Hosking et al., 1994.

CHARACTERISATION OF IRRADIATED HUMAN TUMOR CELL LINES

Since these observations appeared to provide a biological basis for the clinical problem of drug resistance that can occur in previously irradiated tumors, it became important to determine whether this phenotype was unique to rodent cells or whether it represented a more general mechanism of multiple drug resistance resulting from radiation exposure.

Prior radiotherapy has been reported to result in reduced response rates to subsequent chemotherapy in certain patients with cancers of the head and neck, of breast, ovary or testis (cf. review by Hill, 1991). Cell lines established from these various tumor types were therefore selected for study. Logarithmically-growing cultures of each parental line were exposed in vitro to a dose of X-irradiation which resulted in a one log cell kill for 10 or 11 fractions, so that the total radiation dose administered approximated to that used in clinical radiotherapy protocols for each particular histologic tumor type. Detailed characterisation, in terms of cytological, biological and kinetic parameters, revealed no significant differences between the parental cells and their X-irradiated sublines (cf. Hill, 1991).   Since all the cell lines formed colonies their drug and radiation responses were quantitated by clonogenic cell survival assays.

Patterns of Drug Resistance Expressed

Characteristically, in vitro exposure of these various human tumor cell lines to fractionated X-irradiation resulted in the expression of resistance to the Vinca alkaloids and to the epipodophyllotoxins, exemplified by vincristine and etoposide respectively, but not to the anthracyclines, including doxorubicin (see Table 2).   The levels of resistance expressed were modest i.e., 2- to 4-fold, yet proved statistically significant as judged by clonogenic assay.   Similar studies utilising cell lines derived from either a human transitional cell carcinoma of the bladder or, more recently, a colon carcinoma have also provided evidence of 2- to 4-fold levels of resistance to vincristine or to etoposide in the irradiated sublines, without any expression of resistance to doxorubicin (Hill et al., 1988; Hill, 1991).   These result therefore provided direct evidence that human tumor cell drug responses could be influences markedly by exposure in vitro to fractionated X-irradiation.   Noticeably the same pattern of resistance/sensitivity to these drugs was identified in all the lines tested of both human and rodent origin.

 To elucidate the underlying cellular and molecular events associated with these modified drug responses in these irradiated human tumor sublines, we examined in more detail the two ovarian tumor cell lines. Ovarian tumors generally respond initially to chemotherapy, but subsequently develop clinical resistance (Schilder and Ozols, 1992) and prior radiotherapy has been reported to result in reduced response rates in certain ovarian cancers (Young et al., 1982).

P-Glycoprotein Overexpression in Irradiated Human Ovarian Tumor Cells

Working with the JA-T cell lines, parental and X-irradiated cells were xenografted into nude mice. The animals were then treated with a single LD10 dose of vincristine, etoposide or doxorubicin and 48 hours later the surviving clonogenic cells in each tumor were quantitated (Dempke et al., 1992). Significantly fewer colonies grew from the JA-T/P xenografts treated with either vincristine or with etoposide, as opposed to the JA-T/DXR-10 tumors, whilst comparable colony numbers were recorded after doxorubicin treatment. These data suggested that the distinctive multiple drug resistant phenotype identified following exposure to fractionated X-irradiation in vitro is also expressed in vivo. Further support for this finding came from a study by Mattern and his colleagues (Mattern et al., 1991) which reported that after exposing human lung cancer xenografts to fractionated X-irradiation in vivo the irradiated xenografts proved resistant to the Vinca alkaloids.

On examining P-glycoprotein expression in these irradiated human ovarian tumor sublines significant amounts of P-glycoprotein were detectable by Western blotting using the C219 monoclonal antibody, although the protein was undetectable in their respective parental cells. This protein was also cross-reactive with the C494 antibody, indicating that it was the MDR1 gene product which was overexpressed (Hill et al., 1994a). These results were particularly interesting since they showed an ability to detect P-glycoprotein overexpression in cell lines exhibiting only 2- to 4-fold levels of resistance. If these findings are reflected clinically, P-glycoprotein overexpression should be identifiable in certain human tumors after radiotherapy. Despite this overexpression of P-glycoprotein in the SKOV3/DXR-10 cells there was no concomitant increase in P-glycoprotein mRNA, as judged by RNase protection (Hill et al., 1994a). The fact that a signal for MDR1 P-glycoprotein mRNA was not detectable in either the parental or irradiated SKOV3 cell lines precluded any definitive statement that MDR1 mRNA was not overexpressed in the irradiated subline. Indeed, with the recently developed more sensitive cDNA-PCR assay for MDR1 mRNA (Holzmayer et al., 1992) it may prove possible to detect a signal. However, whether such minute levels could contribute significantly to resistance would have to be established.

We next went on to compare the regulation of this resistance-associated protein in our irradiated DXR-10 subline with that in a vincristine-selected 'classical' multidrug-resistant subline, designated SKVCR/O.25. P-glycoprotein was immunoprecipitated at different time intervals from 35S-labelled cellular proteins. The half-life of P-glycoprotein in the SKVCR/0.25 cells was determined as 16 hours, whilst that identified in the SKOV3/DXR-10 cells was considerably longer, i.e. approximately 39 hours (Hill et al., 1994a). Therefore our initial demonstration that P-glycoprotein was regulated by a post-translational increased stability in irradiated CHO cells (McClean and

Hill, 1993), was now confirmed in this irradiated human ovarian tumor subline. The mechanism involved remains to be elucidated, but some recent evidence appears to support our proposal that this might represent a novel drug resistance mechanism, since protein stabilisation has been implicated in regulating N-myc expression in aggressive multidrug-resistant neuroblastoma (Domenech et al., 1993).

Identification of Other Cellular Proteins Upregulated by Radiation Exposure In Vitro

The next question considered was: Does exposure to X-irradiation lead to overexpression of other membrane-associated or cytoplasmic proteins and, if so, does this involve transcriptional or post-translational regulation?

The expression of multidrug resistance in tumor cells in vitro is not only associated with P-glycoprotein overexpression, but also with alterations in many other proteins, as reviewed by McClean and Hill (1992), although their causal role in mediating drug resistance remains to be established in many cases. In our initial studies, using the SKOV3/DXR-10 cells, whilst reduced levels of epidermal growth factor receptors and unchanged levels of topoiosmerase II were identified, there was marginal overexpression of another membrane-associated protein c-erbB2 and significantly elevated levels of the cytoplasmic heat shock protein HSP27 (Hill et al., 1994a). In these latter cases, however, concomitant increases in their respective mRNA levels were also detected, implicating regulation at the transcriptional level. These results therefore imply that regulation by protein stabilisation may be specific for P-glycoprotein in these irradiated tumor cells. Investigations are now underway to quantitate the expression of other proteins implicated in drug resistance in these SKOV-3/DXR-10 cells and also to extend our observations to evaluate our other irradiated human tumor sublines.

CLINICAL IMPLICATIONS OF THESE EXPERIMENTAL DATA

Results from these experimental laboratory-based investigations have provided evidence to suggest that the monitoring of P-glycoprotein in tumor biopsy material for potential prognostic significance should involve quantitation of mRNA expression, but also, and perhaps of more importance, of protein levels. In this respect there is a major requirement for standardization, optimization and quantitation of current immunocytochemical detection methods for P-glycoprotein. Our proposal that different resistance mechanisms may operate or predominate depending on whether tumor cells have been previously exposed to drugs or to X-rays, if confirmed, may also need to be considered in planning and optimizing treatment protocols.

REFERENCES

Bellamy AS and Hill BT (1984): Murine L5178Y cells resulting in altered drug sensitivities from fractionated radiation exposure in vitro. *J Natl Cancer Inst* 72:411-417

Bradley G, Naik M and Ling V (1989): P-glycoprotein expression in multidrug resistant human ovarian carcinoma cell lines. *Cancer Res* 49:2790-2796

Chen Y-H, Mickley LA, Schwartz AM, Acton EM, Hwang J and Foto AT (1990): Characterization of Adriamycin-resistant human breast cancer cells which display overexpression of a novel resistance-related membrane protein. *J Biol Chem* 265:10073-10080

Dalton WS (1990): Reversing multidrug resistance in the laboratory and the clinic. *Proc Am Assoc Cancer Res* 31:520-521

Dempke WCM, Whelan RDH and Hill BT (1992): Expression of resistance to etoposide and vincristine in vitro and in vivo after X-irradiation of ovarian tumor cells. *Anti-Cancer Drugs* 3:395-399

Dhir R and Gros P (1992): Functional analysis of chimeric proteins constructed by exchanging homologous domains of two P-glycoproteins conferring distinct drug resistance profiles. *Biochemistry* 31:6103-6110

Domenech C, Spengler BA, Ross RA and Biedler JL (1993): Prolonged half-life in a multidrug-resistant N-myc-amplified human neurobalstoma cell line. *Proc Am Assoc Cancer Res* 34:16

Futscher BW, Campbell K and Dalton WS (1992): Collateral sensitivity to nitrosoureas in multidrug-resistant cells selected with verapamil. *Cancer Res* 52:5013-5017

Hill BT (1991): Interactions between antitumor agents and radiation and the expression of resistance. *Cancer Treat Rev* 18:149-190

Hill BT (1993): Differing patterns of cross-resistance resulting from exposures to specific antitumor drugs or to radiation in vitro. *Cytotechnol* 12:265-288

Hill BT and McClean S (1994): Characterisation of a novel multidrug resistant subline selected in vitro by exposure to fractionated X-irradiation in the presence of verapamil. *Proc Am Assoc Cancer Res* 35:343

Hill BT, Deuchars K, Hosking LK, Ling V and Whelan RDH (1990): Overexpression of P-glycoprotein in mammalian tumor cell lines after fractionated X-irradiation in vitro. *J Natl Cancer Inst* 82:607-612

Hill BT, Shaw HJ, Dalley VM and Price LA (1984): 24-Hour combination chemotherapy without cisplatin in patients with recurrent or metastatic head and neck cancer. *Am J Clin Oncol* 7:335-340

Hill BT, Whelan RDH, Hosking LK, Shellard SA, Bedford P and Lock RB (1988) Interactions between antitumor drugs and radiation in mammalian tumor cell lines: Differential drug responses and mechanisms of resistance following fractionated X-irradiation or continuous drug exposure in vitro. *NCI Mongr* 6:177-181

Hill BT, Whelan RDH, Hurst HC and McClean S (1994a): Identification of a distinctive P-glycoprotein-mediated resistance phenotype in human ovarian carcinoma cells following their in vitro exposure to fractionated X-irradiation. *Cancer* 73:2990-2999

Hill BT, Whelan RDH, Shellard SA, McClean S and Hosking LK (1994b): Differential cytotoxic effects of docetaxel in a range of mammalian tumor cell lines and certain drug resistant sublines in vitro. *Invest New Drugs* in press

Holzmayer TA, Hilsenbeck S, Von Hoff DD and Roninson IB (1992): Clinical correlates of MDR1 (P-glycoprotein) gene expression in ovarian and small-cell lung carcinomas. *J Natl Cancer Inst* 84:1486-1491

Hosking LK, Whelan RDH, Shellard SA, Davies SL, Hickson ID, Danks MK and Hill BT (1994): Multiple mechanisms of resistance in a series of human testicular teratoma cell lines selected for increasing resistance to etoposide. *Int J Cancer* 57:259-267

Ling V and Thompson LH (1974): Reduced permeability in CHO cells as a mechanisms of resistance to colchicine. *J Cell Physiol* 83:103-116

Lock RB and Hill BT (1988): Differential patterns of anti-tumor drug responses and mechanisms of resistance in a series of independently-derived VP-16-resistant human tumor cell lines. *Int J Cancer* 42:373-381

Maltzman W and Czyzyk L (1984): UV irradiation stimulates levels of p53 tumor antigen in nontransformed mouse cells. *Mol Cell Biol* 4:1689-1694

Mattern J, Efferth T and Volm M (1991): Overexpression of p-glycoprotein in human lung carcinoma xenografts after fractionated irradiation in vivo. *Radiat Res* 127:335-338

McClean S and Hill BT (1992): An overview of membrane, cytosolic and nuclear proteins associated with the expression of resistance to multiple drugs in vitro. *Biochim Biophys Acta* 1114:107 -127.

McClean S and Hill BT (1993): Evidence of post-translational regulation of P-glycoprotein associated with the expression of a distinctive multiple drug resistance phenotype in Chinese hamster ovary cells. *Eur J Cancer* 29A:2243-2248

McClean S and Hill BT (1994): Modified multiple drug resistance phenotype of Chinese hamster ovary cells selected with X-rays and vincristine versus X-rays only. *Br J Cancer* 69:711-716

McClean S, Hosking LK and Hill BT (1992): Dominant expression of multiple drug resistance after in vitro X-irradiation exposure of intraspecific Chinese hamster ovary hybrids. *J Natl Cancer Inst* 85:48-53

McClean S, Whelan RDH, Hosking LK, Hodges GM, Thompson FH, Meyers MB, Schuurhuis GJ and Hill BT (1993a): Characterisation of the P-glycoprotein overexpressing drug resistance phenotype exhibited by Chinese hamster ovary cells following their in vitro exposure to fractionated X-irradiation. *Biochim Biophys Acta* 1177:117-126

McClean S, Hosking LK and Hill BT (1993b): Expression of P-glycoprotein-mediated drug resistance following exposure of Chinese hamster ovary cells to a single X-ray dose of 30Gy. *Int J Radiat Biol* 63:765-773

Riordan JR, Deuchars K, Kartner N, Alon N, Trent J and Ling V (1985): Amplification of P-glycoprotein genes in multi-drug resistant mamalian cell lines. *Nature* 316:817-819

Schilder RJ and Ozols RF (1992): New therapies for ovarian cancer. *Cancer Invest* 10:307-315

Shen DW, Fojo A, Chin JE, Roninson IB, Richert N, Pastan I and Gottesman MM (1986): Human multidrug resistant cell lines: increased mdr1 expression can precede gene amplification. *Science* 232:643-645

Thacker J (1992): Radiation-induced mutation in mammalian cells at low doses and low dose rates. In: *Advances in Radiation Biology*, Nygaard OF, Sinclair WK, Lett JT, eds. San Diego: Academic Press pp 77-121

Trent J, Bell D, Willard H and Ling V (1985): Chromosomal localization in normal human-cells and CHO cells of a sequence derived from P-glycoprotein (PGY1). *Cytogenet Cell Genet* 40:761-762

Whelan RDH and Hill BT (1993): Differential expression of steroid receptors, hsp27, and pS2 in a series of drug resistant human breast tumor cell lines derived following exposure to antitumor drugs or to fractionated X-irradiation. *Breast Cancer Res Treat* 26:23-39

Young RC, Knapp RC and Perez CA (1982): Cancer of the ovary. In: *Cancer Principles and Practice of Oncology*. DeVita VT Jr, Hellman S, Rosenberg SA, eds. Philadelphia: Lippincott pp 884-913

8. TAXOIDS AND MULTIDRUG RESISTANCE

Robert A. Newman and Dominic Fan

INTRODUCTION

Paclitaxel (Taxol®)

Taxol is now recognized as one of the most interesting and promising new drugs derived from natural products to enter clinical trials for the treatment of cancer in many years. Its importance to the international movement to preserve biodiversity has been profound and far-reaching, as it represents proof of the potential value of natural products, and particularly those derived from the rapidly disappearing forests of this planet (Junod 1991). Originally regarded as the tree of death, the toxic constituents of portions of the yew tree were known as long ago as the time of Julius Caesar (Kingston 1994). Tales of poison associated with the bark of the western yew tree (*Taxus brevifolia*), an evergreen tree found in the forests of the Pacific Northwest, were told for many years by native Americans but the antitumor activity of taxol present within the bark itself was discovered only recently (Suffness 1989). The small, slow-growing western yew has little commercial value and it is generally cut and burned as larger more valuable fir, spruce and pine trees are harvested.

Initially, extracts of the bark of the western yew demonstrated useful antileukemic activity against the murine P388 lymphocytic leukemia cell line. The active principle was identified in 1971 by Wani and colleagues

in the laboratory headed by Monroe Wall at Research Triangle Park
(Wani et al. 1971). Further testing revealed notable antitumor activity
against human tumor xenografts but the development of paclitaxel was
suspended for more than a decade because of the lack of convincing
evidence of its superior activity in existing experimental models and
problems in procuring and processing the compound. Preliminary data
suggested that taxol acted as a mitotic inhibitor but it was not until
studies performed by Horwitz in 1979 (Schiff et al. 1979, Schiff and
Horwitz 1980) that the unique mechanism of action of taxol was
discovered and interest in the development of taxol as a potential
anticancer drug was renewed. Impressive bundles of cytoplasmic tubules
in cells treated with taxol were noted by Schiff and Horwitz (1980) which
suggested an effect on tumor cells quite different from that produced by
either vinca alkaloids or colchicine. Their work suggested that, rather
than inhibiting the polymerization of tubulin as did the vinca alkaloids
and agents such as maytansine, taxol stabilized microtubules and actually
promoted their assembly (Schiff et al. 1979). Paclitaxel binds specifically
yet reversibly to microtubules (usually the b subunit to a single set of
high affinity binding sites). Drugs such as colchicine, which
depolymerize microtubules, eliminate paclitaxel binding, thus
corroborating that the presence of microtubules is essential in paclitaxel's
mechanism of action (Schiff et al. 1979; Parness and Horwitz 1981).

The normal balance of assembly and disassembly of microtubules, a
dynamic process under physiologic conditions, is drastically shifted
toward tubule formation in the presence of taxol, with catastrophic effects
on dividing cells. The mechanisms of cell death which result from
stabilization of microtubules are not clear, but it is now realized that
taxol-treated cells cannot form a normal mitotic spindle and thus cannot
continue with normal cell division. Instead, multiple abnormal arrays of
microtubules distributed seemingly randomly around the cytoplasm are
formed (Roberts et al. 1989), representing a unique marker of
taxane-mediated cell injury.

In 1983 the NCI began toxicological studies of paclitaxel and initiated
clinical Phase I trials. Progress of these trials was hampered by
hypersensitivity reactions, which led to the premature closure of some
Phase I studies. As these reactions were observed more commonly with
infusions of shorter duration, a decision was made to continue clinical
trials using a 24-h continuous infusion of paclitaxel with premedication
to lessen the reactions (Weiss et al. 1990, Pazdur et al. 1994). The
decision proved to be fortuitous as excellent activity of paclitaxel against

breast and ovarian cancer has since been observed in numerous clinical cancer centers.

Docetaxel (Taxotere®)

Initial environmental problems with the supply and development of taxol prompted investigators at Rhône-Poulenc Rorer in conjunction with the French Centre National des Recherches Scientifiques to explore alternate taxoid-like compounds. They discovered that taxotere, a compound structurally related to taxol, possessed interesting cytotoxicity and that it could be prepared from 10-deacetyl baccatin III, a noncytotoxic precursor extracted from the needles of the European yew, Taxus baccata L. That precursor is then condensed by esterification with the additional side chain prepared by chemical synthesis (Denis et al. 1988; Mangatal et al. 1989; Colin et al. 1990). This efficient semisynthetic process using a renewable drug source led to extensive preclinical testing. Docetaxel was very active against colon adenocarcinoma models and in the B16 melanoma model caused a total log cell kill 2.7 times greater than that of paclitaxel at equitoxic doses (Bissery et al. 1991). Phase I clinical trials of docetaxel were initiated in 1991 and broad phase II testing was begun in 1992.

Like paclitaxel, docetaxel is a potent inhibitor of cell replication and promotes *in vitro* over-stabilization of microtubules in the absence of GTP (Barasoain et al., 1991; Ringel and Horwitz 1991). Docetaxel has been observed to be more active as a promoter of *in vitro* assembly of stable microtubules in the absence of GTP and as an inhibitor of microtubule depolymerization. Docetaxel is approximately twice as potent as paclitaxel (Gueritte-Voegelein et al. 1991). In addition to having a greater efficacy on tubulin assembly, docetaxel may differ from paclitaxel in its ability to alter certain classes of microtubules, especially Tau-dependent microtubules. Tubulin polymers produced by either the tubulin promoter Tau or by MAP2 disassemble at different rates and efficiencies in the presence of paclitaxel as compared to docetaxel. This finding suggests that the tubulin polymers generated by paclitaxel differ structurally from those generated by docetaxel (Fromes et al. 1992).

Other observed differences in the mechanism(s) of action of docetaxel and. paclitaxel include the fact that paclitaxel alters the number of protofilaments in microtubules but docetaxel does not (Peyrot and Briand 1992). Furthermore, Barasoain et al. (1991) compared docetaxel's ability to promote polymerization of pure tubulin with that of paclitaxel and found that docetaxel induces the polymerization of tubulin in conditions in which paclitaxel cannot. The tubulin critical concentrations of GTP for tubulin polymerization are 0.05 mg/ml and 0.1 mg/ml in the presence of docetaxel and paclitaxel, respectively (Barasoain et al. 1991). This difference in the relative ability to stabilize microtubules may reflect the difference in relative cytotoxicity between these two taxane compounds.

New Taxanes

Both taxol and taxotere can now be synthesized in a semi-synthetic manner from 10-deacetylbaccatin III (10-DAB-III), a taxane found in yew needles. The world's largest supplier of 10-DAB III is Indena, a natural products company in Milan, Italy. Investigators at this company recently discovered 14-hydroxy-10-deacetylbaccatin III, a baccatin compound with an additional hydroxyl group. Because of the additional hydroxyl group, the 14-hydroxy compound has higher water solubility than does 10-DAB III. Analogs derived from the new taxane also have higher water solubility than either paclitaxel or docetaxel, which may make them easier to formulate and administer to humans. One of the most promising 14-hydroxy derived taxane compounds is USBOJ-Tax-1101, which has been shown to be more than three times as active against a human small cell lung cancer cell line, and more than twice as active against a human colon cancer cell line (Borman 1993). The 1101 analog also shows stronger antitumor activity than does taxol against human ovarian and breast cancer cell lines, including those resistant to doxorubicin (Borman 1993).

TAXANE STRUCTURE-ACTIVITY RELATIONSHIPS

The structure activity relationships of taxanes has been well documented (Kingston 1991; Kingston 1993). These studies have provided a still-incomplete but, nevertheless, substantial body of information on structure-activity relationships (Kingston 1994) which is summarized in Figure 1.

Figure 1. Structure-activity relationships of taxol.
(Reprinted from Kingston 1994 with permission)

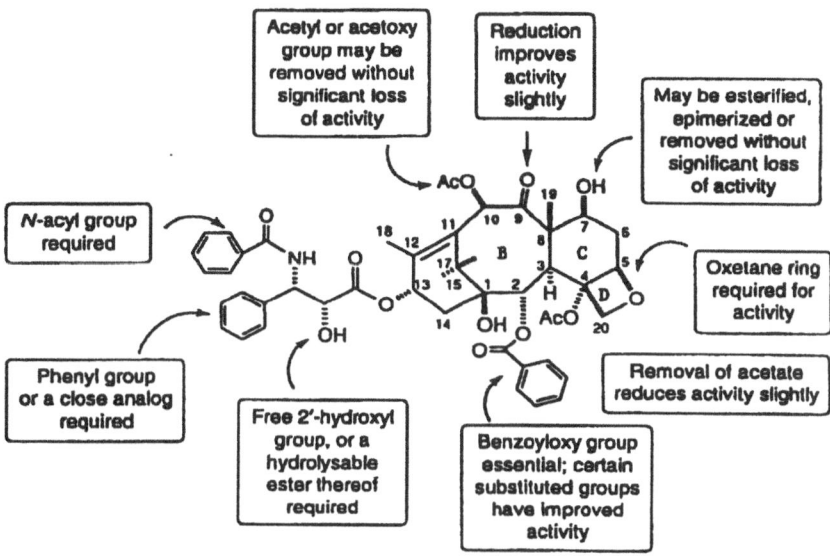

The Diterpenoid Ring System

Taxol can be converted to a rearranged product with a contracted A-ring
(Samaranayake et al. 1991). This A-nor-taxol has a tubulin-assembly
activity that is only three times less than that of taxol although its
cytotoxicity is reduced by orders of magnitude.

The Side Chain

The *N*-benzoyl-b-phenylisoserine side chain of taxol can be cleaved
selectively by various methods to yield baccatin III as the diterpenoid
component. Baccatin III can also be obtained from various Taxus species
such as *T. baccata* (Della Casa de Marcano et al. 1975) and *T.
wallichiana* (Miller et al. 1981), and its analog 10-deacetylbaccatin III
can be obtained in an excellent yield of 0.1% from *T. baccata* needles
(Denis et al. 1988).

Table 1. Characteristics of Selected Resistant Cell Lines With Altered Sensitivity to Taxoids

Cell lines	Selecting drugs	Resistant rate*	P-gp mdr-1	I.C. drug	Altered tubulin	Resistance feature	Resistance reversed by	References
P-gp MDR type								
C1300	Homoharringtonine	214	↑	↓	-		Cremophor EL	Chervinsky et. al. 1993
DXR-10	Fractionated x-ray	3.4	↑		-		-	McClean et. al. 1993
CHO/VCR	Vincristine	2-16	-	↓	no		Verapamil	Brewer et al. 1987
CHO (CH^{R}C5)	Colchicine	54	↑	↓	no		SDZ PSC833, Verapamil	Jachez et. al. 1993
CHO/VinR	Vinblastine	4	-	↓	no			Gupta 1985
P388-DoxR	Doxorubicin	101	↑	↓	no		SDZ PSC833, Verapamil	Jachez et al. 1993, Johnson et al. 1978
P388/DOX	Doxorubicin	187	↑	↓	no	Altered top II activity	-	Riou et al. 1992
J7/TAX-50	Taxol	800	135-kd P-gp	↓	no		-	Horwitz et al. 1986, Roy & Horwitz 1985
HeLa-PurR-27	Puromycin	12.5	-	↓	-		Verapamil	Gupta et al. 1988
DC-3F/9-OH-Ellipticin	9-hydroxy-ellipticine	-	↑	-	-	Overexpress *myc*	-	DeLaporte et al. 1991
K562	Taxol	-	-	-	-	Polyploidy	Verapamil, Nifedipine	Roberts et al. 1990
Caco-2	-	-	↑	-	-			Hunter et al. 1993
Altered Microtubule Function								
H69/VDS,	Vindesine,	11.6	-	-	Yes	Altered acetylation of tubules (H69/Txl)	Verapamil	Ohta et al. 1993,
H69/Txl	Taxol	4.7	-	-	Yes			Ohta et al. 1994
CHO/Tax	Taxol	-	-	-	Yes	Hypersensitive to vincristine	-	Minotti et al. 1991
CHO	Maytansine	2	↑	-	Yes	Hypersensitive to taxol	-	Schibler & Cabral 1985
CHO-Pod^{R1}	Podophyllo-toxin	5	-	-	Yes		-	Gupta 1983

Baccatin III is significantly less active than taxol in both cytotoxicity assays (Wani et al. 1971) and tubulin-assembly assays (Lataste et al. 1984) indicating the importance of the side chain for its activity. Importantly, baccatin III can be converted back to taxol through a variety of methods (Kingston 1994) which have made it possible to elucidate more detailed structure-activity relationships of the side chain portion.

Analogs in which the side chain N-benzoyl group is replaced with other acyl groups have also been prepared. One such analog is docetaxel (Taxotere®). Taxotere has an N-t-butoxycarbonyl group in place of the N-benzoyl group of taxol, and also lacks the 10-acetate group (Gueritte-Voegelein et al. 1991); it is about five times as active as taxol against taxol resistant cells (Ringel and Horwitz 1991). Other modifications at the N-benzoyl position have, however, yielded analogs with diminished activity compared to taxol (Kingston 1994). Therefore, it appears that the activity of taxol and related compounds is highly dependent on side chain substitutions but less so on those examined thus far on the taxane ring system itself.

IN VITRO STUDIES OF TAXANE-MEDIATED CYTOTOXICITY AND RESISTANCE MECHANISMS

MDR-Mediated Mechanisms of Resistance

One mechanism of acquired resistance (to paclitaxel and docetaxel) is characterized by the multidrug resistance (MDR) phenotype related to overproduction of a specific membrane protein. This membrane glycoprotein, which migrates on SDS electrophoretic gels with an apparent molecular weight of 170 kD and is thus known as p-170, acts as an energy-dependent drug efflux pump to maintain intracellular drug concentrations below cytotoxic levels (Gupta 1983; Horwitz et al. 1986). Many cell lines have now been reported which exhibit the MDR phenotype and which contain p-170. Of these, quite a few have been shown to be resistant to paclitaxel irregardless of the particular MDR-related compound against which the resistance was originally developed (see Table 1). One especially resistant cell line J774.2/Taxol (800-fold resistance to taxol), reported by Horwitz et al. (1986) was observed to be cross-resistant to vinca alkaloids and doxorubicin. The use of radiolabelled taxol made it clear that the resistant cells accumulated approximately 10% of the drug found in the sensitive cells (Table 1). This inability to accumulate taxol appears to be an important determinant in understanding the resistant phenotype (Horwitz et al. 1993).

Resistance due to Altered Tubulin Structure/Function

Another reported mechanism of cellular resistance to taxane compounds appears to involve the formation of abnormal tubulin. Cabral et al. (1983, 1986) has reported, for example, that certain Chinese hamster ovary cell lines with acquired taxol resistance possess altered alpha- or beta-tubulin and actually require taxol in their medium for normal growth (Table 1). These resistant cell lines lack normal microtubules in their interpolar mitotic spindles when grown in the absence of taxol resulting in impaired microtubule assembly. Continuous exposure to taxol is required for polymerization to occur normally, thereby promoting the formation of functional microtubules. Interestingly, the taxol-dependent cell lines exhibit an enhanced sensitivity to vinca alkaloids (Cabral et al. 1983). Conversely, at least one cell line whose resistance was raised against continuous exposure to maytansine exhibits a hypersensitivity to taxol (Schibler and Cabral 1985). These findings suggest that certain tumors in humans which become resistant clinically to vinca alkaloid therapy may remain responsive to taxane compounds and, alternatively, those tumors which fail to continue to respond to paclitaxel and docetaxel may develop an enhanced sensitivity to vinca alkaloids and other compounds which act to interfere with microtubule formation. Further clinical testing with both taxane compounds and vinca alkaloids, of course, will have to be done to determine whether the mechanisms of resistance to these compounds observed *in vitro* are similar to those in human tumors.

Reversal of Resistance to Taxoids

Those compounds (e.g. verapamil, SDZ PSC833) that have been shown to be capable of reversing the MDR phenotype in cells in culture, have also been shown to be useful in reverting cell resistance to taxane compounds (see Table 1). To date, however, there has been no direct clinical trial of any of the MDR-reversing agents against specific taxol or taxotere-mediated resistance in humans and, hence, the ultimate utility of these compounds awaits further clinical studies.

Whether specific tubulin defects such as those reported by Cabral et al. (1983) within tumor cells occur within humans being treated with taxanes remains unclear. If they do, it is also unclear how the resistance might be overcome. One suggestion, referred to above, is that taxane-resistant tumors may develop a hypersensitivity to microtubule destabilizing drugs such as vinca alkaloids. Another interesting suggestion has recently been made by Ohta et al. (1994) who have shown that the relative degree of cellular resistance to paclitaxel may depend on the extent of microtubule acetylation. These investigators have shown that their taxol-resistant human small cell lung cancer cell line contained alpha tubulin with an increased extent of acetylation. They have suggested that the extent of alpha tubulin acetylation may directly influence the ability of agents such as paclitaxel to bind to it. If this is true then it may be possible to reduce the extent of tubulin acetylation to revert taxane resistance. Further experimentation on this concept is certainly called for.

IN VIVO STUDIES OF TAXANES

The *in vivo* efficacy of taxol against several transplantable murine leukemias was initially demonstrated by the Division of Cancer Treatment at the National Cancer Institute (Wall and Wani 1967; Wani et al. 1971; Douros and Suffness 1981). Taxol is the first compound of this type to have antineoplastic activity against B16 melanoma, L1210 and P388 leukemia, human MX-1 mammary tumor, CX-1 colon and LX-1 lung tumor xenografts, as well as several primary human tumors of breast, endometrium, ovary, brain, and lung transplanted into athymic nude mice (Douros and Suffness 1978; Fucha and Johnson 1978; Riondel et al. 1986). Superior *in vivo* efficacy of the semisynthetic analog taxotere was documented nearly 2 decades later (Lavelle et al. 1989). Subsequent studies showed marked *in vivo* antitumor activity of taxotere against several experimental murine tumor models, including the B16 melanoma, colon adenocarcinomas C38 and 51/A, pancreatic ductal adenocarcinoma 03 (Bissery et al. 1991), M 109 lung cancer implanted subcutaneously (Fujimoto 1994), and several human xenografts implanted in nude mice (Lavelle et al. 1993). Although taxotere is generally more active than taxol tested in animal models, significant antitumor activity of taxol has been recently demonstrated on two human ovarian carcinoma xenografts (HOC8 and HOC22) transplanted intraperitoneally in nude mice (Nicoletti et al. 1993). Because of their excellent preclinical antitumor activity and their unique mechanism of action, both taxane compounds have entered extensive clinical trials.

CLINICAL STUDIES OF TAXANES

Results of early phase I and phase II clinical trials were discouraging because of the unacceptable levels of toxicities such as hypersensitivity reactions, myelosupression, neurotoxicity, and cardiac toxicity are dose-limiting (Kris et al. 1986; Legha et al. 1986; Wiernik et al. 1987; Rowinsky et al. 1989; Weiss et al. 1990). To better manage clinical toxicities, subsequent clinical studies (Table 2) employ pretreatment of patients with dexamethasone (anti-inflammatory glucocorticoid), diphenhydramine (antihistaminic), famotidine (histamine H2 receptor antagonist), or cimetidine (histamine H2 receptor antagonist) for prophylaxis of hypersensitivity reactions, and controlled administration of granulocyte-colony stimulating factor (G-CSF) for amelioration of myelosuppression (Sarosy et al. 1992). The amounts of clinical efforts have been tremendous and met with encouraging outcome (Table 2). The commonly reported clinical toxicities from these selected studies include hypersensitivity reactions, granulocytopenia, neutropenia, leukopenia, neurotoxicity, mucositis, and alopecia, Significant clinical responses have been seen with refractory cancers of the breast and ovarian treated with taxol or taxotere, and with moderate responses noted also in patients with malignant melanoma and advanced non-small-cell-lung cancer. Unfortunately, the efficacy of taxane compounds for the treatment of renal cell carcinomas and prostate cancer could not be derived (Table 2).

PERSPECTIVES

Oncologists have not had for a long time, since the development of doxorubicin, a new, effective chemotherapeutic agent. The discovery of taxol and its derivatives, their remarkable anticancer activity and the promising clinical trials have instilled hope into clinical oncology for improved management of certain cancers. Although taxol is also associated with the MDR phenotype and unlikely to be able to reverse MDR as a single agent, the unique action of mechanism of taxanes against cellular microtubules and tubulin pools may be used to target a specific compartment of cancer metastases. The vigorous efforts being placed in current clinical trials and chemical modification research may derive workable protocols and critical pharmaceutical information for the effective utilisation of taxoids in the near future.

Table 2. Selected Clinical Trials of Taxol and Taxotere

Cancer	Protocol	Dose	Route	Schedule	Toxicity	CR+PR/Eval.	Center (Reference)
Breast ca.	taxol	250 mg/m²	iv-inf	24h q 3wk	granulocytopenia	14/25	M. D. Anderson Ca. Ctr. (Holmes et al. 1991)
Breast ca.	taxol G-CSF	250 mg/m² 5 μg/kg/d	iv-inf sc	24h q 3wk d3-d10	alopecia	16/26	Mem. Sloan-kettering (Reichman et al. 1993)
Melanoma	taxol	250 mg/m²	iv-inf	24h q 3wk	hypersensitivity neutropenia	4/28	Albert Einstein Ca. Ctr. (Einzig et al. 1991b)
Mixed solid	taxol cis-p	110-200 mg/m² 50/75 mg/m²	iv-inf iv-inf	24h q 3wk 1 mg/min	neutropenia neurotoxicity	10/44	Johns Hopkins Oncol. Ctr. (Rowinsky et al. 1991)
Mixed solid	taxol	225 mg/m²	iv-inf	6h q 3wk	myelotoxicity	4/31	UTHSC-San Antonio (Brown et al. 1991)
Mixed solid	taxol	5-36 mg/m²	iv-inf	120h q 3wk	leukopenia	1/20	Dana Farber Ca. Inst. (Spriggs and Tondini 1992)
Mixed solid	taxotere	1-14 mg/m²	iv-inf	1hx5d q3wk	granulocytopenia	7/39	M. D. Anderson Ca. Ctr. (Pazdur et al. 1992)
Mixed solid	taxotere	10-90 mg/m²	iv-inf	24h q 3wk	neutropenia mucositis	0/30	Beatson Oncol. Ctr. Scotland (Bissett et al. 1993)
Mixed solid	taxol cis-p G-CSF	135-250 mg/m² 75 mg/m² 5 μg/kg/d	iv-inf iv-inf sc	24h q 3wk	neuropathy	9/24	Johns Hopkins Oncol. Ctr. (Rowinsky et al. 1993)
Mixed solid (pediatric)	taxol	200-420 mg/m²	iv-inf	24h q 3wk	myelotoxicity neurotoxicity	3/31	St. Jude Child. Res. Hosp. (Hurwitz et al. 1993)
Mixed solid	taxotere	100-115 mg/m²	iv-inf	2/6h q 3wk	neutropenia	5/58	UTHSC-San Antonio (Burris et al. 1993)
Mixed solid	taxotere	5-115 mg/m²	iv-inf	1-2h q 2-3wk	neutropenia	4/65	Hopital Saint-Louis, France (Extra et al. 1993)
Mixed solid	taxol G-CSF	250-300 mg/m² 5 μg/kg/d	iv-inf sc	3h q 3wk 9-14d	myelotoxicity neuropathy	4/35	U. Wisconsin Comp. Ca. Ctr. (Schiller et al. 1994)

Table 2. Selected Clinical Trials of Taxol and Taxotere. (continued)

Cancer	Protocol	Dose	Route	Schedule	Toxicity	CR+PR/Eval.	Center (Reference)
NSCLC	taxol	250 mg/m^2	iv-inf	24h q 3wk	leukopenia	5/24	U. Rochester Ca. Ctr. (Chang et al. 1993)
NSCLC	taxol	200 mg/m^2	iv-inf	24h q 3wk	granulocytopenia	6/25	M. D. Anderson Ca. Ctr. (Murphy et al. 1993)
Ovarian ca.	taxol	180-250 mg/m^2	iv-inf	24h q 3wk	myelotoxicity	6/30	Albert Einstein Ca. Ctr. (Einzig et al. 1992)
Ovarian ca.	taxol	25-175 mg/m^2	IP	q 3-4wk	abdominal pain leukopenia	6/24	Mem. Sloan-kettering (Markman et al. 1992)
Ovarian ca.	taxol G-CSF	170-300 mg/m^2 10 µg/kg/d	iv-inf sc	8h q 3wk	neuropathy	5/14	NCI-NIH, Bethesda (Sarosy et al. 1992)
Ovarian ca.	taxol	250 mg/m^2	iv-inf	24h q 3wk	leukopenia	21/43	FDA, Rockville (Jamis et al. 1993)
Ovarian ca.	taxol	135 mg/m^2	iv-inf	24h q 3wk	leukopenia	220/1000	NCI-NIH, Rockville (Trimble et al. 1993)
Ovarian ca.	taxol G-CSF	135 mg/m^2 5 µg/kg/d	iv-inf sc	24h q 3wk thru d-18	neutropenia	6/22	Roswell Mem. Park Ca. Inst. (Baker et al. 1993)
Ovarian ca.	taxol	135/175 mg/m^2	iv-inf	3h q 3wk 24h q 3wk	neutropenia	53/286	Netherlands Ca. Inst. (ten-Bokkel-Huinink et al. 1993)
Ovarian ca.	taxol	135-175 mg/m^2	iv-inf	3h & 24h	leukopenia	6/38	Beilinson Med. Ctr., Israel (Sulkes et al. 1994)
Ovarian ca.	taxol C-CSF	250 mg/m^2 10 µg/kg/d	iv-inf sc	24h q 3wk	neuropathy	21/44	NCI-NIH, Bethesda (Kohn et al. 1994)
Prostate ca.	taxol	135-170 mg/m^2	iv-inf	24h q 3wk	leukopenia	1/23	Indiana U. Ned. Ctr. (Roth et al. 1993)
Renal ca.	taxol	250 mg/m^2	iv-inf	24h q 3wk	neutropenia	0/18	Albert Einstein Ca. Ctr. (Einzig et al. 1991a)
Renal ca.	taxotere	100 mg/m^2	iv-inf	1 hr q3wk	neutropenia hypersensitivity	0/18	London Regional Ca. Ctr. (Mertens et al. 1994)

REFERENCES

Baker TR, Piver MS, Hempling RE (1993): Response to Taxol chemotherapy in resistant ovarian carcinoma. *Eur J Gynaecol Oncol* 14:449-454

Barasoain I, De Ines C, Diaz F, Andreu JM, Peyrot V, Leynadier D, Garcia P, Briand C, De Sousa G, Rahmani R (1991): Interaction of tubulin and cellular microtubules with Taxotere (RP 56976), a new semisynthetic analog of taxol. *Proc Amer Assoc Cancer Res* 32:329

Bissery MC, Guenard D, Gueritte VF, Lavelle F (1991): Experimental antitumor activity of taxotere (RP 56976, NSC 628503), a taxol analogue. *Cancer Res* 51:4845-4852

Bissett D, Setanoians A, Cassidy J, Graham MA, Chadwick GA, Wilson P, Auzannet V, Le BN, Kaye SB, Kerr DJ (1993): Phase I and pharmacokinetic study of taxotere (RP 56976) administered as a 24-hour infusion. *Cancer Res* 53:523-527

Borman S (1993): New family of taxol, taxotere analogs developed. *Chemistry and Engineering News* (magazine) pp 36-37

Brewer F, Warr JR (1987): Verapamil reversal of vincristine resistance and cross-resistance patterns of vincristine-resistant chinese hamster ovary cells. *Cancer Treat Rep* 71:353-359

Brown T, Havlin K, Weiss G, Cagnola J, Koeller J, Kuhn J, Rizzo J, Craig J, Phillips J, Von HD (1991): A phase I trial of taxol given by a 6-hour intravenous infusion. *J Clin Oncol* 9:1261-1267

Burris H, Irvin R, Kuhn J, Kalter S, Smith L, Shaffer D, Fields S, Weiss G, Eckardt J, Rodriguez G, et al (1993): Phase I clinical trial of taxotere administered as either a 2-hour or 6-hour intravenous infusion. *J Clin Oncol* 11:950-958

Cabral F, Wible L, Brenner S, Brinkley BR (1983): Taxol-requiring mutant of Chinese hamster ovary cells with impaired mitotic spindle assembly. *J Cell Biol* 97: 30-39

Cabral F, Brady RC, Schibler MJ (1986): A mechanism of cellular resistance to drugs that interfere with microtubule assembly. *Ann NY Acad Sci* 466: 745-756

Chang AY, Kim K, Glick J, Anderson T, Karp D, Johnson D (1993): Phase II study of taxol, merbarone, and piroxantrone in stage IV non-small-cell lung cancer: The Eastern Cooperative Oncology Group Results 'see comments:. *J Natl Cancer Inst* 85:388-394

Chervinsky D, Brecher ML, Hoelcle MJ (1993): Cremophor-EL enhances taxol efficacy in a multidrug resistant C1300 neuroblastoma cell line. *Anticancer Res* 13:93-96

Colin M, Guenard D, Gueritte-Voegelein F (1990): Process for preparing derivatives of baccatin III and of 10-deacetyl baccatin III. *U.S. Patent* 4924012, granted May 8, 1990

DeLaporte C, Larsen AK, Dautry F, Jacquemin-Sablon A (1991): Influence of *myc* overexpression on the phenotype properties of chinese hamster lung cells resistant to antitumor agents. *Exp Cell Res* 197:176-182

Della Casa de Marcano DP, Halsall TG (1975): Structures of some taxane diterpenoids, baccatins-III, -IV, -VI, and -VII and 1-dehydroxybaccatin-IV, possessing an oxetan ring. *J Chem Soc Chem Commun* 15:365-366

Denis JN, Greene AE, Guenard D, Gueritte-Voegelein F, Mangatal L, Potier P (1988): A highly efficient, practical approach to natural taxol. *J Am Chem Soc* 110:5917-5919

Douros J, Suffness M (1978): New natural products of interest under development at the National Cancer Institute. *Cancer Chemother Pharmacol* 1:91-100

Douros J, Suffness M (1981): New natural products under development at the National Cancer Institute. *Recent Results Cancer Res* 76:153-175

Einzig AI, Gorowski E, Sasloff J, Wiernik PH (1991a): Phase II trial of taxol in patients with metastatic renal cell carcinoma. *Cancer Invest* 9:133-136

Einzig AI, Hochster H, Wiernik PH, Trump DL, Dutcher JP, Garowski E, Sasloff J, Smith TJ (1991b): A phase II study of taxol in patients with malignant melanoma. *Invest New Drugs* 9:59-64

Einzig AI, Wiernik PH, Sasloff J, Runowicz CD, Goldberg GL (1992): Phase II study and long-term follow-up of patients treated with taxol for advanced ovarian adenocarcinoma. *J Clin Oncol* 10:1748-1753

Extra JM, Rousseau F, Bruno R, Clavel M, Le BN, Marty M (1993): Phase I and pharmacokinetic study of Taxotere (RP 56976; NSC 628503) given as a short intravenous infusion. *Cancer Res* 53:1037-1042

Fromes Y, Gounon P, Bissery MC, Fellous A (1992): Differential effects of taxol or taxotere on Tau and MAP2 containing microtubules. *Proc Amer Assoc Cancer Res* 33:551

Fucha DA, Johnson RK (1978): Cytologic evidence that taxol, an antineoplastic agent from Taxus brevifolia, acts as a mitotic spindle poison. *Cancer Treat Rep* 62:1219-1222

Fujimoto S (1994): Schedule dependency of i.v.-paclitaxel against SC-M 109 mouse lung cancer. *Gan To Kagaku Ryoho* 21:671-677

Gupta RS (1983): Taxol resistant mutants of Chinese hamster ovary cells: genetic biochemical, and cross-resistant studies. *J Cell Physiol* 114:137-144

Gupta RS (1985): Cross-resistance of vinblastine and taxol-resistant mutants of chinese hamster ovary cells to other anticancer agents. *Cancer Treat Rep* 69:515-521

Gupta RS, Murray W, Gupta R (1988): Cross resistance patterns toward anticancer drugs of a human carcinoma multidrug-resistant cell line. *Br J Cancer* 58:441-447

Gueritte-Voegelein F, Guenard D, Lavelle F, Le Goff MT, Mangatal L, Potier P (1991): Relationships between the structure of taxol analogues and their antimitotic activity. *J Med Chem* 34:992-998

Holmes FA, Walters RS, Theriault RL, Forman AD, Newton LK, Raber MN, Buzdar AU, Frye DK, Hortobagyi GN (1991): Phase II trial of taxol, an active drug in the treatment of metastatic breast cancer. *J Natl Cancer Inst* 83:1797-1805

Horwitz SB, Lothstein L, Manfredi JJ, Mellado W, Parness J, Roy SN, Schiff PB, Sorbara L, Zehab R (1986): Taxol: mechanisms of action and resistance. *Ann N Y Acad Sci* 466:733-744

Horwitz SB, Cohen D, Rao S, Ringel I, Shen H-J, Yang C-P (1993): Taxol: mechanisms of action and resistance. *J Natl Cancer Inst Monographs* 15: 55-61

Hunter J, Jepson MA, Tsuruo T, Simmons NL, Hirst BH (1993): Functional expression of P-glycoprotein in apical membranes of human intestinal Caco-2 cells. *J Biol Chem* 268:14991-14997

Hurwitz CA, Relling MV, Weitman SD, Ravindranath Y, Vietti TJ, Strother DR, Ragab AH, Pratt CB (1993): Phase I trial of paclitaxel in children with refractory solid tumors: a Pediatric Oncology Group Study. *J Clin Oncol* 11:2324-2329

Jachez B, Nordmann R, Loor F (1993): Restoration of taxol sensitivity of multidrug-resistant cells by the cyclosporine SDZ PSC833 and the cyclopeptide SDZ 280-466. *J Natl Cancer Inst* 85:478-483

Jamis DCA, Klecker RW, Sarosy G, Reed E, Collins JM (1993): Steady-state plasma concentrations and effects of taxol for a 250 mg/m2 dose in combination with granulocyte-colony stimulating factor in patients with ovarian cancer. *Cancer Chemother Pharmacol* 33:48-52

Johnson RK, Chitnis MP, Embrey WM, Gregory EB (1978): In vivo characteristics of resistance and cross-resistance of an adriamycin-resistant subline of P388 leukemia. *Cancer Treat Rep* 62:1535-1547

Junod T (1991): Tree of hope. *Life* (magazine) 15:71-76

Kingston DGI (1991): The chemistry of taxol. *Pharm Ther* 52:1-34

Kingston DGI, Molinero AA, Rimoldi JM (1993): In: *Progress in the Chemistry of Organic Natural Products,* (eds. W Herz, GW Kirby, RE Moore, W Steglich, C Tamm, vol. 6, pp. 1-206, Springer-Verlag

Kingston DGI (1994): Taxol: the chemistry and structure-activity relationships of a novel anticancer agent. *Trends in Biotechnology* 12:222-227

Kohn EC, Sarosy G, Bicher A, Link C, Christian M, Steinberg SM, Rothenberg M, Adamo DO, Davis P, Ognibene FP, et al (1994): Dose-intense taxol: high response rate in patients with platinum-resistant recurrent ovarian cancer. *J Natl Cancer Inst* 86:18-24

Kris MG, O'Connell JP, Gralla RJ, Wertheim MS, Parente RM, Schiff PB, Young CW (1986): Phase I trial of taxol given as a 3-hour infusion every 21 days. *Cancer Treat Rep* 70:605-607

Lataste H, Senilh V, Wright M, Guenard D, Potier P (1984): Relationships between the structure of taxol and baccatine III derivatives and their in vitro action on the disassembly of mammalian brain and Physarum amoebal microtubules. *Proc Natl Acad Sci USA* 81:4090-4094

Lavelle F, Fizames C, Gueritte-Voegelein F, Guénard D, Potier P (1989): Experimental properties of RP 56976, a taxol derivative. *Proc Amer Assoc Cancer Res* 30:2254

Lavelle F, Gueritte VF, Guenard D (1993): Taxotere: from yew's needles to clinical practice:. *Bull Cancer (Paris)* 80:326-338

Legha SS, Tenney DM, Krakoff IR (1986): Phase I study of taxol using a 5-day intermittent schedule. *J Clin Oncol* 4:762-766

Mangatal L, Adeline MT, Gueenard D, Gueritte-Voegelein F, Potier P (1989): Application of the vicinal oxyamination reaction with asymmetric induction to teh hemisynthesis of taxol and analogues. *Tetrahedron* 45:4177-4190

Markman M, Rowinsky E, Hakes T, Reichman B, Jones W, Lewis JLJ, Rubin S, Curtin J, Barakat R, Phillips M, et al (1992): Phase I trial of intraperitoneal taxol: a Gynecoloic Oncology Group study. *J Clin Oncol* 10:1485-1491

McClean S, Whelan RDH, Hosking LK, Hodges GM, Thompson FH, Meyers MB, Schuurhuis GJ, Hill BT (1993): Characterization of the P-glycoprotein over-expressing drug resistance phenotype exhibited by Chinese hamster ovary cells following their in vitro exposure to fractionated x-irradiation. *Biochim Biophys Acta* 1177:117-126

Mertens WC, Eisenhauer EA, Jolivet J, Ernst S, Moore M, Muldal A (1994): Docetaxel in advanced renal carcinoma. A phase II trial of the National Cancer Institute of Canada Clinical Trials Group. *Ann Oncol* 5:185-187

Miller RW, Powell RG, Smith CR Jr, Arnold E, Clardy J (1981): Antileukemic alkaloids from Taxus wallichiana Zucc. *J Org Chem* 46:1469-1474

Minotti AM, Barlow SB, Cabral F (1991): Resistance to antimitotic drugs in Chinese hamster ovary cells correlates with changes in the level of polymerized tubulin. *J Biol Chem* 266:3987-3994

Murphy WK, Fossella FV, Winn RJ, Shin DM, Hynes HE, Gross HM, Davilla E, Leimert J, Dhingra H, Raber MN, et al (1993): Phase II study of taxol in patients with untreated advanced non-small-cell lung cancer. *J Natl Cancer Inst* 85:384-388

Nicoletti MI, Lucchini V, Massazza G, Abbott BJ, DIncalci M, Giavazzi R (1993): Antitumor activity of taxol (NSC-125973) in human ovarian carcinomas growing in the peritoneal cavity of nude mice. *Ann Oncol* 4:151-155

Ohta S, Nishio K, Kubo S, Nishio M, Ohmori T, Takahashi T, Saijo N (1993): Characterization of a vindesine-resistant human small cell lung cancer cell line. *Br J Cancer* 68:74-79

Ohta S, Nishio K, Kubota N, Ohmori T, Funayama Y, Ohira T, Nakajima H, Adachi M, Saijo N (1994): Characterization of a Taxol-resistant human small-cell lung cancer cell line. *Jpn J Cancer Res* 85:290-297

Parness J, Horwitz SB (1981): Taxol binds to polymerized tubulin in vitro. *J Cell Biol* 91:479-481

Pazdur R, Kudelka AP, Kavanagh JJ, Cohen PR, Raber MN (1993): The taxoids: paclitaxel (Taxol) and docetaxel (Taxotere). *Cancer Treat Rev* 19:351-386

Pazdur R, Newman RA, Newman BM, Fuentes A, Benvenuto J, Bready B, Moore DJ, Jaiyesimi I, Vreeland F, Bayssas MM, et al (1992): Phase I trial of Taxotere: five-day schedule. *J Natl Cancer Inst* 84:1781-1788

Peyrot V, Briand C (1992): Biophysical characterization of the assembly of purified tubulin induced by taxol and Taxotere (RP 56976). *Second Interface of Clinical and Laboratory Responses to Anticancer Drugs: Drugs and Microtubules*, Marseille, France, (Abstract S22)

Reichman BS, Seidman AD, Crown JP, Heelan R, Hakes TB, Lebwohl DE, Gilewski TA, Surbone A, Currie V, Hudis CA, et al (1993): Paclitaxel and recombinant human granulocyte colony-stimulating factor as initial chemotherapy for metastatic breast cancer. *J Clin Oncol* 11:1943-1951

Ringel I, Horwitz SB (1991): Studies with RP 56976 (Taxotere): a semisynthetic analogue of taxol. *J Natl Cancer Inst* 84:1781-1788

Riondel J, Jacrot M, Picot F, Beriel H, Mouriquand C, Potier P (1986): Therapeutic response to taxol of six human tumors xenografted into nude mice. *Cancer Chemother Pharmacol* 17:137-142

Riou J-F, Naudin A, Lavelle F (1992): Effects of Taxotere on murine and human tumor cell lines. *Biochem Biophys Res Commun* 187:164-170

Roberts JR, Allison DC, Donehower RC, Rowinsky EK (1990): Development of polyploidization in taxol-resiatnt human leukemia cells in vitro. *Cancer Res* 50:710-716

Roberts JR, Rowinsky EK, Donehower RC, Robertson J, Allison DC (1989): Demonstration of the cell cycle positions of taxol-induced 'asters' and 'bundles' by sequential measurements of tubulin immunofluoresence, DNA content, and autoradiographic labeling of taxol-sensitive and -resistant cells. *J Histochem Cytochem* 37:1659-1665

Roth BJ, Yeap BY, Wilding G, Kasimis B, McLeod D, Loehrer PJ (1993): Taxol in advanced, hormone-refractory carcinoma of the prostate. A phase II trial of the Eastern Cooperative Oncology Group. *Cancer* 72:2457-2460

Rowinsky EK, Burke PJ, Karp JE, Tucker RW, Ettinger DS, Donehower RC (1989): Phase I and pharmacodynamic study of taxol in refractory acute leukemias. *Cancer Res* 49:4640-4647

Rowinsky EK, Chaudhry V, Forastiere AA, Sartorius SE, Ettinger DS, Grochow LB, Lubejko BG, Cornblath DR, Donehower RC (1993): Phase I and pharmacologic study of paclitaxel and cisplatin with granulocyte colony-stimulating factor: neuromuscular toxicity is dose-limiting. *J Clin Oncol* 11:2010-2020

Rowinsky EK, Gilbert MR, McGuire WP, Noe DA, Grochow LB, Forastiere AA, Ettinger DS, Lubejko BG, Clark B, Sartorius SE, et al (1991): Sequences of taxol and cisplatin: a phase I and pharmacologic study. *J Clin Oncol* 9:1692-1703

Roy SN, Horwitz SB (1985): A phosphoglycoprotein associated with taxol resistance in J774.2 cells. *Cancer Res* 45:3856-3863

Sarosy G, Kohn E, Stone DA, Rothenberg M, Jacob J, Adamo DO, Ognibene FP, Cunnion RE, Reed E (1992): Phase I study of taxol and granulocyte colony-stimulating factor in patients with refractory ovarian cancer. *J Clin Oncol* 10:1165-1170

Samaranayake G, Magri NF, Jitrangsri C, Kingston DGI (1991): Modified taxols. 5. Reaction of taxol with electrophilic reagents, and preparation of a rearranged taxol derivative with tubulin assembly activity. *J Org Chem* 56:5114-5119

Schibler MJ, Cabral F (1985): Maytansine-resistant mutants of chinese hamster ovary cells with an alteration in b-tubulin. *Can J Biochem Cell Biol* 63:503-510

Schiff PB, Fant J, Horwitz SB (1979): Promotion of microtubule assembly in vitro by taxol. *Nature* 277:665-667

Schiff PB, Horwitz SB (1980): Taxol stabilizes microtubules in mouse fibroblast cells. *Proc Natl Acad Sci USA* 77:1561-1565

Schiller JH, Storer B, Tutsch K, Arzoomanian R, Alberti D, Feierabend C, Spriggs D (1994): Phase I trial of 3-hour infusion of paclitaxel with or without granulocyte colony-stimulating factor in patients with advanced cancer. *J Clin Oncol* 12:241-248

Spriggs DR, Tondini C (1992): Taxol administered as a 120 hour infusion. *Invest New Drugs* 10:275-278

Suffness M (1989): Development of antitumor natural products at the National Cancer Institute: Gann Monog. *Cancer Res* 36:21-44

Sulkes A, Beller U, Peretz T, Shacter J, Hornreich G, McDaniel C, Winograd B (1994): Taxol: initial Israeli experience with a novel anticancer agent. *Isr J Med Sci* 30:70-78

ten-Bokkel-Huinink WW, Eisenhauer E, Swenerton K (1993): Preliminary evaluation of a multicenter, randomized comparative study of TAXOL (paclitaxel) dose and infusion length in platinum-treated ovarian cancer. Canadian-European Taxol Cooperative Trial Group. *Cancer Treat Rev* 19 (Suppl C):79-86

Trimble EL, Adams JD, Vena D, Hawkins MJ, Friedman MA, Fisherman JS, Christian MC, Canetta R, Onetto N, Hayn R, et al (1993): Paclitaxel for platinum-refractory ovarian cancer: results from the first 1,000 patients registered to National Cancer Institute Treatment Referral Center 9103. *J Clin Oncol* 11:2405-2410

Wall ME, Wani C (1967): Recent progress in plant anti-tumor agents. *The 153rd American Chemical Society National Meeting,* Abstract M-006

Wani MC, Taylor HI, Wall ME, Coggon P, McPhail AT (1971): Plant antitumor agents. VI. The isolation and structure of taxol, a novel antileukemic and antitumor agent from Taxus brevifolia. *J Am Chem Soc* 93:2325-2327

Weiss RB, Donehower RC, Wiernik PH, Ohnuma T, Gralla RJ, Trump DL, Baker JRJ, Van Echo DA, Von Hoff DD, Leyland Jones B (1990): Hypersensitivity reactions from taxol. *J Clin Oncol* 8:1263-1268

Wiernik PH, Schwartz EL, Strauman JJ, Dutcher JP, Lipton RB, Paietta E (1987): Phase I clinical and pharmacokinetic study of taxol. *Cancer Res* 47:2486-2493

9. THE CONTRIBUTION OF PROTEIN KINASE C TO MULTIPLE DRUG RESISTANCE IN CANCER

Catherine A. O'Brian, Nancy E. Ward, Krishna P. Gupta, and Karen R. Gravitt

INTRODUCTION

The use of combination chemotherapy in cancer treatment to address the heterogeneous nature of tumor cell populations has long been accepted as a standard practice. The acquisition of resistance to chemotherapeutic agents by malignant tumor cell populations during cancer therapy presents a formidable barrier to efforts underway to successfully manage the disease (Gottesman and Pastan, 1993). This has been the driving force behind the search for agents that can reverse clinical drug resistance in cancer therapy. In recent years, the heterogeneous nature of drug resistance mechanisms acquired by cancer cell populations during chemotherapy and innate in certain untreated cancers has become evident (Gottesman and Pastan, 1993; Fan et al., 1994; Kellen, 1994; Beck, 1989). For example, drug resistance mechanisms in cancer cell populations have been found to involve to various extents glutathione-S-transferases (Chapter 2), the multidrug resistance-associated protein (MRP) (Chapter 5), topoisomerases (Chapters 7 and 8), the oncogene Bcl-2 (Chapter 12), the drug-efflux pump P-glycoprotein (Endicott and Ling, 1989), and protein kinase C (PKC). This suggests that a combination of agents that antagonize distinct drug resistance mechanisms may be required to reverse clinical drug resistance in cancer and improve the ultimate therapeutic outcome for the patient. Rational design of strategies for the reversal of drug resistance in clinical cancer will require an understanding of the molecular events that underlie the major drug resistance mechanisms operative in the disease.

Protein kinase C (PKC) is an isozyme family with at least ten mammalian members (Table 1) (Lester and Epand, 1992; Kuo, 1994). Largely as a result of the discovery that phorbol-ester tumor promoters are specific activators of PKC (Castagna et al., 1982), PKC was initially recognized for its critical role in cell growth and differentiation. It is now clear that PKC is also an essential component of signal-transduction pathways involved in specialized processes such as muscle contraction and neurotransmission (Nishikawa and Hidaka, 1994; Conn and Sweatt, 1994; Kikkawa et al., 1989). Consideration of PKC as a target in cancer therapy is predicated on recent observations that PKC phosphorylates and modulates the activities of several proteins that are directly responsible for drug resistance in cancer, including glutathione-S-transferase, topoisomerases, and P-glycoprotein (Table 2). This chapter focuses on the contribution of PKC to P-glycoprotein-mediated multidrug resistance (MDR) in cancer cells. Evidence that PKC regulates the drug efflux activity of P-glycoprotein will be discussed, and the potential value of drugs that target PKC as reversal agents of drug resistance in clinical cancer will considered.

Table 1. The Protein Kinase C (PKC) Isozyme Family[a]

Name of Subfamily	Activating Cofactors	Members
Common PKC (cPKC)	Ca^{2+}, PS[b], phorbol ester	α, β_1, β_2, γ
Novel PKC (nPKC)	PS, phorbol ester	δ, ε, η, Θ
Atypical PKC(aPKC)	PS, ?[c]	ζ, λ, ι

[a]The PKC isozyme family is divided into three subfamilies based on structural homology. Shown are the distinct cofactor requirements associated with each subfamily (Asaoka et al., 1992; Dekker and Parker, 1994). [b]PS denotes phosphatidylserine. [c]Phosphatidylinositol (3,4,5)-triphosphate (PIP$_3$) is a candidate activating cofactor for the atypical PKC subfamily (Nakanishi et al., 1993).

Table 2. Enzymes and Transporter Proteins Implicated in Drug Resistance in Cancer that are Phosphorylated and Functionally Modified by Protein Kinase C(PKC).

PKC Substrate	Effect of PKC-Catalyzed Phosphorylation	Reference
Glutathione-S-Transferase	n.d.[1]	(Taniguchi and Pyerin, 1989)
P-Glycoprotein	activation[2]	(Chambers et al., 1993; Orr et al., 1993)
Topoisomerase I[3]	activation	(Pommier et al., 1990)
Topoisomerase II[3]	activation	(DeVore et al., 1992; Corbett et al., 1993)

[1]The effect of phosphorylation on transferase activity was not measured but a decreased affinity for bilirubin was noted for the phosphorylated enzyme.
[2]PKC-catalyzed phosphorylation of P-glycoprotein is associated with enhanced cellular drug efflux levels (Chambers et al., 1992) but direct activation of P-glycoprotein transporter function by PKC has not been demonstrated. [3]Drug resistance that is related to decreased topoisomerase II activity or expression in cancer cells is termed atypical MDR (atMDR); resistance phenotypes associated with a reduction in topoisomerase I activity have also been observed (Beck, 1989; Chen and Beck, 1993; Gudkov et al., 1993). PKC-catalyzed phosphorylation sensitizes topoisomerase I to camptothecin (Pommier et al., 1990), and PKC-catalyzed phosphorylation of topoisomerase II appears to provide cells resistance against topoisomerase II poisons by reducing their levels of drug-induced DNA cleavage products (DeVore et al., 1992).

EFFECTS OF MODULATION OF PROTEIN KINASE C ACTIVITY ON MULTIDRUG RESISTANCE IN CANCER CELLS

The hallmark of P-glycoprotein-mediated MDR is a sharp reduction in the intracellular accumulation of cytotoxic drugs due to the drug efflux activity of the pump (Endicott and Ling, 1989). A potential role for PKC in P-glycoprotein-mediated MDR was suggested by early observations that specific phorbol-ester PKC activators transiently protect human carcinoma KB cells from several cytotoxic drugs (Ferguson and Cheng, 1987) and human leukemic cells from colchicine (O'Connor, 1985), and that they also induce a reduction in [^{3}H] vincristine and [^{14}C] daunorubicin accumulation in murine leukemic P388 cells (Ido et al., 1986; Kessel, 1988).   The discovery that specific phorbol-ester PKC activators induce resistance in human breast cancer cells to multiple cytotoxic drugs that are P-glycoprotein substrates in association with a reduction in the intracellular accumulation of the drugs (Fine et al., 1988) provided the first definitive evidence that PKC plays an important role in P-glycoprotein-mediated MDR.   In that report, the induction of drug resistance in drug-sensitive human breast cancer MCF7 cells and the enhancement of MDR in Adriamycin-selected MCF7-MDR cells by phorbol esters were both antagonized by the MDR reversal agent verapamil, consistent with the hypothesized role for PKC in MDR (Fine et al., 1988).   These findings have been extended to several cell lines, and the magnitude of the phorbol ester effect is generally a 2-4-fold increase in the IC_{50} values of cytotoxic drugs (reviewed in O'Brian et al., in press).

SN-1,2-diacylglycerol is a second messenger that activates PKC by the same mechanism as phorbol esters (Kikkawa et al., 1989).   A synthetic diacylglycerol has been shown to potently reduce the accumulation of multiple cytotoxic drugs that are P-glycoprotein substrates in human colon cancer KM12L4a cells (Dong et al., 1991), providing evidence that aberrant production of diacylglycerol may be a contributing factor in drug resistance in cancer.   At least eight members of the PKC isozyme family are phorbol ester-dependent (Table 1).   Phorbol ester activation of the isozyme PKC-α has been shown to trigger the induction of MDR in KM12L4a cells, in studies that measured the induction of resistance by the isozyme-selective PKC activator thymeleatoxin and determined the PKC isozyme composition of the cells (Gravitt et al., in press).

Various   PKC inhibitors have been shown to restore drug accumulation in MDR cancer cells (Table 3) and to partially reverse the MDR phenotype (Table 4).   Although the mechanistic significance of these observations is limited by the nonselective nature of the majority of the inhibitors examined, the inhibitors do suggest new avenues that merit exploration for the development of novel MDR reversal agents.

Table 3. Restoration of Drug Accumulation in MDR Tumor Cells by Protein Kinase C Inhibitors.

PKC Inhibitor	Cell Line[1]	Reference
Calphostin C	Ls 180Vb20 MCF7-TH SW620 Ad300 KB-V1	Bates et al., 1993 Chambers et al., 1992
H7	CH^RC5	Epand and Stafford, 1993
NA382	P388/ADR AH66 K562/ADR	Miyamoto et al., 1993
N-myristoylated pseudosubstrate peptide	MCF7/MDR	Gupta, KP, et al., 1994
Safingol	MCF7-MDR	Sachs et al., 1994
SR33557	P388/ADR	Jaffrezou et al., 1991
Staurosporine	SW620 Ad300 KB-V1 CH^RC5 P388/ADR K562/ADR	Bates et al., 1993 Chambers et al., 1992 Epand and Stafford, 1993 Miyamoto et al., 1993 Sato et al., 1990

[1]Ls180Vb20 is a vinblastine-selected human colon cancer cell line, MCF7-TH is an Adriamycin-selected human breast cancer cell line, SW620 Ad300 is an Adriamycin-selected human colon cancer cell line, KB-V1 is a vinblastine-selected human nasopharyngeal line, CH^RC5 is a colchicine-selected Chinese hamster ovary line, MCF7-MDR is an Adriamycin-selected human breast cancer cell line, P388/ADR is an Adriamycin-selected murine leukemic line, K562/ADR is an Adriamycin selected human leukemia line and AH66 is a rat hepatoma line.

Table 4. Partial Reversal of Multidrug Resistance by Protein Kinase C (PKC) Inhibitors

PKC Inhibitor	Cell Line[a]	Reference
Cardiotoxin	K562/0A200	(Zheng et al., 1994)
CGP41251[b]	MCF7-MDR UV-2237-ADR[R]	(Fan et al., 1994)
Chlorpromazine	KB-Ch[R]-24	(Akiyama et al., 1986)
H7[c]	LoVoC1.7 UV-2237M-ADR[R] KM12L4a	(Dolfini et al., 1993) (O'Brian et al., 1989) (Dong et al., 1991)
NA-382[b]	K562/ADR	(Miyamoto et al., 1993)
N-myristoyl-RKRTLRRL	UV-2237M-ADR[R]	(O'Brian et al., 1991b)
safingol[d]	MCF7-MDR	(Sachs et al., 1994)
SR33557	P388/ADR	(Jaffrezou et al., 1991)
Staurosporine	S180-A10	(Posada et al., 1989)
Tamoxifen	CHO-ADR[R]	(Chatterjee and Harris, 1990)
	CH[R]C5	(Kang and Perry, 1993)
Trifluoperazine	KB-CH[R]-24	(Akiyama et al., 1986)

[a]K562/0A200 is an okadaic acid-selected human leukemic line, MCF7-MDR is an Adriamycin-selected human breast cancer line, UV-2237M-ADR[R] is an Adriamycin-selected murine fibrosarcoma line, KB-Ch[R]-24 is a colchicine-selected human epidermoid cell line, LoVoC1.7 and KM12L4a are human colon cancer cell lines, K562/ADR is an Adriamycin-selected human leukemic line, P388/ADR is an Adriamycin-selected murine leukemic cell line, S180-A10 is an Adriamycin-selected murine sarcoma cell line, CHO-ADR[R] is an Adriamycin-selected Chinese hamster ovary cell line, and ChRC5 is a colchicine-selected Chinese hamster ovary cell line. [b]CGP41251 and NA-382 are staurosporine analogs, [c]H7 is an isoquinolinesulfonamide, and [d]safingol is a sphingosine analog.

PROTEIN KINASE C ISOZYME EXPRESSION IN MULTIDRUG RESISTANT CANCER CELLS

Elevated PKC activity levels have been observed in several Adriamycin- and vinblastine-selected MDR tumor cell lines (Palayoor et al., 1987; Aquino et al., 1988; Fine et al., 1988; Chambers et al., 1990b). A direct correlation between the level of PKC activity and MDR was noted in a series of drug-sensitive, moderately resistant, and highly resistant Adriamycin-selected MDR murine fibrosarcoma cell lines (O'Brian et al., 1989).

Examination of PKC isozyme expression in paired drug-sensitive and MDR tumor cell lines has revealed that elevated PKC activity levels in MDR tumor cells generally reflect PKC isozyme overexpression. PKC-α overexpression is often a feature of Adriamycin-selected MDR cell lines (Table 5). PKC-α overexpression has been shown to occur at the level of the message in the MDR cell lines KB-A10 (Posada et al., 1989), MCF7-MDR (Blobe et al., 1993) and P388/ADR (Gupta S et al., 1994). Overexpression of PKC-α protein in MCF7-MDR cells is most pronounced in the nuclear fraction (Lee et al., 1992). In association with PKC-α overexpression, overexpression of PKC-ß and its message has been observed in P388/ADR cells (Gupta S et al., 1994) and loss of PKC-δ and PKC-ε has been noted in MCF7-MDR cells (Blobe et al., 1993). Loss of PKC-ε in MCF7-MDR appears to be secondary to PKC-α overexpression, because PKC-ε expression is partially restored after transfection of the cells with antisense PKC-α (Ahmad and Glazer, 1993).

Table 5. PKC Isozyme Overexpression in Cytotoxic Drug-Selected Multidrug Resistant (MDR) Cells.

Cell Line[a]	Selecting Agent	Overexpressed Isozyme	Fold Over-Expression	Reference
P388/ADR	ADR	cPKC-α	2	(Gollapudi et al.,
		cPKC-ß	2	1992; Gupta S et al., 1994)
MCF7-MDR	ADR	cPKC-α	30	(Blobe et al., 1993; Lee et al., 1992)
HL60/ADR	ADR	cPKC-γ	Not expressed in parental line	(Aquino et al., 1990)
UV-2237M-ADR[R]	ADR	cPKC-α	2	(O'Brian et al., 1991a)
KB-A10	ADR	cPKC-α	3	(Posada et al., 1989)

[a]The cell lines are murine leukemia P388/ADR, human breast cancer MCF7-MDR, human promyelocytic leukemia HL60/ADR, murine fibrosarcoma UV-2237M-ADR[R], and human nasopharyngeal KB-A10.

In contrast with the results described above, an MDR leukemic K562 cell line that was selected with the protein phosphatase inhibitor okadaic acid showed no alteration in PKC isozyme expression other than loss of PKC-ε (Zheng et al., 1994), suggesting that nPKC-ε may modulate MDR. In addition, the MDR cell line HL60/ADR has been reported to have a normal level of PKC-α expression and to overexpress PKC-γ (Aquino et al., 1990). Taken together, these studies demonstrate a strong association between overexpression of the common PKC (cPKC) isozyme subfamily (Table I) and the MDR phenotype of Adriamycin-selected tumor cells. To determine the generality of this phenomenon, PKC isozyme expression should be further analyzed in MDR tumor cells selected with other cytotoxic drugs.

Table 6. Effects of Engineering Specific Alterations in Protein Kinase C (PKC) Isozyme Expression on Multidrug Resistance (MDR)

Cell Line[1]	Transfected Gene	Effect on PKC Isozyme Expression	Effect on MDR	Reference
MCF7	PKC-α	Increased α	No effect	(Yu et al.,
BC-19	PKC-α	Increased α	Induction of MDR	1991)
Rat 6	PKC-ß$_1$	Increased ß$_1$	Induction of MDR	(Fan et al., 1992)
BC-19	PKC-γ	Increased γ, Decreased ε	No effect	(Ahmad et al., 1992)
MCF7-MDR	Antisense PKC-α	Decreased α, Increased ε	Partial Reversal	(Ahmad and Glazer, 1993)

[1]MCF7 is a human breast cancer cell line, BC-19 is an *mdr*-1 transfected MCF7 variant, Rat 6 is a rat embryo fibroblast line, and MCF7-MDR is an Adriamycin-selected variant of MCF7.

To directly test the effect of altered PKC isozyme expression on MDR, specific alterations in PKC isozyme expression have been engineered into cells by transfection with constructs encoding the PKC isozymes or the corresponding anti-sense cDNA's (Table 6). Overexpression of PKC-ß$_1$ alone was sufficient to induce a modest but significant MDR phenotype in a rat fibroblast line (Fan et al., 1992). In contrast, PKC-α overexpression did not affect the chemosensitivity of MCF7 cells, unless the cells were first transfected with *mdr1*, the gene encoding P-glycoprotein (Yu et al., 1991). In both cases, induction of resistance by PKC isozyme overexpression was associated with a reduced level of intracellular drug accumulation (Fan et al., 1992; Yu et al., 1991). In the PKC isozyme family, PKC-γ is closely related to PKC-α and PKC-ß (Table 1). Despite this relatedness, in studies of PKC-γ transfectants, it was found that overexpression of PKC-γ had no effect on the chemosensitivity of the *mdr-1* transfected MCF7 subline BC19; PKC-γ was also without effect on drug accumulation in the cells (Ahmad et al., 1992).

The induction of MDR by overexpression of PKC-α in BC19 cells (Yu et al., 1991) and the elevated level of PKC-α expression in MCF7 MDR cells (Lee et al., 1992; Blobe et al., 1993) suggest that antagonism of PKC-α expression should partially reverse MDR in MCF7-MDR cells. This has been shown to be the case in a study of antisense PKC-α-transfected MCF7-MDR cells (Ahmad and Glazer, 1993). However, the effects of anti-sense PKC-α expression on intracellular drug accumulation and drug resistance were modest, suggesting that more efficient expression systems for full-length anti-sense PKC-α or anti-sense PKC-α oligonucleotides are needed to achieve potent reversal of the MDR phenotype in the cells (Ahmad and Glazer, 1993).

PHOSPHORYLATION OF P-GLYCOPROTEIN BY PROTEIN KINASE C

A number of PKC substrates may mediate effects of the enzyme on MDR. These substrates include P-glycoprotein (Chambers et al., 1990b), glutathione S-transferase (Taniguchi and Pyerin, 1989), topoisomerase I (Pommier et al., 1990), topoisomerase II (Corbett et al., 1993), raf (Cornwell and Smith, 1993; Kolch et al., 1993; Egan and Weinberg, 1993), vinculin (Aquino et al., 1988), and the heat shock proteins pp27a and pp27b (Regazzi et al., 1988; Issandou et al., 1988; Darbon et al., 1990; Fine et al., 1988). The importance of PKC-catalyzed P-glycoprotein phosphorylation as a contributing factor in MDR has been established in studies described below. However, the contribution of other PKC-catalyzed phosphorylation events to MDR has not yet been determined. The overexpression of nuclear PKC-α in MDR human breast cancer cells (Lee et al., 1992) strongly suggests that phosphorylation of nuclear proteins by PKC also plays an important role in MDR. The role of nuclear PKC in MDR should be examined.

P-glycoprotein is phosphorylated by multiple protein kinases, including PKC (Chambers et al., 1990b), cAMP-dependent protein kinase (Mellado and Horwitz, 1987), and the membrane-associated protein kinase PK-1 (Staats et al., 1990), but only PKC-catalyzed P-glycoprotein phosphorylation has been linked to alterations in the function of the drug-efflux pump. Although modulation of the drug-efflux activity of isolated P-glycoprotein by PKC has not been demonstrated, activation of PKC in MDR tumor cells is tightly linked to P-glycoprotein phosphorylation concomitant with a precipitous drop in intracellular drug retention

(Chambers et al., 1990a; Chambers et al., 1992; Bates et al., 1992; Bates et al., 1993). The converse phenomenon has also been observed, *i.e.*, inhibition of PKC in MDR tumor cells is associated with decreased P-glycoprotein phosphorylation and enhanced intracellular drug retention (Chambers et al., 1992; Bates et al., 1993).

Alterations in P-glycoprotein drug efflux activity induced by modulating PKC activity in MDR tumor cells appear to result from direct phosphorylation of P-glycoprotein by PKC, because the sites of P-glycoprotein that are phosphorylated in MDR tumor cells upon PKC activation are the same sites that are phosphorylated in isolated P-glycoprotein by purified PKC (Chambers et al., 1990b; 1992). Furthermore, PKC appears to be the predominant protein kinase responsible for basal P-glycoprotein phosphorylation, because similar sites of P-glycoprotein are phosphorylated in MDR tumor cells, whether or not the cells are treated with phorbol-ester PKC activators (Chambers et al., 1990b; 1992). Finally, phosphorylation of P-glycoprotein at these sites is also enhanced by treating cells with the protein phosphatase inhibitor okadaic acid, providing evidence that protein phosphatases 1 and 2a dephosphorylate the drug-efflux pump at PKC phosphorylation sites (Chambers et al., 1992). PKC phosphorylation sites in murine and human P-glycoprotein have been identified in the linker region between the two homologous halves of P-glycoprotein, which is analogous to the R domain of the cystic fibrosis conductance regulator (Orr et al., 1993; Chambers et al., 1993).

Several lines of evidence implicate PKC-α as the PKC isozyme that phosphorylates P-glycoprotein. Increased P-glycoprotein phosphorylation observed in MCF7-MDR cells is associated with PKC-α overexpression and loss of nPKC-δ and nPKC-ε (Blobe et al., 1993). Transfection of BC19 cells with PKC-α increased P-glycoprotein phosphorylation, but transfection of the cells with the closely related isozyme PKC-γ had no effect on the phosphorylation of the drug efflux pump (Yu et al., 1991; Ahmad et al., 1992). P-glycoprotein phosphorylation was antagonized when BC19 cells were transfected with anti-sense PKC-α cDNA (Ahmad and Glazer, 1993). While it is clear from these studies that P-glycoprotein is a PKC-α substrate, it is premature to conclude that other members of this extensive isozyme family do not phosphorylate P-glycoprotein.

CONCLUSIONS

It is now clear that PKC activation induces or enhances MDR in a broad range of tumor cell types through its phosphorylation and activation of the drug efflux pump P-glycoprotein and possibly other proteins that mediate drug resistance mechanisms in tumor cells, e.g., topoisomerase II. There is also evidence that the isozyme responsible for the contribution of PKC to MDR is PKC-α, and the hypothesis that selective inhibition of PKC-α may chemosenistize tumor cells to anticancer therapy should be tested. Strategies need to be devised to selectively inhibit PKC-α in tumor cells. Transfection of cells with dominant-negative PKC-α mutants (Dekker and Parker, 1994) and treatment of cells with PKC-α antisense oligonucleotides and with PKC-α inhibitor peptides that are based on the autoinhibitory pseudosubstrate sequence in the regulatory domain of PKC-α are likely to be the definitive experiments. In fact, an N-myristoylated PKC-α pseudosubstrate peptide has already been shown to restore drug retention in MDR human breast cancer cells (Gupta KP, et al., 1994), and the peptide chemosensitizes the cells to the cytotoxic effects of Adriamycin and vincristine (Gupta KP, and O'Brian CA, manuscript in preparation).

ACKNOWLEDGMENTS

Supported by NCI Grant CA52460, Robert A. Welch Foundation Grant G1141, and an award from the Sid W. Richardson Foundation. We thank Patherine Greenwood for expert preparation of the manuscript.

REFERENCES

Ahmad S, Glazer RI (1993): Expression of the antisense cDNA for protein kinase C-α attenuates resistance in doxorubicin-resistant MCF-7 breast carcioma cells. *Molec Pharmacol* 43:858-862
Ahmad S, Trepel JB, Ohno S, Suzuki K, Tsuruo T, Glazer RI (1992): Role of protein kinase C in the modulation of multidrug resistance: expression of the atypical γ isoform of protein kinase C does not confer increased resistance to doxorubicin. *Molec Pharmacol* 42:1004-1009

Akiyama S, Shiraishi N, Kuratomi Y, Nakagawa M, Kuwano M (1986): Circumvention of multiple-drug resistance in human cancer cells by thioridazine, trifluoperazine, and chlorpromazine. *J Natl Canc Inst* 76:839-844

Aquino A, Hartman KD, Knode MC, Grant S, Huang K-P, Niu C-H, Glazer RI (1988): Role of protein kinase C in phosphorylation of vinculin in Adriamycin-resistant HL-60 leukemia cells. *Cancer Res* 48:3324-3329

Aquino A, Warren BS, Omichinski J, Hartman KD, Glazer RI (1990): Protein kinase C-γ is present in Adriamycin-resistant HL-60 leukemia cells. *Biochem Biophys Res Commun* 166:723-728

Asaoka Y, Nakamura S, Yoshida K, Nishizuka Y (1992): Protein kinase C, calcium and phospholipid degradation. *Trends Biochem Sci* 17:414-417

Bates SE, Currier SJ, Alvarez M, Fojo AT (1992): Modulation of P-glycoprotein phosphorylation and drug transport by sodium butyrate. *Biochem* 31:6366-6372

Bates SE, Lee JS, Dickstein B, Spolyar M, Fojo AT (1993): Differential modulation of P-glycoprotein transport by protein kinase inhibition. *Biochem* 32:9156-9164

Beck WT (1989): Unknotting the complexities of multidrug resistance: The involvement of DNA topoisomerases in drug action and resistance. *J Natl Cancer Inst* 81:1683-1685

Blobe GC, Sachs CW, Khan WA, Fabbro D, Stabel S, Wetsel WC, Obeid LM, Fine RL, Hannun YA (1993): Selective regulation of expression of protein kinase C (PKC) isoenzymes in multidrug-resistant MCF7 cells. *J Biol Chem* 268:658-664

Castagna M, Takai Y, Kaibuchi K, Sano K, Kikkawa U, Nishizuka Y (1982): Direct activation of calcium-activated, phospholipid-dependent protein kinase by tumor-promoting phorbol esters. *J Biol Chem* 257:7847-7851

Chambers TC, Chalikonda I, Eilon G (1990a): Correlation of protein kinase C translocation, P-glycoprotein phosphorylation, and reduced drug accumulation in multidrug resistant human KB cells. *Biochem Biophys Res Commun* 169:253-259

Chambers TC, McAvoy EM, Jacobs JW, Eilon G (1990b): Protein kinase C phosphorylates P-glycoprotein in multidrug resistant human KB carcinoma cells. *J Biol Chem* 265:7679-7686

Chambers TC, Pohl J, Raynor RL, Kuo JF (1993): Identification of specific sites in human P-glycoprotein phosphorylated by protein kinase C. *J Biol Chem* 268:4592-4595

Chambers TC, Zheng B, Kuo JF (1992): Regulation by phorbol ester and protein kinase C inhibitors, and by a protein phosphatase inhibitor (okadaic acid), of P-glycoprotein phosphorylation and relationship to drug accumulation in multidrug resistant human KB cells. *Molec Pharmacol* 41:1008-1015

Chatterjee M, Harris AL (1990): Reversal of acquired resistance to Adriamycin in CHO cells by tamoxifen and 4-hydroxy tamoxifen: Role of drug interaction with alpha 1 acid glycoprotein. *Br J Cancer* 62:712-717

Chen M, Beck WT (1993): Teniposide resistant CEM cells, which express mutant DNA topoisomerase IIα, when treated with non-complex-stabilizing inhibitors of the enzyme, display no cross-resistance and reveal aberrant functions of the mutant enzyme. *Cancer Res* 53:5946-5953

Conn PJ, Sweatt JD (1994): Protein kinase C in the nervous system. *In: Protein Kinase C* (JF Kuo, Editor), Oxford Univ. Press, New York, pp 199-235

Corbett AH, Fernald AW, Osheroff N (1993): Protein kinase C modulates the catalytic activity of topoisomerase II by enhancing the rate of ATP hydrolysis: Evidence for a common mechanism of regulation by phosphorylation. *Biochemistry* 32:2090-2096

Cornwell MM, Smith DE (1993): A signal transduction pathway for activation of the mdr1 promoter involves the proto-oncogene c-raf kinase. *J Biol Chem* 268:15347-15350

Darbon JM, Issandou M, Tournier JF, Bayard F (1990): The respective 27kDa and 28kDa protein kinase C substrates in vascular endothelial and MCF-7 cells are most probably heat shock proteins. *Biochem Biophys Res Commun* 168:527-536

Dekker LV, Parker PJ (1994): Protein kinase C - a question of specificity. *Trends Biochem Scis* 19:73-77

DeVore RF, Corbett AH, Osheroff N (1992): Phosphorylation of topoisomerase II by casein kinase II and protein kinase C: effects on enzyme-mediated DNA cleavage/religation and sensitivity to the antineoplastic drugs etoposide and 4'-(9-acridinylamino)methane-sulfon-*m*-aniside. *Cancer Res* 52:2156-2161

Dolfini E, Dasdia T, Perletti G, Romagnoni M, Piccinini F (1993): Analysis of calcium dependent protein kinase C isozymes in intrinsically resistant cloned lines of LoVo cells: Reversal of resistance by kinase inhibitor 1-(5-isoquinolinylsulfonyl) 2-methylpiperazine. *Anticancer Res* 13:1123-1128

Dong Z, Ward NE, Fan D, Gupta KP, O'Brian CA (1991): *In vitro* model for intrinsic drug resistance: Effects of protein kinase C activators on the chemosensitivity of cultured human colon cancer cells. *Molec Pharmacol* 39:563-569

Egan SE, Weinberg RA (1993): The pathway to signal achievement. *Nature* 365:781-783

Epand RM, Stafford AR (1993): Protein kinases and multidrug resistance. *The Cancer J* 6:154-157

Endicott JA, Ling V (1989): The biochemistry of P-glycoprotein-mediated multidrug resistance. *Annu Review Biochem* 58:137-171

Fan D, Beltran P, O'Brian CA (1994): Reversal of multidrug resistance. *In: Reversal of Multidrug Resistance in Cancer*. (JA Kellen, Editor), CRC Press, Boca Raton, pp 93-125

Fan D, Fidler IJ, Ward NE, Seid C, Earnest LE, Housey GM, O'Brian, CA (1992): Stable expression of a cDNA encoding rat brain protein kinase C-ß₁ confers a multidrug-resistant phenotype on rat fibroblasts. *Anticancer Res* 12:661-668

Fan D, Regenass U, Kaufmann H, Beltran PJ, Campbell TE, Fidler IJ (1994): The protein kinase C (PKC) inhibitor staurosporine derivative CGP41251 enhances the *in vitro* cytotoxicity of doxorubicin (DOX) against multidrug resistant (MDR) murine fibrosarcoma, murine colon carcinoma, and human breast carcinoma cells. *Proc Am Assoc Cancer Res* 35:446

Ferguson PJ, Cheng Y (1987): Transient protection of cultured human cells against antitumor agents by 12-0-tetradecanoylphorbol-13-acetate. *Cancer Res* 47:433-441

Fine RL, Patel J, Chabner BA (1988): Phorbol esters induce multidrug resistance in human breast cancer cells. *Proc Natl Acad Sci USA* 85:582-586

Gollapudi S, Patel K, Jain V, Gupta S (1992): Protein kinase C isoforms in multidrug resistant P388/ADR cells: a possible role in daunorubicin transport. *Cancer Let* 62:69-75

Gottesman MM, Pastan I (1993): Biochemistry of multidrug resistance mediated by the multidrug transporter. *Annu Review Biochem* 62:385-427

Gravitt KR, Ward NE, Fan D, Skibber JM, Levin B, O'Brian CA (1994): Evidence that protein kinase C-α activation is a critical event in phorbol ester-induced multiple drug resistance in human colon cancer cells. *Biochem Pharmacol*, in press

Gudkov AV, Zelnick CR, Kazarov AR, Thimmapaya R, Suttle DP, Beck WT, Roninson IB (1993): Isolation of genetic suppressor elements, inducing resistance to topoisomerase II-interactive cytotoxic drugs, from human topoisomerase II cDNA. *Proc Natl Acad Sci* 90:3231-3235

Gupta KP, Ward NE, Gravitt KR, O'Brian CA (1994): Restoration of drug accumulation in multidrug-resistant (MDR) human breast cancer MCF7 cells by an N-myristoylated pseudosubstrate peptide and an *N*-myristoylated peptide substrate analog of protein kinase C. *Proc Am Assoc Cancer Res* 35:2654

Gupta S, Kim C, Qin Y, Gollapudi S (1994): Expression of protein kinase C isozymes in multidrug resistant murine leukemia P388/ADR cells. *Intl J Oncology* 4:311-315

Ido M, Asao T, Sakurai M, Inagaki M, Saito M, Hidaka H (1986): An inhibitor of protein kinase C, 1-(5-isoquinolinylsulfonyl)-2-methylpiperazine (H7) inhibits TPA-induced reduction of vincristine uptake from P388 murine leukemic cell. *Leukemia Res* 10:1063-1069

Issandou M, Bayard F, Darbon JM (1988): Inhibition of MCF7 cell growth by 12-0-tetradecanoylphorbol-13-acetate and 1,2-dioctanoyl-sn-glycerol: Distinct effects on protein kinase C activity. *Cancer Res* 48:6943-6950

Jaffrezou J-P, Herbert J-M, Levade T, Gau M-N, Chatelain P, Laurent G (1991): Reversal of multidrug resistance by calcium channel blocker SR33557 without photoaffinity labeling of P-glycoprotein. *J Biol Chem* 266:19858-19864

Kessel D (1988): Effects of phorbol esters on doxorubicin transport systems. *Biochem Pharmacol* 37:2297-2299

Kang Y, Perry RR (1993): Modulatory effects of tamoxifen and recombinant human α-interferon on doxorubicin resistance. *Cancer Res* 53:3040-3045

Kellen JA (1994): Multidrug resistance. *In: Reversal of Multidrug Resistance in Cancer* (JA Kellen, Editor), CRC Press, Boca Raton, pp 1-19

Kikkawa U, Kishimoto A, Nishizuka Y (1989): The protein kinase C family: heterogeneity and its implications. *Annu Rev Biochem* 58:31-44

Kolch W, Heidecker G, Kochs G, Hummel R, Vahidi H, Mischak H, Finkenzeller G, Marme D, Rapp UR (1993): Protein kinase C-α activates raf-1 by direct phosphorylation. *Nature* 364:249-252

Kuo JF, Editor (1994): *Protein Kinase C*, Oxford University Press, New York

Lee SA, Karaszkiewicz JW, Anderson WB (1992): Elevated level of nuclear protein kinase C in multidrug-resistant MCF-7 human breast carcinoma cells. *Cancer Res* 52:3750-3759

Lester DS, Epand RM, Editors (1992): *Protein Kinase C: Current Concepts and Future Perspectives,* Ellis Horwood Press, New York

Mellado W and Horwitz SB (1987): Phosphorylation of the multidrug resistance associated glycoprotein. *Biochemistry* 26:6900-6904

Miyamoto K, Inoko K, Wakusawa S, Kajita S, Hasegawa T, Takagi K, Koyama M (1993): Inhibition of multidrug resistance by a new staurosporine derivative, NA-382, *in vitro* and *in vivo. Cancer Res* 53:1555-1559

Nakanishi H, Brewer KA, Exton JH (1993): Activation of the ζ isozyme of protein kinase C by phosphatidylinositol 3, 4, 5-trisphosphate. *J Biol Chem* 268:13-16

Nishikawa M, Hidaka H (1994): Protein kinase C in smooth muscle. In *Protein Kinase C* (JF Kuo, Editor), pp 236-248. New York: Oxford University Press

O'Brian CA, Fan D, Ward NE, Seid C, Fidler IJ (1989): Level of protein kinase C activity correlates directly with resistance to Adriamycin in murine fibrosarcoma cells. *FEBS Letts* 246:78-72

O'Brian CA, Fan D, Ward NE, Dong Z, Iwamoto L, Gupta KP, Earnest LE, Fidler IJ (1991a): Transient enhancement of multidrug resistance by the bile acid deoxycholate in murine fibrosarcoma cells *in vitro. Biochem Pharmacol* 41:797-806

O'Brian CA, Ward NE, Gravitt KR, Fan D (1994): The role of protein kinase C in multidrug resistance. In *Anticancer Drug Resistance: Adv in Molec and Clin Res* (LJ Goldstein, RF Ozols, Editors), Kluwer Acad. Publishers, Norwell in press

O'Brian CA, Ward NE, Liskamp RM, de Bont DB, Earnest LE, van Boom JH, Fan D (1991b): A novel, *N*-myristylated synthetic octapeptide inhibits protein kinase C activity and partially reverses murine fibrosarcoma cell resistance to Adriamycin. *Investig New Drugs* 9:169-179

O'Connor TWE (1985): Phorbol ester-induced loss of colchicine ultrasensitivity in chronic lymphocytic leukemia cells. *Leukemia Res* 9:885-895

Orr GA, Han EKH, Browne PC, Nieves E, O'Conner BM, Yang CPH, Horwitz SB (1993): Identification of the major phosphorylation domain of murine mdr 1b P-glycoprotein. *J Biol Chem* 268:25054-25062

Palayoor ST, Stein JM, Hait WN (1987): Inhibition of protein kinase C by antineoplastic agents: Implications for drug resistance. *Biochem Biophys Res Commun* 148:718-725

Pommier Y, Kerrigan D, Hartman KD, Glazer RI (1990): Phosphorylation of DNA topoisomerase I and activation by protein kinase C. *J Biol Chem* 265:9418-9422

Posada JA, McKeegan EM, Worthington KF, Morin MJ, Jaken S, Tritton TR (1989): Human multidrug resistant KB cells overexpress protein kinase C: Involvement in drug resistance. *Cancer Commun* 1:285-292

Regazzi R, Eppenberger U, Fabbro D (1988): The 27,000 daltons stress proteins are phosphorylated by protein kinase C during the tumor promoter-mediated growth inhibition of human mammary carcinoma cells. *Biochem Biophys Res Comm* 152:62-68

Sachs CW, Safa A, Fine RL (1994): Inhibition of protein kinase C by safingol is associated with chemosensitization of multidrug resistant MCF7 cells. *Proc Am Assoc Cancer Res* 35:447

Sato W, Yusa K, Naito M, Tsuruo T (1990): Staurosporine, a potent inhibitor of C-kinase, enhances drug accumulation in multidrug-resistant cells. *Biochem Biophys Res Commun* 173:1252-1257

Staats J, Marquadt D, Center MS (1990): Characterization of a membrane-associated protein kinase of multidrug resistant HL60 cells which phosphorylates P-glycoprotein. *J Biol Chem* 265:4084-4090

Taniguchi H, Pyerin W (1989): Glutathione S-transferase is an *in vitro* substrate of Ca^{++} phospholipid-dependent protein kinase (protein kinase C). *Biochem Biophys Res Commun* 162:903-907

Yu G, Ahmad S, Aquino A, Fairchild CR, Trepel JB, Ohno S, Suzuki K, Tsuruo T, Cowan KH, Glazer RI (1991): Transfection with protein kinase Cα confers increased multidrug resistance to MCF-7 cells expressing P-glycoprotein. *Cancer Commun* 3:181-189

Zheng B, Chambers TC, Raynor RL, Markham PN, Gebel HM, Vogler WR, Kuo JF (1994): Human leukemia K562 cell mutant (K562/0A200) selected for resistance to okadaic acid (protein phosphatase inhibitor) lacks protein kinase C-ε, exhibits multidrug resistance phenotype, and expresses drug pump P-glycoprotein. *J Biol Chem* 269:12332-12338

10. BCL-2 AND CHEMORESISTANCE IN CANCER

John C. Reed

INTRODUCTION

Programmed cell death is a physiological process that plays a critical role in the regulation of tissue homeostasis by ensuring that the rate at which new cells are produced in the body through cell division is offset by a commensurate rate of cell loss. Though largely overlooked until recently, it is now becoming increasing appreciated that disturbances in the physiological cell death process that prevent or delay normal cell turnover can be just as important to the pathogenesis of cancer as abnormalities in the regulation of the cell cycle. Perhaps of even greater importance for the clinical oncologist is the recent realization that defects in the cell death pathway are important not only for the origins of cancer, but also may markedly influence our ability to treat it. This is because nearly all chemotherapeutic drugs, as well as radiation, ultimately tap into endogenous physiological pathways for cell death in order to kill cancer cells. Consequently, the loss of genes required for cell death or the over-activation of genes that block it can render tumor cells relatively more resistant to the cytotoxic effects of a broad spectrum of anti-cancer drugs. Knowledge about the genes involved in the regulation of physiological cell death and the alterations that can occur in at least some of them in cancer, therefore, is beginning to contribute useful prognostic information and to suggest approaches for the development of new therapeutics.

The bcl-2 gene, a key regulator of cell death pathways

The first realization that defects in the cell death pathway could contribute to the development of human neoplasia came from the discovery of a gene involved frequently in non-Hodgkin's lymphomas, called *bcl-2* for "B- cell lymphoma-2" (Tsujimoto et al., 1986). In ~90% of follicular small cleaved-cell non-Hodgkin's lymphomas, as well as ~30% of more aggressive B-cell lymphomas, chromosomal translocations move the *bcl-2* gene from its normal location on chromosome 18 into juxtaposition with the immunoglobulin (Ig) heavy-chain gene locus on chromosome 14, probably as the result of errors in the normal DNA recombination mechanisms that cut and splice together the V, D, and J gene segments to create functional Ig genes during B-cell differentiation in the bone marrow (Tsujimoto et al., 1988; Weiss et al., 1987; Zelenetz et al., 1991). The resulting t(14;18) translocations place the *bcl-2* gene under the influence of powerful transcriptional enhancers associated with the Ig locus, thus dysregulating the expression of *bcl-2* (Reed et al., 1989). Because the protein encoded by the *bcl-2* gene blocks programmed cell death, B-cells containing a t(14;18) translocation enjoy a selective survival advantage relative to their normal counterparts, and begin to clonally expand without necessarily experiencing an increase in their doubling times. Given that the average life-span of B-cells is only 5 to 7 days, it becomes immediately obvious how a genetic alteration that prevents cell death can impact on the homeostatic mechanisms that control the number of these cells in the body.

Bcl-2 blocks a common pathway for cell death

A variety of experimental observations have pointed to *bcl-2* as a critical regulator of the cell death process. Studies of Bcl-2 function using gene transfer approaches in mammalian cells, for example, have demonstrated that over-production of this oncoprotein can render cells relatively more resistant to induction of apoptosis by a wide variety of stimuli (reviewed by Reed, 1994). Among the experimental situations in which Bcl-2 has been shown to provide protection from cell death are: (i) growth factor deprivation from hemopoietic, lymphoid, and fibroblastic cells; (ii) neurotrophic factor withdrawal from neurons; (iii) UV and g- radiation; (iv) heat-shock; (v) some types of cytotoxic lymphokines (Tumor Necrosis Factor); (vi) Calcium ionophores; (vii) some types of viruses; (viii) excitotoxic neurotransmitters such as L-glutamate; and (ix) agents that induce free-radical production. This broad range of stimuli, with their numerous biochemical mechanisms of action in cells, suggests that Bcl-2 functions at a distal point in a pathway leading to cell death. There have been reported some scenarios, however, where gene transfer-mediated elevations in Bcl-2 protein levels have failed to protect against cell death. Furthermore, it some cases, the cell death process was clearly consistent with apoptosis as opposed to necrosis, such as with antigen receptor-induced apoptosis in some B- and T- lymphocyte cell lines (Cuende et al., 1993; Gottschalk et al., 1994; Makover et al., 1991). Though these data have often been used to argue for the existance of *bcl-2-* independent pathways that regulate apoptosis, it is also possible that the mechanisms involved in cell death induction did indeed involve the *bcl-2* pathway but that the mere over-production of the Bcl-2 protein was insufficient to provide protection for a variety reasons, including (i) absence of partner proteins that Bcl-2 may require to fulfill its mission as a cell death blocker, (ii) presence of high levels of proteins that inhibit Bcl-2, or (iii) stimulation of post- translational modifications of the Bcl-2 protein that impair its function.

Mechanisms of bcl-2 oncogene activation

In addition to its involvement in lymphomas, relatively high levels of Bcl-2 protein have been detected by flow-cytometric and immunoblotting methods in ~20% of patients with acute myelogenous leukemia (AML) and ~70% with chronic lymphocytic leukemia (CLL) (Campos et al., 1993; Hanada et al., 1993).   Moreover, in solid tumors, immunohistochemical analysis of Bcl-2 protein levels has suggested that alterations in either the levels or patterns of expression of *bcl-2*, or both, can occur in a variety of tumor types including adenocarcinoma of the prostate, colon, and stomach, squamous carcinoma of the lung, neuroblastomas, and undifferentiated nasopharyngeal cancers (Bronner et al., 1994; Castle et al., 1993; Colombel et al., 1993; Lu et al., 1993; McDonnell et al., 1992; Pezzella et al., 1993; Reed et al., 1991; Krajewski, et al., 1994).   Unlike many B-cell lymphomas that contain t(14;18) chromosomes, however, rarely are these high levels of Bcl-2 protein production associated with translocations or other structural alterations to the *bcl-2* gene.   Thus, additional mechanisms besides chromosomal translocations appear to be capable of leading to high levels of Bcl-2 protein production in many types of cancer.

One mechanism that may play a role in *bcl-2* gene dysregulation in solid tumors as well as some types of leukemia is loss of the tumor suppressor p53. The p53 gene encodes a DNA-binding protein that functions at least in part as a transcription factor to induce cell cycle arrest and apoptosis, particularly in response to DNA damage induced by chemotherapeutic drugs and radiation (Vogelstein and Kinzler, 1992). Production of DNA strand breaks by radiation and other means, for example, has been shown to result in increases in the levels of p53 protein in cells and elevations in p53 transcriptional activity (Zhan et al., 1993). Loss of p53 occurs in over half of all human cancers and has been correlated with worse prognosis for patients with several types of cancers. In vitro gene transfer studies have shown that cultured cell lines which lack functional p53 exhibit increased resistance to induction of apoptosis by multiple anticancer drugs and radiation (Lowe et al., 1993). Furthermore, transgenic animals with homozygous disruptions of their p53 genes [p53 "knock-out" mice], experience less radiation-induced apoptosis in the small intestine compared to normal littermate control animals (Merrit et al., 1992). In addition, thymocytes isolated from p53 knock-out mice have impaired apoptotic responses to induction of apoptosis by g-irradiation and topoismerase inhibitors, relative to p53-expressing control animals (Clarke et al., 1993; Lowe et al., 1993). Taken together, these observations have suggested that p53 plays an important role in a DNA damage and repair pathway that helps to maintain genomic stability by arresting cells with DNA damage at the G_1/S-border before errors in the DNA become fixed through DNA replication and by inducing cell suicide in cases were the damage to DNA is too excessive for accurate repair.

Though considerable progress towards understanding the mechanisms by which p53 induces cell cycle arrest has been made with the finding that p53 induces expression of a gene (*waf-1/cdi-1*) that interferes with the function of cyclins required for G_1>S phase transition (reviewed in Marx, 1993), until recently little was known about how p53 triggers apoptosis. Recently however we discovered that gene transfer-mediated elevations in p53 activity can lead to rapid down-regulation of *bcl-2* gene expression (Miyashita et al., 1994). Furthermore, we have mapped a p53 negative response element in the *bcl-2* gene by use of reporter gene assays (Miyashita et al., 1994). Finally, in p53 knock-out mice, Bcl-2 protein levels were discovered to be elevated in some tissues such as prostate, thymus, and spleen (Miyashita et al., 1994). Thus, loss of p53 can lead to increases in Bcl-2 protein levels in some tissues in vivo.

However, not all tissues have evidence of Bcl-2 over-production in p53 deficient mice, suggesting that tissue-specific regulatory factors also play an important role in the regulation of this gene in vivo.

In addition to potential regulation of *bcl-2* gene transcription by p53, the activity of the *bcl-2* gene is additionally modulated at the protein level by an opposing protein Bax, which shares 21% amino-acid identity with the Bcl-2 protein and which can bind to Bcl-2 and neutralize its ability to block cell death (Oltvai et al., 1993). Thus, loss of *bax* expression could be tantamount to over-production of Bcl-2. Recent work in our lab indicates that the p53 tumor suppressor can regulate the expression of *bax* in at least some tissues (Miyashita et al., 1994), thus further strengthening the connection between p53 loss in human cancers and mechanisms for dysregulation of both *bcl-2* gene and protein function. Moreover, we have identified a p53-binding site in the human *bax* gene promoter and have shown through reporter gene assays that p53 can *trans-* activate the *bax* promoter (Miyashita and Reed, manuscript in preparation). Of note, when gene transfer approaches were used to maintain high levels of Bcl-2 protein production in leukemic cells despite induction of p53, apoptosis was partially prevented (Selvakumaran et al., 1994). These latter findings therefore strongly suggest that a direct cause-and-effect relation exists between apoptosis-induction by p53 and the ability to p53 to regulate the expression of *bcl-2, bax,* or both of these genes, at least in some types of cells. Of note, *bcl-2-* transfected cells which are resistant to p53-induced apoptosis still undergo p53- mediated cell cycle arrest (Ryan et al., 1994; Selvakumaran et al., 1994; Wang et al., 1993), demonstrating that the anti- proliferative and apoptotic functions of p53 are separable.

Bcl-2 and Chemoresistance

Using gene transfer methods to over-express *bcl-2* in leukemia and solid tumor cell lines that contained low levels of Bcl-2 protein, as well as antisense approaches to reduce the levels of Bcl-2 protein in t(14;18)-containing lymphoma cell lines that contained high levels of this protein, we and others have shown that the levels of Bcl-2 protein correlate with relative sensitivity or resistance to a wide spectrum of chemotherapeutic drugs as well as g- irradiation (Campos et al., 1994; Collins et al., 1992; Dole et al., 1994; Epperly et al., 1994; Fisher et al., 1993; Griffiths et al., 1994; Hanada et al., 1993; Kamesaki et al., 1993; Kitada et al., 1994; Miyashita and Reed, 1992; Miyashita and Reed,

1993; Reed et al., 1994; Sentman et al., 1991; Siegel et al., 1992; Strasser et al., 1991; Walton et al., 1993). Included among the drugs that Bcl-2 has been experimentally shown to render cells more resistant to killing by are: dexamethasone, cytosine arabinoside (Ara-C), methotrexate, cyclophosphamide, adriamycin, daunomycin, 5-fluoro-deoxy-uridine, 2-chlorodeoxyadenosine, fludarabine, taxol, etoposide (VP-16), camptothecin, nitrogen mustards, mitoxantrone, cisplatin, vincristine and some retinoids. The extent to which gene transfer-mediated elevations in Bcl-2 protein levels provide protection from the cytotoxic effects of these drugs varies, depending on the particular drug and the cell line, but can be as much as 4 or more logs (10,000x) or as little as half a log (0.5x). When translated to clinical situations, however, even a half-log of protection may be highly significant, given that most attempts to employ so-called "high-dose" aggressive chemotherapy involve a mere doubling of the concentrations of drugs.

The observation that Bcl-2 provides protection against such a wide variety of drugs which have markedly diverse mechanisms of action suggests that they all utilize the same final common pathway for ultimately inducing cell death and that Bcl-2 is a regulator of this pathway. Indeed, several studies have provided evidence that chemotherapeutic drugs, as well as g-radiation, when administered in vitro to tumor cell lines induce cell death through mechanisms consistent with apoptosis as opposed to necrosis (Eastman, 1990; Kaufman, 1989). Furthermore, the data argue that despite the diversity of their biochemical mechanisms of action, all of these drugs have in common the ability to active the programmed cell death pathway at some point that lies upstream of Bcl-2.

The drug resistance imparted to cancer cells by elevated levels of Bcl-2 protein differs from all other previously described forms of chemoresistance. Traditionally, pharmacologist have thought of the chemoresistance problem in cancer in terms of four major issues: (i) problems with delivery of drug to the target, such as occurs when the *mdr-1* gene product, P-glycoprotein, is over-produced in the plasma membrane of cancer cells and pumps drugs out of the cell or when a drug is metabolized to an inactive product; (ii) modification of the drug target, an example of which is amplification of the gene for dihydrofolate reductase which often occurs following exposure to methotrexate; (iii) increased rates of repair of damage to DNA or other structures; and (iv) diminished rates of drug-induced damage to DNA or other macromolecules, as can occur for some drugs when glutathione levels are elevated in tumors. Bcl-2, in contrast, appears to act through a different mechanism.

Studies from several laboratories (Fisher et al, 1993; Kamesaki et al., 1993; Walton, et al., 1993) have shown that Bcl-2 does not prevent entry of drugs into cells (contrast with *mdr-1* over-expression). Bcl-2 also does not alter the extent to which drugs induce damage to DNA or the rate at which cells repair damaged DNA. Furthermore, no effects have been found of Bcl-2 on nucleotide pools or rates of cell cycling, which represent additional variables which can influence the relative sensitivity of cells to anticancer drugs. Similarly, though Bcl-2 was reported to produce elevations in intracellular glutathione levels in one neural cell line (Kane et al., 1993), this has not been observed in several other tumor and leukemia lines, indicating that no consistent relation of Bcl-2 to this intracellular antioxidant exists (Hockenbery et al., 1993 and unpublished data). It appears therefore that in the setting of Bcl-2 over-production, drugs still enter cells and induce damage, but this damage is somehow ineffectively translated into signals for cell death. In fact, it has been shown that anticancer drugs can still induce cell cycle arrest when Bcl-2 is present at high levels, but the cells typically fail to die or do so at markedly slower rates compared to control transfected cells (Fisher et al., 1993; Kamesaki et al., 1993; Miyashita et al., 1992; Miyashita and Reed, 1993). Thus, Bcl-2 can convert anticancer drugs from cytotoxic to cytostatic. Furthermore, when drugs are removed from cultures, a scenario that is analogous to the cessation of drugs that occurs clinically between cycles of chemotherapy, *bcl-2* expressing cells can often reinitiate cell growth at higher rates than their control counterparts, based on clonigenic cell assays (Kamesaki et al., 1993; Miyashita and Reed, 1992). Presumably, therefore, because they do not die as easily when exposed to drugs, cells with elevated levels of Bcl-2 protein are able to survive through the period of drug treatment and then repair drug-induced damage and resume their proliferation when drugs are withdrawn. Taken together, these observations suggest that Bcl-2 defines a new category of drug- resistance gene, i.e., those that regulate the physiological cell death pathway.

Though it is far from clear how Bcl-2 renders tumor cells relatively more resistant to the cytotoxic effects of nearly all chemotherapeutic drugs, the link between p53 and regulation of *bcl-2* and *bax* gene expression suggests a possible explanation. Since most anticancer drugs have in common the ability to either directly or indirectly induce DNA damage, which in turn would be expected to result in elevations in p53 transcriptional activity, it could be that the protective effects of Bcl-2 reflect its capacity to interfere with a p53-regulated pathway leading to apoptotic cell death. Moreover, at least one of the participants in this p53-dependent cell death pathway might be Bax, thus explaining the ability of Bcl-2 to abrogate drug-induced apoptosis. This hypothesis most likely represents an over simplification of the complex processes involved in drug-induced apoptosis and exceptions to the proposed model clearly exist, such as glucocorticoids which are potent inducers of apoptosis that do not dependent on p53 for their action (Clarke et al., 1993; Lowe et al., 1993) but which nevertheless are still prevented from inducing apoptosis by Bcl-2 (Miyashita and Reed, 1992; Miyashita and Reed, 1993; Sentman et al., 1991; Siegel et al., 1992; Strasser et al., 1991).

Though speculative, the connection between p53 and regulation of *bax* gene expression may provide insights into the clinical behavior of some types of cancer. For example, the ability of p53 to induce expression of *bax* may explain the somewhat paradoxical observation that patients with follicular lymphomas typically respond well to therapy at least initially, despite the high levels of Bcl-2 in these neoplasms caused by t(14;18) translocations. In this regard, though relapse occurs almost invariably, many patients can be induced into partial or complete clinical remissions a few times, often by use of the same drug regimen. Eventually, however, most patients experience transformation of their disease to an unresponsive state. The initial sensitivity of these tumors could theoretically be explained by induction of increases in p53 protein levels and transcriptional activity as a result of drug- induced damage to DNA (Zhan et al., 1993). This would in turn induce increases in *bax* gene expression, resulting in a temporary neutralization of Bcl-2 protein function by formation of Bcl-2/Bax protein heterodimers. Eventually, this p53-Bax pathway for induction of apoptosis may fail for a variety of reasons, including (i) loss of p53 expression or function, (ii) mutations in the *bax* gene, or (iii) other mechanisms resulting in an non-responsive state where the ratio of Bcl-2 to Bax remains high. Consistent with this idea, p53 gene mutations have previously been associated with histological transformation of follicular lymphomas (Lo Coco et al., 1993; Sander et al., 1993).

In vivo effects of Bcl-2 on chemo- and radiosensitivity

The effects of the Bcl-2 protein on chemosensitivity and radiosensitivity in vivo have been investigated using *bcl-2* transgenic mice, where Bcl-2 protein was over-produced in either B- or T-cells through use of tissue-specific transcriptional enhancers. In animals in which the human Bcl-2 protein was produced in thymocytes, for example, marked resistance to induction of cell death by in vivo administration of glucocorticoids and by exposure to g-radiation was observed relative to non-transgenic littermate controls (Sentman et al., 1991; Siegel et al., 1992; Strasser et al., 1991). In another approach, the in vivo effects of *bcl-2* were examined in murine bone marrow cells that had been transducted with a recombinant *bcl-2* retrovirus and transplanted into irradiated mice. Significantly less myelosuppression in response to VP16 (etoposide) was seen in mice that received *bcl-2* virus transduced bone marrow cells compared to animals whose hemopoietic cells contained a negative control virus (Kondo et al., 1994). Taken together, therefore, these animal studies provide evidence in support of an important role for Bcl-2 in regulating the in vivo resistance of at least some kinds of hemopoietic and lymphoid cells to chemotherapeutic drugs and radiation.

In addition to animal experiments, a variety of attempts have been made to correlate alterations in either *bcl-2* gene structure or expression with clinical outcome in patients with non-Hodgkin's lymphomas (NHLs) and other types of cancer. Nearly all of these studies, however, suffer from small sample size, non-uniform treatment of patients, or both. In addition, several technical issues must be considered when interpreting these data. For example, with studies that have relied on cytogenetic techniques to detect t(14;18) chromosomes, false-positives can occur due to failure to obtain mitoses from the tumor cells or poor quality chromosomal morphology. Similarly, use of PCR and conventional Southern blotting methods to detect rearrangements of the *bcl-2* gene fails to identify ~20% and ~10% of t(14;18) chromosomes, respectively, because of variations in chromosomal breakpoints (Zelenetz et al., 1991). Finally, with immunohistochemical evaluations of Bcl-2 protein, reviewer subjectivity may contribute to differences in interpretation of the data, as well as technical issues such as effects of fixation on preservation of epitopes and differences in the sensitivity of various antibodies. Some interesting trends can nevertheless be gleaned from the literature available to date from correlations of *bcl-2* with patient outcome.

a.) Lymphomas: In two studies of patients with NHLs having diffuse histology with a large cell component (DLCL), an association was found between *bcl-2* gene rearrangements and shorter survival, shorter disease-free survival (DFS), or failure to achieve a complete remission (CR)

(Offit et al., 1989; Yunis et al., 1989). The data approached statistical significance (P=0.07) in a third study of DLCL but the patient follow-up time in this case was short (2 year survival data) (Offit et al., 1991). Though *bcl-2* status was not of prognostic significance in 5 other reports involving patients with aggressive histology NHL (Gascoyne et al., 1994; Jacobson et al., 1993; Offit et al., 1991; Piris et al., 1994; Romaguera, et al., 1993), in one study the combination of p53 and Bcl-2 immunostaining data defined a subgroup of patients at high risk for death (Piris et al., 1994). As discussed above, therefore, the interplay between p53 and regulation of both of the *bcl-2* and *bax* genes may have been a contributor to the particularly poor prognosis observed for these patients. In addition, in several of the studies where the correlation between *bcl-2* and survival did not reach statistical significance, there was a tendency for patients with evidence of *bcl-2* gene activation to relapse or die sooner. For example, the 3 year survival for patients with *bcl-2* positive tumors was only 45% compared to 75% in a report by Romaguera et al, and the time to treatment failure was shorter for patients with Bcl-2-positive tumors (48% vs 11%) in a study by Jacobson et al. Similarly, survival at 5 yrs was shorter for patients with Bcl-2-positive DLCL (35% vs 46%) in the report a Piris et al. as well as in a study by Offit et al.

In patients with follicular lymphomas, Yunis et al. reported a significant association between *bcl-2* gene rearrangements and both failure to achieve CR and reduced survival in cases where the histology included a large-cell component (FLCL) (Yunis et al., 1989). Conversely, in an analysis of patients with low-grade NHLs (follicular small-cleaved cell and follicular mixed cell), *bcl-2* status was not of prognostic significance (Pezzella et al., 1992). One limitation of this latter study, however, was that the size of the *bcl-2*-negative group was small, since >85% of low-grade NHLs contain a t(14;18). Taken together, with the data on patients with DCLC lymphomas, these data suggest a trend towards a clinically significant role for *bcl-2* gene activation in poor outcome in patients with some types of lymphomas.

b.) Other types of cancers: In addition to lymphomas, suggestions of an association between *bcl-2* and poor responses to therapy have been found in patients with acute myelogenous leukemia (AML), where the presence of $\geq 20\%$ of Bcl-2-positive cells correlated with failure to achieve CR and shorter survival (Campos et al., 1993), as well as in men with adenocarcinoma of the prostate where Bcl-2-positive immunostaining was correlated with failure to response to anti-androgen therapy (McDonnell et al., 1992). Interestingly, in another report where a cross-sectional analysis of prostate cancers was preformed, positive Bcl-2 immunostaining was found in 100% of hormone-independent cancers (Colombel et al., 1993), again suggesting an association between elevations in Bcl-2 protein production and poor response to hormonal therapy. Though no survival data were available, Bcl-2 immunostaining was also positively correlated with unfavorable histology and *N-myc* gene amplification in one study of children and infants with neuroblastoma (Castle et al., 1993). In addition, while no correlation between Bcl-2 immunostaining and histology or *N-myc* was noted by Krajewski et al., elevated Bcl-2 immunostaining was seen in residual nests of viable tumor cells in 4 of 5 patients after therapy suggesting that Bcl-2 may be cytoprotective. Correlations of Bcl-2 immunostaining with survival in a study of women with lymph node-negative breast cancer and of patients with squamous cell carcinoma of the lung paradoxically suggested an inverse correlation between Bcl-2 and poor outcome (Pezzella et al., 1993; Silvestrini et al., 1994). In these studies, however, the treatment was primarily or even exclusively surgical, with only some patients receiving local regional radiotherapy as opposed to systemic chemotherapy. Thus, the relevance of these findings in breast and lung cancers may be limited, where the role of *bcl-2* as a clinically significant modulator of chemosensitivity is concerned.

Taken together, these clinical correlative studies of *bcl-2* status in non-Hodgkin's lymphomas, leukemias, and solid tumors suggest, but fall far short of proving, that *bcl-2* may be a clinically relevant prognostic indicator of patient responses to chemotherapy. However, given the importance of interactions of the Bcl-2 protein with other proteins such as Bax, and the observation that additional genes have now been identified that represent homologs of Bcl-2 (reviewed in Reed, 1994), it may be insufficient to assess only Bcl-2 protein levels in tumors. Further studies involving larger groups of patients that received uniform treatment, therefore, are required before any firm conclusions can be drawn as to the usefulness of Bcl-2 as a prognostic indicator, when used either alone or in combination with other laboratory tests such as p53 or Bax immunostaining.

The Bcl-2 protein

The predicted amino-acid sequence of the Bcl-2 protein has failed to provide any clues about the biochemical action of this protein that blocks cell death. In all species examined thus far, the protein has a molecular mass of ~25 to 26-kDa and contains a stretch of hydrophobic amino-acids near its C- terminus that constitutes a transmembrane domain (reviewed in Reed, 1994). The intracellular membranes into which Bcl-2 inserts are highly interesting. A combination of subcellular fractionation, immunofluorescence confocal, laser-scanning, and electron microscopic methods have provided conclusive evidence that Bcl-2 is associated with mitochondria, specifically the outer mitochondrial membrane, as opposed to the inner membrane where many of the steps of oxidative phosphorylation occur (de Jong et al., 1994; Jacobson et al., 1993; Krajewski et al., 1993). Bcl-2 immunoreactivity in the outer membrane of mitochondria is not uniformly distributed, but rather is patchy in its distribution-- a property which is suggestive of proteins that associate with the mitochondrial junctional complexes where the inner and outer membranes come into contact and where various transport phenomenon occur (de Jong et al., 1994; Krajewski et al., 1993). In addition to the mitochondrial outer membrane, much of the Bcl-2 protein is found in the nuclear envelope. Similar to the situation with mitochondria, electron microscopic data suggest that the Bcl-2 protein is non-uniformly distributed in the nuclear envelope in a punctate pattern that is reminiscent of nuclear pore complexes where the inner and outer nuclear membranes come into contact and where transport between nucleus and cytosol of protein, RNA, and possibly ions occurs (de Jong et al., 1994; Krajewski et al., 1993). Bcl-2 is also found in at least parts of the endoplasmic reticulum.

Though the functional significance of the unusual intracellular distribution of the Bcl-2 protein remains unclear, the possible association of Bcl-2 with mitochondrial junctional complexes (MJCs) and nuclear pore complexes (NPCs) raises some possibilities. The nucleus and mitochondria have several features in common, including the fact that both contain DNA. Thus, at least part of Bcl-2's role may be to protect this DNA from damage. Both the nucleus and mitochondria are also the only intracellular organelles that have an outer and an inner membrane. The MJCs and NPCs where these membranes come into contact are the sites of transport of macromolecules and possibly some ions into and out of these organelles. Evidence supporting a role for Bcl-2 in regulating some aspect of protein transport in the nuclear envelope, has been obtained by Meikrantz, et al., who reported reduced ratios of nuclear to cytosolic cdc-2 and cdk-2 kinase in HeLa cells transfected with *bcl-2* expression plasmids. Ryan, et al. also found that translocation of the p53 protein from cytosol into the nucleus was prevented by co-transfection of a mouse leukemia line with the combination of *bcl-2* and *c-myc* expression vectors. These findings suggest that Bcl-2 may either directly or indirectly influence the trafficking of proteins into the nucleus. On the other hand, however, Jacobson, et al. have shown that Bcl-2 can protect the cytoplasm of enucleated cells from "apoptosis," suggesting that the presence of a nucleus is not essential for Bcl-2 action (Jacobson et al., 1994).

Another possible functional implication of the intracellular locations of the Bcl-2 protein is suggested by data showing that Bcl-2 can influence intracellular Ca^{2+} homeostasis (Baffy et al., 1993). Using an IL-3-dependent hemopoietic cell line as a model for apoptosis induced by growth factor withdrawal, a striking loss of Ca^{2+} from the endoplasmic reticulum (ER) was seen in control cells prior to apoptosis, whereas ER pools of Ca^{2+} were maintained in the normal range in cells over-producing Bcl-2. Conversely, estimates of mitochondrial Ca^{2+} pools suggested that elevations occur in the amounts of releasable Ca^{2+} in mitochondria and that Bcl-2 prevents the accumulation of Ca^{2+} in this organelle. A functional connection between dysregulation of intracellular Ca^{2+} and apoptosis has been well-established by experimentation involving use of Ca^{2+} ionophores and other agents, including the observation that apoptosis is induced by thapsigargin and other drugs that poison the Ca^{2+}-ATPase of the ER and result in massive loss of Ca^{2+} from this organelle (Lam et al., 1993). Similarly, gene transfer- mediated elevations in calbindin-D, a Ca^{2+} binding protein that resides in the lumen of the ER, have been shown to delay the onset of apoptosis in a glucocorticoid-treated lymphoid cell line, arguing that increasing the ability of the ER to sequester Ca^{2+} protects against apoptosis (Dowd et al., 1992). The presence of Bcl-2 in nuclear and ER membranes, therefore, may have some relevance to the fact that most of the Ca^{2+} in cells is sequestered in the lumen of the ER which is contiguous with the space between the inner and outer nuclear membranes. Furthermore, in most types of cells, the mitochondria represent the next largest intracellular storage site for Ca^{2+}, again suggesting that Bcl-2 is at least located in the right places to function either directly or indirectly act as a regulator of intracellular Ca^{2+} homeostasis.

Finally, it has been suggested that Bcl-2 may function in an antioxidant pathway, based on the finding that Bcl-2 prevents induction of cell death induced by agents that either result in oxygen free radical production or that deplete intracellular glutathione, and on the observation that over-expression of certain antioxidant enzymes such as forms of superoxide dismutase (SOD) or glutathione peroxidase can also render cells more resistant to induction of cell death analogous to Bcl-2. Bcl-2 also prevents the accumulation of lipid peroxides in some models of cell death, suggesting that Bcl-2 somehow nullifies damage to membranes by reactive oxygen species (Hockenbery et al., 1993; Kane et al., 1993). The relevance of these findings to the intracellular locations of the Bcl-2 protein could be that mitochondrial, ER and plasma membranes are the major sites of free-radical generation in cells.

Bcl-2-binding proteins

Several proteins have now been identified which are capable of specifically interacting with Bcl-2. One of the more interesting revelations to come from these studies is that Bcl-2 can interact with a family of proteins that are homologous to itself. At present, 5 homologs of Bcl-2 have been reported, including Bax, Bcl-X, Mcl-1, A1, and Bap-1 (reviewed in Reed, 1994). Some of these proteins have additional forms that arise through alternative splicing mechanisms. Among these are the Bcl-X-L and Bcl-X-S proteins which have opposing functions. Bcl-X-L is a blocker of cell death analogous to Bcl-2, whereas the Bcl-X-S protein acts as an antagonist of Bcl-2 which accelerates apoptotic cell death (Boise et al., 1993). In addition to Bcl-X-S, the Bax protein has been shown to function as an inducer of rather than protector from cell death (Oltvai et al., 1993). Moreover, viral homologs of Bcl-2 have been discovered (Cleary, et al., 1986; Neilan, et al., 1993). At least one of these, the BHRF-1 protein of Epstein Barr Virus (EBV), can block cell death in mammalian cells (Henderson, et al., 1993; Takayama, et al., 1994). [See Table 1 for summary]. Though the role of these cellular and viral homologs of Bcl-2 in tumorigenesis and chemoresistance has yet to be examined in detail, we have found at least one example of a leukemia cell line that over-produced Bcl-X-L protein in association with acquisition of broad-spectrum resistance to anticancer drugs (Kühl et al., 1994). Thus, it will be of interest in the future to explore the expression of other members of the *bcl-2* gene family in human cancers.

Table 1. The known members of the Bcl-2 protein family are listed, including those identified in mammalian species (human, mouse, rat), the nematode (*C.Elegans*), and viruses. The function of these proteins as determined by gene transfer experiments is indicated, where known. In some cases, the function of these proteins has only preliminarily been explored (unpublished data) or is inferred by structural comparisons with other members of the family.

BCL-2 PROTEIN FAMILY

Bcl-2	blocker	mammalian
Bcl-X-L	blocker	mammalian
Bcl-X-S	inducer	mammalian
Bax	inducer	mammalian
Mcl-1	blocker(?)	mammalian
A1	blocker(?)	mammalian
BAP-1	inducer(?)	mammalian
Ced-9	blocker	nematode
BHRF-1	blocker	viral [EBV]
E1b 19-kDa	blocker	viral [Adenovirus]
LMW5-HL	?	viral [African Swine]

The discovery of a family of homologous proteins that are capable of interacting with each other suggests that the activities of Bcl-2 and these homologous proteins can be modulated by protein-protein dimerization or multimerization. Indeed, the cell death inducing proteins Bax and Bcl-X-S have been shown to bind to Bcl-2, suggesting that these protein-protein interactions modulate the activity of the Bcl-2 protein (Oltvai et al., 1993; Sato et al., 1994). Preliminary data, however, suggest that Bax and Bcl-X-S function in different ways to accelerate cell death. In this regard, we have recently proposed a model in which we envision Bax (probably in the form of a homodimer or multimer) as an activator or enhancer of the apoptotic cell death pathway (Sato et al., 1994). Binding of Bcl-2 to Bax neutralizes the activity of Bax and protects from cell death. The same is presumably true for Bcl-X-L and probably Mcl-1, which at least in yeast can bind to and neutralize the toxicity imparted by expression of Bax (Sato et al., 1994). Conversely, Bcl-X-S is able to bind to Bcl-2 but not Bax. It therefore may act as a Bcl-2 antagonist by binding to Bcl-2 and sequestering the Bcl-2 protein so that it cannot interact with and functionally neutralize Bax. At least some elements of this proposed model have been confirmed in mammalian cells. For example, it has been shown that mutants of Bcl-2 which fail to heterodimerize with Bax but which can still homodimerize with wild-type Bcl-2 are incapable of blocking apoptosis (Yin et al., 1994). Thus, the data available to date suggest that Bax is an effector protein that amplifies or triggers the cell death pathway and that Bcl-2 is a regulator of Bax which suppresses its function. However, Bcl-2 may also have activities irrespective of Bax, given that the human Bcl-2 protein can restore growth under aerobic conditions to mutant strains of yeast having defects in antioxidant enzymes (Kane, et al., 1993).

In addition to homologs of Bcl-2, other types of proteins have been identified that can bind to Bcl-2. Among these are p23-R-Ras, a member of the Ras family of low-molecular weight GTPases (Fernandez et al., 1993); p72- Raf-1, a serine/threonine-specific protein kinase (Wang et al., 1994); and BAG-1 (Bcl-2- associated AthanoGene-1), a novel protein that we have identified which has little homology to other known proteins and that may define a new category of anti-cell death genes ("athanogenes" from the Greek word for the opposite of death, *athanos*) (S. Takayama, et al. manuscript in preparation). Based on co-transfection experiments performed in mammalian cells, Raf-1 and BAG-1 appear to function in cooperation with Bcl-2, protecting cells from apoptosis. How the interactions of BAG-1 and Raf-1 with Bcl-2 facilitate its ability to block cell death, however, remains to be defined. One possibility concerns the unusual locations where the Bcl-2 protein resides in cells, making it tempting to speculate that Bcl-2 may help to target signal transducing proteins such as Raf-1 and R-Ras to locations where they can come into contact with unique regulatory proteins or substrates which they might not otherwise meet. Until these interactions of Bcl-2 with Raf-1, R-Ras, and BAG-1 are somehow related to its ability to dimerize with Bax and other members of the Bcl-2 protein family, however, our vision at the biochemical level of how Bcl-2 regulates cell death will remain clouded.

Implications for the treatment of cancer

Though much work remains to be done, rapidly emerging data are beginning to suggest some novel approaches to the treatment of cancers in which *bcl-2* is expressed at high levels. For example, the interaction of Bcl-2 with the Bax protein appears to be critical for Bcl-2 to protect cells from cell death, suggesting that it may be possible to develop pharmaceuticals that could disrupt Bcl-2/Bax interactions and thus abrogate Bcl-2 protein function. Alternatively, antisense oligonucleotides have been employed in vitro for down- regulating Bcl-2 protein levels in lymphoma cell lines and AML cells, demonstrating that decreases in *bcl-2* gene expression can enhance sensitivity to chemotherapeutic drugs (Campos et al., 1994; Kitada et al., 1994).   An alternative approach to modulating *bcl-2* gene expression in cancer cells is suggested by the observations that certain lymphokines and retinoids can regulate the expression of this apoptosis-blocking gene and in turn influence sensitivity to anticancer drugs (Bradbury et al., 1994; Lotem and Sachs, 1994; Naumovski and Cleary, 1994; Selvakumaran et al., 1994).   In the short term, therefore, lymphokines, lymphokine antagonists, or retinoids could be explored for their ability to lower the levels of *bcl-2* expression in some types of cancer in vivo and thus render these malignant cells more sensitive to induction of apoptosis by chemotherapeutic drugs and radiation.

CONCLUSIONS

Essentially all chemotherapeutic drugs available to date, as well as radiation, ultimately rely on elements of the physiological cell death pathway for triggering the death of tumor cells. Defects in the genetic pathway that controls this cell death process therefore can figure prominently not only in the origins of cancer, but also in problems with its treatment.   Over-production of the Bcl-2 protein constitutes a novel mechanism of chemoresistance in cancer.   With improved knowledge at the molecular level of the actions of Bcl-2 and related proteins and of the mechanisms that regulate the expression of the genes that encode these proteins, it may eventually be possible to develop novel treatments for cancer that specifically seek to modulate the physiological cell death pathway as opposed to nearly all currently available drugs which are targeted at some aspect of the cell division cycle.

ACKNOWLEDGEMENTS

The author wishes to acknowledge the intense dedication of all those in our laboratory and elsewhere who contributed to the data described here, and the generous support of the American Cancer Society, Leukemia Society of America, the Council for Tobacco Research, and the National Cancer Institute.

REFERENCES

Baffy G, Miyashita T, Williamson JR and Reed JC (1993): Apoptosis induced
    by withdrawal of Interleukin-3 [IL-3] from an IL-3-dependent
    hematopoietic cell line is associated with repartitioning of intracellular
    calcium and is blocked by enforced bcl-2 oncoprotein production. *J Biol
    Chem* 268:6511-6519
Boise LH, González-Garcia M, Postema CE, Ding L, Lindsten T, Turka A, Mao
    X, Nunez G and Thompson CB (1993): bcl-x, a bcl-2 related gene that
    functions as a dominant regulator of apoptotic cell death. *Cell* 74:597-608
Bradbury D, Zhu Y-M and Russel N (1994): Regulation of Bcl-2 expression and
    apoptosis in acute myeloblastic leukaemia cells by granulocyte-
    macrophage colony-stimulating factor. *Leukemia* 8:786-791
Bronner M, Culin C, Reed JC and Furth EE (1994): Bcl-2 proto-oncogene and
    the gastrointestinal epithelial tumor progression model. *Amer J Pathol*, in
    press
Campos L, Roualult J-P, Sabido O, Oriol P, Roubi N, Vasselon C, Archimbaud
    E, Magaud J-P and Guyotat (1993): High expression of bcl-2 protein in
    acute myeloid leukemia cells is associated with poor response to
    chemotherapy. *Blood* 81:3091-3096
Campos L, Sabido O, Rouault J-P, and Guyatat D (1994): Effects of BCL-2
    antisense oligodeoxynucleotides on in vitro proliferation and survival of
    normal marrow progenitors and leukemic cells. *Blood* 84:595-600
Clarke AR, Purdie CA, Harison DJ, Morris RG, Bird CC, Hooper ML and
    Wyllie AH (1993): Thymocyte apoptosis induced by p53-dependent and
    independent pathways. *Nature* 362:849-852
Castle VP, Heidelberger KP, Bromberg J, Ou X, Dole M and Nunez G (1993):
    Expression of the apoptosis-suppressing protein bcl-2, in neuroblastoma
    is associated with unfavorable histology and N-*myc* amplification. *Am J
    Pathology* 143:1543-1550
Cleary ML, Smith SD and Sklar J (1986): Cloning and structural analysis of
    cDNAs for bcl-2 and a hybrid bcl-2/immunoglobulin transcript resulting
    from the t(14;18) translocation. *Cell* 47:19-28
Colombel M, Symmans F, Gil S, O'Toole KM, Chopin D, Benson M, Olsson
    CA, Korsmeyer S and Buttyan R (1993): Detection of the apoptosis-
    suppressing oncoprotein bcl-2 in hormone-refractory human prostate
    cancers. *Am J Pathology* 143:390-400
Collins MKL, Marvel J, Malde P and Lopez-Rivas A (1992): Interleukin 3
    protects murine bone marrow cells from apoptosis induced by DNA
    damaging agents. *J Exp Med* 176:1043-1051
Cuende E, Alés-Martínez JE, Ding L, Gónzalez-García M, Martinez A and
    Nunez G (1993): Programmed cell death by bcl-2-dependent and
    independent mechanisms in B lymphoma cells. *EMBO J* 12:1555-1560

de Jong D, Prins FA, Mason DY, Reed JC, van Ommen GB, and Kluin PM (1994): Subcellular localization of the *bcl-2* protein in malignant and normal lymphoid cells. *Cancer Res* 54:256-260

Dole M, Nuñez G, Merchant AK, Maybaum J, Rode CK, Block CA and Castle VP (1994): Bcl-2 inhibits chemotherapy-induced apoptosis in neuroblastoma. *Cancer Res* 54:3253-3259

Dowd DR, MacDonald PN, Komm BS, Haussler MR and Miesfeld RL (1992): Stable expression of the calbindin-D28K complementary DNA interferes with the apoptotic pathway in lymphocytes. *Mol Endocrinol* 6:1843-1848

Eastman A (1990): Activation of programmed cell death by anticancer agents: *cis*-platin as a model system. *Cancer Cells* (Cold Spring Harbor) 2:275-280

Epperly MW, Santucci MA, Reed JC, Shields D, Halloran A, and Greenberger JS Expression of the human Bcl-2 transgene increases the radiation resistance of a hematopoietic progenitor cell line. *Rad Oncology Invest,* in press

Fernandez MJ and Bischoff JR (1993): Bcl-2 associates with the ras-related protein R-ras p23. *Nature* 366:274-275

Fisher TC, Milner AE, Gregory CD, Jackman AL, Aherne GW, Hartley JA, Dive C and Hickman JA (1993): *bcl-2* modulation of apoptosis induced by anticancer drugs: resistance to thymidylate stress is independent of classical resistance pathways. *Cancer Res* 53:3321-3326

Gascoyne R, Adomat S, Toleher A, Horsman D and Connors JM (1994): Prognostic relevance of the Bcl-2 translocation in diffuse large cell lymphomas. *Modern Pathol* 7:A630

Gottschalk AR, Boise LH, Thompson CB and Quintáns J (1994): Identification of immunosuppressant-induced apoptosis in a murine B-cell line and its prevention by bcl-x but not *bcl-2*. *Proc Natl Acad Sci USA* 91:7350-7354

Griffiths SD, Goodhead DT, Marsden SJ, Wright EG, Krajewski S, Reed JC, Korsmeyer SJ and Greaves M (1994): Interleukin 7-dependent B lymphocyte precursor cells are ultrasensitive to apoptosis. *J Exp Med* 179:1789-1797

Hanada M, Delia D, Aiello A, Stadtmauer E and Reed JC (1993): *bcl-2* gene hypomethylation and high-level expression in B-cell chronic lymphocytic leukemia. *Blood* 82:1820-1828

Hanada M, Krajewski S, Tanaka S, Cazals-Hatem D, Spengler BA, Ross RA, Biedler JL and Reed JC (1993): Production of the p26-Bcl-2 protein in human neuroblastoma cell lines correlates with neuroblastic differentiation and resistance to chemotherapy. *Cancer Res* 53:4978-4986

Henderson S, Huen D, Rowe M, Dawson C, Johnson G and Rickinson A (1993): Epstein-Barr virus-coded BHRF1 protein, a viral homologue of Bcl-2, protects human B cells from programmed cell death. *Proc Natl Acad Sci USA* 90:8479-8483

Hockenbery D, Oltvai Z, Yin X-M, Milliman C and Korsmeyer SJ (1993): Bcl-2. functions in an antioxidant pathway to prevent apoptosis. *Cell* 75:241-251

Jacobson JO, Wilkes BM, Kwiatkowski DJ, Medeiros LJ, Aisenberg AC and Harris NL (1993): *bcl-2* rearrangements in *De Novo* diffuse large cell lymphoma. *Cancer* 72:231-236

Jacobson MD, Burne JF, King MP, Miyashita T, Reed JC and Raff MC (1993): Apoptosis and Bcl-2 protein in cells without mitochondrial DNA. *Nature* 361:365-368

Jacobson MD, Burne JF and Raff MC (1994): Programmed cell death and Bcl-2 protection in the absence of a nucleus. *EMBO J* 13:1899-1910

Kaufmann SH (1989): Induction of endonucleolytic DNA cleavage in human acute myelogenous leukemia cells by etoposide, camptothecin, and other cytotoxic anticancer drugs: A cautionary note. *Cancer Res* 49:5870-5878

Kamesaki S, Kamesaki H, Jorgensen TJ, Tanizawa A, Pommier Y and Cossman J (1993): *bcl-2* protein inhibits etoposide-induced apoptosis through its effects on events subsequent to topoisomerase II-induced DNA strand breaks and their repair. *Cancer Res* 53:4251-4256

Kane DJ, Sarafin TA, Auton S, Hahn H, Gralla FB, Valentine JC, Ord T and Bredesen DE (1993): Bcl-2 inhibition of neural cell death: decreased generation of reactive oxygen species. *Science* 262:1274-1276

Kitada S, Takayama S, DeRiel K, Tanaka S and Reed JC (1994): Reversal of chemoresistance of lymphoma cells by antisense-mediated reduction of *bcl-2* gene expression. *Antisense Res & Dev* 4:71-79

Kondo S, Yin D, Morimura T, Oda Y, Kikuchi H and Takeuchi J (1994): Transfection with a *bcl-2* expression vector protects transplanted bone marrow from chemotherapy-induced myelosuppression. *Cancer Res* 54:2928-2933

Krajewski S, Chatten J, Hanada M, Womer R and Reed JC Immunohistochemical analysis of Bcl-2 oncoprotein in human neuroblastoma: Correlations with tumor cell differentiation and N-myc protein. *Lab Invest*, in press

Krajewski S, Tanaka S, Takayama S, Schibler MJ, Fenton W and Reed JC (1993): Investigations of the subcellular distribution of the BCL-2 oncoprotein: residence in the nuclear envelope, endoplasmic reticulum, and outer mitochondrial membranes. *Cancer Res* 53:4701-4714

Kühl J-S, Krajewski S, Durán GE, Reed JC and Sikic B (1994): A spontaneously resistant variant of murine P388 leukemia with broad cross-resistance to cytotoxins and overexpression of the long form of the Bcl-X protein. Submitted

Lam M, Dubyak G and Distelhorst CW (1993): Effect of glucocorticosteroid treatment on intracellular calcium homeostasis in mouse lymphoma cells. *Mol Endocrinol* 7:686-693

Lo Coco F, Gaidano G, Louie DC, Offit K, Chaganti RSK and Dalla-Favera R (1993): p53 mutations are associated with histologic transformation of follicular lymphoma. *Blood* 82:2289-2295

Lotem J and Sachs L (1994): Control of sensitivity to induction of apoptosis in myeloid leukemic cells by differentiation and *bcl-2* dependent and independent pathways. *Cell Growth Differ* 5:321-327

Lowe SW, Ruley HE, Jacks T and Houseman DE (1993): p53-dependent apoptosis modulates the cytotoxicity of anticancer agents. *Cell* 74:957-967

Lowe SW, Schmitt EM, Smith SW, Osborne BA and Jacks T (1993): p53 is required for radiation-induced apoptosis in mouse thymocytes. *Nature.* 362:847-849

Lu Q-L, Elia G, Lucas S and Thomas JA (1993): Bcl-2 proto-oncogene expression in Epstein-Barr-Virus associated nasopharyngeal carcinoma. *Int J Cancer* 53:29-35

Makover D, Cuddy M, Bradley K, Alpers J, Sukhatme V and Reed J (1991): Phorbol ester-mediated inhibition of growth and regulation of proto-oncogene expression in the human T cell leukemia line JURKAT. *Oncogene* 6:455-460

Marx J (1993): How p53 suppresses cell growth. *Science* 262:1644-1645

McDonnell TJ, Troncoso P, Brisbay SM, Logothetis C, Chung LWK, Hsieh J-T, Tu S-M and Campbell ML (1992): Expression of the protooncogene *bcl-2* in the prostate and its association with emergence of androgen-independent prostate cancer. *Cancer Res* 52:6940-6944

Meikrantz W, Gisselbrecht S, Tam SW and Schlegel R (1994): Activation of cyclin A-dependent protein kinases during apoptosis. *Proc Natl Acad Sci USA* 91:3754-3758

Merritt AJ, Potten CS, Kemp CJ, Hickman JA, Balmain A, Lane DP and Hall PA (1994): The role of p53 in spontaneous and radiation-induced apoptosis in the gastrointestinal tract of normal and p53-deficient mice. *Cancer Res* 54:614-617

Miyashita T and Reed JC (1992): BCL-2 gene transfer increases relative resistance of S49.1 and WEHI7.2 lymphoid cells to cell death and DNA fragmentation induced by glucocorticoids and multiple chemotherapeutic drugs. *Cancer Res* 52:5407-5411

Miyashita T and Reed JC (1993): Bcl-2 oncoprotein blocks chemotherapy-induced apoptosis in a human leukemia cell line. *Blood* 81:151-157

Miyashita T, Harigai M, Hanada M and Reed JC (1994): Identification of a p53-dependent negative response element in the *bcl-2* gene. *Cancer Res* 54:3131-3135

Miyashita T, Krajewski S, Krajewska M, Wang HG, Lin HK, Hoffman B, Lieberman D and Reed JC (1994): Tumor suppressor p53 is a regulator of *bcl-2* and *bax* gene expression in vitro and in vivo. *Oncogene* 9:1799-1805

Naumovski L and Cleary ML (1994): Bcl-2 inhibits apoptosis associated with terminal differentiation of HL-60 myeloid leukemia cells. *Blood* 83:2261-2267

Neilan J, Lu Z, Afonso C, Kutish G, Sussman M and Rock DL (1993): An African Swine Fever virus gene with similarity to the *bcl-2* proto-oncogene and the Epstein Barr virus gene BHRF-1. *J Virol* 67:4341-4394

Offit K, Koduru PRK, Hollis R, Filippa D, Jhanwar SC, Clarkson BC and Chaganti RSK (1989): 18q21 rearrangement in diffuse large cell lymphoma: incidence and clinical significance. *Br J Haematol* 72:178-183

Offit K, Wong G, Filippa DA, Tao Y and Chaganti RSK (1991): Cytogenetic analysis of 434 consecutively ascertained specimens of non-Hodgkin's lymphoma: clinical correlations. *Blood* 77:1508-1515

Oltvai Z, Milliman C and Korsmeyer SJ (1993): Bcl-2 heterodimerizes in vivo with a conserved homolog, Bax, that accelerates programmed cell death. *Cell* 74:609-619

Pezzella F, Jones M, Ralfkiaer E, Ersboll J, Gatter KC and Mason DY (1992): Evaluation of *bcl-2* protein expression and 14;18 translocation as prognostic markers in follicular lymphoma. *Br J Cancer* 65:87-89

Pezzella F, Turley H, Kuzu I, Tungekar MF, Dunnill MS, Pierce CB, Harris A, Gatter KC and Mason DY (1993): *bcl-2* protein in non-small-cell lung carcinoma. *New England J Med* 329:690-694

Piris MA, Pezella F, Martinez-Montero JC, Orradre JL, Villuendas R, Sanchez-Beato M, Cuena R, Cruz MA, Martinez B, Garrido MC, Gatter K, Aiello A, Delia D, Giardini R and Rilke F (1994): p53 and *bcl-2* expression in high-grade B-cell lymphomas: correlation with survival time. *Br J Cancer* 69:337-341

Reed JC (1994): Bcl-2 and the regulation of programmed cell death. *J Cell Biol* 124:1-6

Reed JC, Kitada S, Takayama S and Miyashita T (1994): Regulation of chemoresistance by the *bcl-2* oncoprotein in non-Hodgkin's lymphoma and lymphocytic leukemia cell lines. *Annals of Oncology* 5:S61-S65

Reed J, Meister L, Cuddy M, Geyer C and Pleasure D (1991): Differential expression of the BCL-2 proto-oncogene in neuroblastomas and other human neural tumors. *Cancer Res* 51:6529-6538

Reed J, Tsujimoto Y, Epstein S, Cuddy M, Slabiak T, Nowell P and Croce C (1989): Regulation of *bcl-2* gene expression in lymphoid cell lines. containing t(14;18) or normal #18 chromosomes. *Oncogene Res* 4:271-282

Romaguera JE, Pugh W, Luthra R, Goodacre A and Cabanillas F (1993): The clinical relevance of t(14;18)/Bcl-2 rearrangement and Del 6q in diffuse large cell lymphoma and immunoblastic lymphoma. *Annals Oncology* 4:51-54

Ryan JJ, Prochownik E, Gottlieb CA, Apel IJ, Merino R, Nuñez G and Clarke MF (1994): c-*myc* anc *bcl-2* modulates p53 function by altering p53 subcellular trafficking during the cell cycle. *Proc Natl Acad Sci USA* 91:5878-5882

Sander CA, Yano T, Clark HM, Harris C, Longo DL, Jaffe ES and Raffeld M (1993): p53 mutation is associated with progression in follicular lymphomas. *Blood* 82:1994-2004

Sato T, Hanada M, Bodrug S, Irie S, Iwama N, Boise L, Thompson C, Fong L, Wang H-G and Reed JC (1994): Interactions among members of the *bcl-2* protein family analyzed with a yeast two-hybrid system. *Proc Natl Acad Sci USA*, in press

Selvakumaran M, Lin H-K, Miyashita T, Wang HG, Krajewski S, Reed JC, Hoffman B and Liebermann D (1994): Immediate early up-regulation of bax expression by p53 but not TGFb1: a paradigm for distinct apoptotic pathways. *Oncogene* 9:1791-1798

Sentman CL, Shutter JR, Hockenbery D, Kanagawa O and Korsmeyer SJ (1991): *bcl-2* inhibits multiple forms of apoptosis but not negative selection in thymocytes. *Cell* 67:879-888

Siegel R, Katsumata M, Miyashita T, Louie D, Greene M and Reed JC (1992): Inhibition of thymocyte apoptosis and negative antigenic selection in *bcl-2* transgenic mice. *Proc Natl Acad Sci USA* 89:7003-7007

Silvestrini R, Veneroni S, Daidone MG, Benini E, Boracchi P, Mezzetti M, Di Fronzo G, Rilke F and Veronesi U (1994): The *bcl-2* protein: a prognostic indicator strongly related to p53 protein in lymph node-negative breast cancer patients. *J Natl Cancer Inst* 86:499-504

Strasser A, Harris AW and Cory S (1991): Bcl-2 transgene inhibits T cell death and perturbs thymic self-censorship. *Cell* 67:889-899

Takayama S, Cazals-Hatem DL, Kitada S, Tanaka S, Miyashita T, Hovey LR, Huen D, Rickinson A, Veerapandian P, Krajewski S, Saito K and Reed JC (1994): Evolutionary conservation of function among mammalian, avian, and viral homologs of the Bcl-2 oncoprotein: structure-function implications. *DNA & Cell Biol* 13:679-692

Tsujimoto Y and Croce CM (1986): Analysis of the structure, transcripts, and protein products of *bcl-2*, the gene involved in human follicular lymphoma. *Proc Natl Acad Sci USA* 83:5214-5218

Tsujimoto Y, Louie E, Bashir MM and Croce CM (1988): The reciprocal partners of both the t(14;18) and t(11;14) translocations involved in B-cell neoplasms are rearranged by the same mechanism. *Oncogene* 2:347-351

Vogelstein B and Kinzler KW (1992): p53 function and dysfunction. *Cell* 70:523-526

Walton WI, Whysong D, O'Connor PM, Hockenbery D, Korsmeyer SJ and Kohn KW (1993): Constitutive expression of human Bcl-2 modulates mitrogen mustard and camptothecin induced apoptosis. *Cancer Res* 53:1853-1861

Wang H-G, Miyashita T, Takayama S, Sato T, Torigoe T, Krajewski S, Tanaka S, Hovey L III, Troppmair J, Rapp UR and Reed JC (1994): Apoptosis regulation by interaction of Bcl-2 protein and Raf-1 kinase. *Oncogene* 9:2751-2756

Wang Y, Szekely L, Okan I, Klein G and Wiman KG (1993): Wild-type p53-triggered apoptosis is inhibited by *bcl-2* in a v-*myc*-induced T-cell lymphoma line. *Oncogene* 8:3427-3431

Weiss LM, Warnke RA, Sklar J and Cleary ML (1987): Molecular analysis of the t(14;18) chromosomal translocation in malignant lymphomas. *N Engl J Med* 317:1185-1189

Yin X-M, Oltvai ZN and Korsmeyer SJ (1994): BH1 and BH2 domains of Bcl-2 are required for inhibition of apoptosis and heterodimerization with Bax. *Nature* 369:321-333

Yunis JJ, Mayer MG, Arensen MA, Aeppli DP, Oken MM and Frizzera G (1989): Bcl-2 and other genomic alterations in the prognosis of large-cell lymphomas. *N Engl J Med* 320:1047-1054

Zelenetz AD, Chu G, Galili N, Bangs CD, Horning SJ, Donlon TA, Cleary ML and Levy R (1991): Enhanced detecion of the t(14;18) translocation in malignant lymphoma using pulsed-field gel electrophoresis. *Blood* 178:1552-1560

Zhan Q, Carrier F and Fornace Jr AJ (1993): Induction of cellular p53 activity by DNA-damaging agents and growth arrest. *Mol Cell Biol* 13:4242-4250

11. MOLECULAR INTERRELATIONSHIPS IN MULTIDRUG RESISTANCE

John A. Kellen

> .... how can we possibly have come so far,
> and yet still have so far to go?
> Asleigh Brilliant (paraphrased)

The prospect of understanding the molecular basis of malignant growth is full of promises: genetic alterations, involved in transformation, play a role in cancerogenesis and are the mainspring of the infinite capabilities of cancer cells to attain immortality. Genetic changes lead to altered gene products, which in turn may involve drug transport (in, as well as out of cells) and metabolism, changes in drug targets and repair of drug-induced damage (Dalton, 1991).

Immortalisation, an escape from necrosis or apoptosis (the natural fate of all "healthy" cells), is now attributed to oncogenes which interfere with the differentiation process (Gonos and Spandidos, 1993). Increased cell division, one of the common denominators of malignancy, results in the accumulation of genetic errors. Of course, the term error is used from the point of view of the accepted, orderly conduct, expected from normal cells; for the cancer cell, it is an *ad hoc*, optimal solution permitting uncontrolled "joie de vivre" (Preston-Martin et al., 1990). The normal, "unselfish" growth and behaviour of cell populations is tightly regulated by intercellular signalling; malignant cells, in general, have decreased cell-cell communication (Mesnil et al., 1993). The reader is refered to the elegant editorial by Heppner (1989) on tumor cell societies. On careful analysis, it contains a chilling truth. Tumor populations are notoriously heterogeneous, variable and unstable: interference with their internal equilibrium (by targeted cell kill, with any therapeutic modality) stimulates the eventual dominance of surviving subpopulations. Chemotherapy, especially non-curative intervention (which is so far the most frequent) provides a stimulus to diversity which, in the long term, leads to multidrug resistance. This is not intended to preach therapeutic nihilism, but is is quietly accepted that the host of at least a few forms of cancer (cervix *in situ*, some prostate tumors) does reasonably well when left alone.   It is another argument in favour of individualized chemotherapy, aimed at cells whose phenotype has been identified at the molecular level, with additional intervention capable to correct the simultaneous induction of MDR.

Several excellent reviews of the genetic basis of multidrug resistance are available (Kane, 1991; Pauly, 1992 a,b).   A series of articles by Goldie and Coldman (1989) presents, in a mathematical approach, a somatic mutation theory of drug resistance. Even if this theory (like any other model) has not achieved universal acceptance, it contains aspects which are very useful in the clinic. The authors rightly claim that the term "resistance" is a relational statement which does not connote absolute insensitivity. Resistance obviously depends on the concentration of the drug(s) used - which supports the more recent trend to strive for extremely high levels of chemotherapeutics used under hemopoietic and other protection.

Although the players in the MDR game have become increasingly known, there is a lack of systematic studies linking proto-ontogene amplification or gene mutations to the resistance phenomenon. In view of the genomic instability in cancer, the probability of linked gene alterations is great; also, metastatic cell lines have a greater capacity to generate cell variants (including those with the MDR phenotype).   In general, the progression of a tumor leads to increased cellular diversity (Wani et al., 1994). Perhaps the best insight into the interplay between oncogenes and drug resistance is related to the *mdr* system and the tumor suppressor gene p53.   The *mdr1* gene is very efficient in synthesizing relative large amounts of protein and is easily selectable (Kane et al., 1989,1991). The emergence of MDR is frequently, but not exclusively, associated with tumor progression and bad prognosis; so is the amplification of several proto-oncogenes (*c-erbB2*, *bcl-2*, *HER-2/neu*, *ras*, *raf*, *c-myc*, *c-fos*, *c-jun* and probably others).   In human ovarian carcinoma (A2780), platinum-resistant cells show higher basal levels of h-*ras*, vimentin and XPc expression; at low platinum doses, c*myc* and h-*ras* still increased (DeMars et al., 1994). Several cytotoxic drugs enhance

A list of activated oncogenes and their reflection on MDR is presented in Table 1.

Table 1. Proto-oncogenes and their correlations with various MDR phenotypes.

Proto-oncogene amplification	References	Comments
dhfr	Wani et al., 1994	methotrexate resistance
erb2	Matsumura et al., 1994 Lemoine et al., 1993 Johnston et al., 1992	Topo II deletion drug activating enzymes expression enhanced by tamoxifen
HER-*2/neu*	Tsai et al., 1993 a,b	marker for intrinsic MDR
Ha-*ras*	Keith et al., 1991 Kadoyama et al., 1989 Bristow et al., 1994	causes P-gp and GST-pi expression " & resistance to radiation
c-myc	Kadoyama et al., 1989 Scanlon et al., 1989	causes MDR involved in Pt-resistance
c-fos	Scanlon et al., 1989	involved in Pt-resistance
c-jun	Volm, 1993 Robert et al., 1992	causes P-gp expression
bcl-2	Kamesaki et al., 1993	inhibits apoptosis

the mRNA expression of oncogenes (c-*fos*, c-Ha-*ras*) and activate transcription of c-*jun* (Kashani-Sabet et al., 1991, Rubin et al., 1991 and 1992).

At this time, the role of the tumor suppressor p53 related to the MDR phenotype has been studied most. Mutation of this highly conserved protein is associated with cellular transformation; mutant p53 protein(s) act in a dominant negative manner.A multifunctional role of p53 (both wild and mutant) is gaining acceptance. Mutant p53 cooperates with *ras*

(Deppert, 1993) and may not have merely lost its tumor suppressor function, but actively contributes to malignant transformation (Baudier et al., 1992, Miyashita et al., 1994). The promotor of the human *mdr1* gene was shown to be the target for the *c-Ha-ras-1* oncogene and the mutant p53, whereas the wild-type p53 specifically represses *mdr1* (Chin et al., 1992, Zastawny et al., 1993). Coamplification of linked genes (such as the genes for ornithine decarboxylase and ribonucleotide reductase, Heby et al., 1994) may be one of the mechanisms in the development of cross-resistance to drugs.   Both *ras* and the mutant version of p53 are able to turn on the *mdr1* gene in some cells that did not express P-glycoprotein (Gottesman, 1992). Since the human *mdr1* promotor lacks a p53 consensus binding sequence, it has been suggested that mutant p53 affects *mdr1* expression by interaction in combination with other nucleoproteins or by inducing additional transcriptional regulatory factors (Goldsmith et al., 1994). Expression of *mdr1* appears to be associated with oncogene activation and funtional loss of tumor suppressor gene(s) (Liu et al., 1994). However, mutant p53 is not considered a major determinant of *mdr1* regulation, at least not in myeloplastic disorders (Preudhomme et al., 1993). The role of p53 in drug resistance is indirectly supported by the observation that recombinant adenovirus-mediated transfer of the wild-type p53 gene into the human NSCLC H358 cell line (which has a homozygous deletion of p53) results in markedly increased cellular sensitivity to cisplatin (Fujiwara et al., 1994). There is also an intriguing indication that there might be a relationship between p53 and Topo II beta, which is preferentially expressed in cells at growth plateau. High Topo II beta, together with low p53, may be markers of slowly proliferating tumors (Prosperi et al., 1992).

The *ras* family of oncogenes is found mutated in many tumors. NIH3T3 cells, transformed by *ras*, show increased resistance to both cisplatin and radiation (Kasid et al., 1989, Burt et al., 1988). Transformed primary rate epithelial cells become increasingly resistant to doxorubicin and vinblastin; transformation is followed by enhanced expression of the *mdr1* and GST-pi genes (Coles et al., 1990). Elevated transcripts of *C-H-ras*, *c-fos* and *c-myc* have been observed in cisplatin resistance (Scanlon et al., 1989, Sklar, 1988). *C-erb B2* transcriptional regulatory sequences also couple to genes which control several drug-activating enzymes, which may play a role in the detoxification rate of some chemotherapeuticals. Last but not least, *bcl-2* is being increasingly blamed for its interference with apoptotic pathways which are essentially accelerated by some cytotoxic agents (see Chapter 11).

Oncogenes have now been catalogued and pigeon-holed in great detail (Yamamoto, 1993) and we are gaining some insight into the interplay between them and tumor suppressor genes. Once this interplay is well understood, we should be able to replace and restore deleted functions and quell undersirable alterations. Obviously, as yet unidentified mechanisms exist which cause over-expression of certain genes in tumors without genetic alterations. Remote and apparently unrelated gene(s) may influence oncogenic regulation of the stability of oncogene mRNA (Spandidos and Anderson, 1989). DNA is biologically designed to be a highly reactive; a substance which that does not react with DNA will react with nothing at all (Rüdiger, 1990). One could (in theory) avoid or evade all environmental carcinogens and still switch on oncogenes by endogenous compounds.

Finally, the use of gene transfer can be envisaged as another promising tool to change "genetic predestination", which we grudgingly come to accept at least in some cancers. Two interesting avenues are opening: certain cells (such as marrow stem and T cells) could be imparted with drug resistance, which would permit heroic dosage of cytotoxic drugs. Suppression of *mdr* amplification in the tumor cells themselves is another path in this direction.

All the above should remind us of a well-worn cliché about the group of blind men trying to describe an elephant by touch: some features are understood in some detail, but the greater picture avoids us. Cancer is caused and maintained by genetic damage, a well accepted truism. Even the term damage is a subjective reductionism; it is appropriate to direct the reader to some views and hypotheses which may sound heretic, but offer a refreshing alternative. One, by Chigira (1993) considers malignant cells simply as "selfish" in an otherwise altruistic cell society; another, by Blumenthal (1992), regards cancer as the result of a "well planned and coordinated physiological response". Indeed, we have barely scratched (to use another cliché) the tip of the genetic iceberg.

REFERENCES

Baudier J, Delphin C, Grunwald D, Khochbin S, Lawrence JJ (1992): Characterization of the tumor suppressor protein p53 as a protein kinase C substrate and a S100b-binding protein. *Proc Natl Acad Sci US* 89:11627-11631

Blumenthal EZ (1992): Could Cancer be a Physiological Phenomenon Rather Than a Pathological Misfortune? *Med Hypotheses* 39:41-48

Bristow RG, Jang A, Peacock J, Chung S, Benchimol S, Hill RP (1994): Mutant p53 increases radioresistance in rat embryo fibroblasts simultaneously transfected with HPV16-E7 and/or activated H-*ras*. *Oncogene* 9:1527-1536

Burt RK, Garfield S, Johnson K, Thorgeirsson SS (1988): Transformation of rat liver epithelial cells with v-H-*ras* or c-*raf* causes expression of *mdr-1*, glutathione-S-transferase and increased resistance to cytotoxic chemicals. *Carcinogenesis* 9:2329-2332

Chigira M (1993): Selfish cells in altruistic cell society: A theoretical oncology (Review). *Int J Oncol* 3:441-455

Chin K-V, Ueda K, Pastan I, Gottesman MM (1992): Modulation of Activity of the Promoter of the Human *mdr1* Gene by *ras* and p53. *Science* 255:459-462

Coles B, Ketterer B (1990): The role of glutathione and glutathione transferases in chemical carcinogenesis. *Crit Rev in Biochem and Molec Biology* 25:47-70

Dalton WS (1991): Clinical and laboratory approach to drug resistance. *Curr Opinion in Oncol* 3:1043-1048

DeMars L, Li J, Fowler W, Chaney S (1994): Platinum-Inducible Gene Expression and Platinum Resistance. Abstr., 25th Ann Meet Soc Gynecol Oncol, Feb 6-9, Orlando, FL

Deppert W (1993): p53: Oncogene, Tumor Suppressor, or Both? *In: Molecular Diagnostics in Cancer* (ed. Wagener/Neumann), pp 27-29. Heidelberg: Springer-Verlag

Ferrandis E, Da Silva J, Riou G, Benard I (1994): Coactivation of the *mdr1* and *myc-n* genes in Human neuroblastoma Cells during the Metastatic Process in the Nude Mouse. *Cancer Res* 54:2256-2261

Fujiwara T, Grimm EA, Mukhopadhyay T, Zhang W-W, Owen-Schaub LB, Roth JA (1994): Induction of Chemosensitivity in Human Lung Cancer Cells *In Vivo* by Adenovirus-mediated Transfer of the Wild Type *p53* Gene. *Cancer Res* 54:2287-2291

Goldsmith ME, Madden MJ, Gudas JM, Cowan KH (1994): Effect of wild type p53 on transient human multidrug resistance gene expression in a p53

Gonos ES, Spandidos DA: Oncogenes in cellular Immortalisation and Differentiation (Review). *Anticancer Res* 13:1117-1122

Goldie JH, Coldman AJ (1989): The Somatic Mutation Theory of Drug Resistance: The "Goldie-Coldman" Hypothesis Revisited. *Principles & Pract of Oncol* 3:4-12

Gottesman MM (1992): Tumor Cell Trick May Save Patients From Ravages of Chemotherapy. 16th R & H Rosenthal Fnd Award Lecture, AACR Annual Meeting

Haldar S, Negrini M, Monne M, Sabbioni S, Croce CM (1994): Down-Regulation of *bcl-2* by p53 in Breast Cancer Cells. *Cancer Res* 53:2095-2097

Heby O, Ask A, Persson L, Brorsson A, Frostesjö L, Holm I: Development of resistance to hydoxyurea during treatment of human cancer cells with alpha-difluoromethylornithine. A result of coamplification of genes for ornithine decarboxylase and ribonucleotide reductase. *Proc AACR* 35:9

Heppner GH (1989): Tumor Cell Societies. *JNCI* 81:648-649

Johnston SRD, Salter J, MacLennan KA, Sacks NM, McKinna JA, Smith IE, Dowsett M (1992): Short-term tamoxifen induces the cytoplasmic expression of *c-erbB2* and *bcl-2* in ER-positive human primary breast cancer. *The Breast* 1:166

Kadoyama C, Birrer M, Dosaka H, Lai S, Venzon D, Gazdar A (1989): Transfection with *H-ras* or *c-myc* proto-oncogenes results in induction of the multidrug resistant phenotype. *Proc AACR* 30:501

Kamesaki S, Kamesaki H, Jorgensen TJ, Tanizawa A, Pommier Y, Cossman J (1993): *bcl-2* Protein Inhibits Etoposide-induced Apoptosis through Its Effect on Events Subsequent to Topoisomerase II-induced DNA Strand Breaks and Their Repair. *Cancer Res* 53:4251-4256

Kane SE, Reinhard DH, Fordis CM, Pastan I, Gottesman MM (1989): A new vector using the human multidrug resistance gene as a selectable marker enables overexpression of foreign genes in eukaryotic cells. *Gene* 84:439-446

Kane SE (1991): HIgh-level expression of foreign genes in mammalian cells. *Genet Engineering* 13:167-182

Kashani-Sabet M, Wang W, Scalon KJ (1991): Cyclosporin A supressess cisplatin-induced c-*fos* gene expression in ovarian carcinoma cells. *J Biol Chem* 265:11285-11288

Keith WN, Brown R (1991): Carcinogenesis and the Response of Tumours to Anticancer Drugs. *Anticancer Res* 11:1739-1744

Lemoine NR, Sikora K (1993): Interventional Genetics and cancer treatment. *Brit Med J* 306:665-666

Liu B, Nguyen KT, Ueda K, Chin K-V (1994): Transactivation of the Human Multidrug Resistance (mdr1) Gene Promoter by p53 Mutants. *Proc AACR* 35:345

Matsumura K, Isola J, Chew K, Henderson C, Smith HS, Harris AL, Hickson ID, WAldman F (1994): Topoisomerase II alpha deletion as well as amplification associated with *erb*B2 amplification in breast cancer. *Proc AACR* 35:454

Mesnil M, Yamasaki H (1993): Cell-Cell Communication and Growth Control of Normal and Cancer Cells: Evidence and Hypothesis. *Molecul Carcinogen* 7:14-17

Miyashita T, Krajewski S, Krajewska M, Wang HG, Lin HK, Lieberman DA, Hoffman B, Reed JC (1994): Tumor suppressor p53 is a regulator of *bcl-2* and *bax* gene expression *in vitro* and *in vivo*. *Oncogene* 9:1799-1804

Pauly M, Ries F, Dicato M (1992a): Genetic Aspects of Multidrug Resistance. *Path Res Pract* 188:804-807

Pauly M, Reis F, Dicato M (1992b): The Genetic Basis of Multidrug Resistance. *Path Res Parct* 188:804-807

Preston-Martin S, Pike MC, Ross RK, Jones PA, Henderson BE (1990): Increased Cell Division as a cause of Human Cancer. *Cancer Res* 50:7415-7412

Preudhomme C, Lepelley P, Vachee A, Soenen V, Quesnel B, Cosson A, Fenaux P (1993): Relationship between p53 Gene Mutations and Multidrug Resistance (mdr1) Gene Expression in Myelodysplastic Syndromes. *Leukemia* 7:1888-1890

Prosperi E, Oliani C, Negri C, Mazzini G, Astaldi-Ricotti G, Bottiroli G (1992): Topoisomerase II and p53 expression in human ovarian tumors. *Anticancer Res* 12:209

Robert J, Barra Y, Riou JF (1992): Résistance aux médicaments anticancéreux. *Quelques lignes de force dans les recherches actuelles* Bull Cancer 79:1025-1030

Rubin E, Kharbanda S, Gunji H, Kufe D (1991): Activation of the c-*jun* proto-oncogene in human myeloid leukemia cells treated with etoposide. *Mol Pharmacol* 39:697-701

Rubin E, Kharbanda S, Gunji H, Kufe D (1992): Cis-diaminochloroplatinum (II) induces c-*jun* expression in human myeloid luekemia cells: Potential involvement of a protein kinase C-dependent signalling pathway. *Cancer Res* 52:878-882

Rüdiger HW (1990): Endogenous carcinogens: implications of an emerging concept. *Mut Res* 238:173-174

Scanlon KJ, Kashani-Sabet M, Miyachi H, Sowers LC, Rossi J (1989): Molecular basis of cis-platin resistance in human carcinomas: Model systems and patients. *Anticancer Res* 9:1301-1312

Sklar M (1988): Increased resistance to cis-diaminedichlor-o-platinum (II) in NIH3T3 cells transformed by *ras* oncogenes. *Cancer Res* 48:793-797

Spandidos DA, Anderson MLM (1989): Oncogenes and onco-suppressor genes: their involvement in cancer. *J Path* 157:

Tsai Ch-M, Chang K-T, Perng R-P, Mitsudomi T, Chen M-H, Kadoyama Ch, Gazdar AF (1993): Correlation of Intrinsic Chemoresistance of Non-Small-Cell Lung Cancer Cell Lines with*HER-2/neu* Gene Expression but Not With *ras* Gene Mutations. *JNCI* 85:897-901

Volm M (1993): P-Glycoprotein Associated Expression of c-*fos* and c-*jun* Products in Human Lung Carcinomas. *Anticancer Res* 13:375-378

Wani MA, Xu X, Stambrook PJ (1994): Increased Methotrexate Resistance and
    dhfr Gene Amplification as a Consequence of Induced *Ha-ras* Expression in
    NIH3T3 Cells. *Cancer Res* 54:2504-2508
Yamamoto T (1993): Molecular Basis of Cancer: Oncogenes and Tumor
    Suppressor Genes. *Microbiol Immunol* 37:11-22
Zastawny RL, Salvino R, Chen J, Benchimol S, Ling V (1993): The core
    promoter of the P-glycoprotein gene is sufficient to confer differential
    responsiveness to wild-type and mutant p53. *Oncogene* 8:1529-1535

12. MECHANISMS OF CISPLATIN RESISTANCE AND ITS REVERSAL IN HUMAN TUMORS

Hironori Ishida, Hiroshi Kijima, Yukinori Ohta, Mohammed Kashani-Sabet, and Kevin J. Scanlon

Despite tremendous strides in understanding the molecular basis of cancer (Weinberg, 1989), treatment of human cancer is still limited by the toxicity of chemotherapeutic agents and the development of intrinsic or acquired resistance to these drugs. *cis*-diamminedichloroplatinum (II) (cisplatin) is one of the most widely-used anticancer agents, active in the treatment of ovarian, testicular, head-and-neck, non-small cell lung and brain tumors, among others (Rosenberg, 1985). However, the rapid development of resistance to cisplatin represents an important challenge to clinicians and laboratory investigators alike. Therefore, understanding the biochemical and molecular basis of cisplatin resistance may potentially result in the development of rational approaches to circumvent this problem. At the core of understanding cisplatin resistance lies the realization of both the similarities and differences between the mechanisms of cisplatin action and resistance and that of other chemotherapeutic agents. Cisplatin-resistant cells display a unique cross-resistance pattern to multiple agents, including anti-metabolites such as 5-fluorouracil and methotrexate, DNA polymerase inhibitors such as azidothymidine (AZT), and topoisomerase inhibitors such as camptothecin and etoposide. This "atypical" multidrug resistance is both phenotypically and molecularly distinct from the "classical" multidrug resistance which may involve overexpression of the MDR-1 gene (Gottesman and Pastan, 1993).

A cursory review of the literature in cisplatin resistance quickly points to a potentially confusing array of mechanisms purported to be involved in this process, most of them seemingly disparate and unrelated. Recent advances in the workings of signal transduction in normal and cancer cells have led to a more cohesive picture of cellular pathways involved in the response to extracellular agents (e.g., growth factors, tumor promoters, viruses, and chemotherapeutic agents). This in turn has merged seemingly independent biochemical processes activated in response to various stimuli. An important molecular mechanism in cisplatin resistance concerns the c-*fos* proto-oncogene. The Fos protein dimerizes with the c-*jun* gene product to drive many important cell processes by transcriptional activation of AP-1-responsive genes (reviewed by Ransone and Verma, 1990). Numerous AP-1-responsive genes have been identified which participate in DNA synthesis and repair processes and which have been implicated in cisplatin resistance (Scanlon et al., 1991a). These include metallothionein, DNA polymerase β, thymidylate synthase, topoisomerase II, and glutathione-S-transferase. Furthermore, the Fos/Jun heterodimers are thought to mediate the effects of H-*ras* activation following growth factor activation (Boguski and McCormick, 1993). And protein kinase C is a known participant in cellular signalling pathways leading to the activation of c-*fos* gene expression (Ransone and Verma, 1990).

The goal of this review is to discuss mechanisms of resistance to cisplatin by developing a clear picture which connects as many of these mechanisms as possible. Glutathione, metallothionein, oncogene expression, protein kinase C, DNA repair, the folate pathway, and DNA polymerases and topoisomerases, all of which have been implicated in cisplatin resistance, can be presented and viewed as part of a complex interrelated cellular network. The review will initially discuss work done in human *in vitro* and *in vivo* model systems, differing in its focus from that of several recent reviews on cisplatin and its analogs (Johnson et al., 1993, 1994; Farrell, 1993; Muggia, 1993; Timmer-Bosscha et al., 1992). Next, strategies employed to circumvent the aforementioned resistance to cisplatin at the biochemical and molecular level will be reviewed. Finally, the potential applications of these studies to gene therapy of cancer will be discussed.

MECHANISMS OF CISPLATIN RESISTANCE

It has been well established that intracellular cisplatin binds to DNA, and that these cisplatin-DNA adducts contribute to cellular toxicity (Fram, 1992). As chemotherapeutic resistance to cisplatin has been investigated in detail, it has become obvious that there are multiple mechanisms of cisplatin resistance (Fram, 1992; Perez et al., 1993). These include (1) alterations in cisplatin transport, (2) enhanced detoxification mechanisms, (3) increased repair or tolerance of DNA damage, (4) alterations in signal transduction, and (5) alterations in mitochondrial membrane potential.

Cisplatin Transport

Decreased intracellular cisplatin accumulation, resulting from decreased influx or increased efflux of cisplatin, has been shown in many, but not all, cisplatin-resistant tumor cell lines (Andrews and Howell, 1990). However, the decreased level of accumulation does not correlate with the level of cisplatin resistance. Therefore, the resistance to cisplatin may be determined not only by the decreased accumulation of cisplatin, but also other molecular mechanisms.

Several reports have shown that cisplatin enters cells through passive diffusion (Gale et al., 1973; Ogawa et al., 1975). Despite the evidence of passive diffusion, the data supporting an active transporter for cisplatin has been increasing. Properties of amino acid transport systems were altered in K562 human leukemia cells resistant to cisplatin (Shionoya et al., 1986). The sodium-dependent uptake for methylaminoisobutyric acid was significantly inhibited by threonine in the K562 sensitive cell line, while the uptake was minimally inhibited in the K562 cell subline resistant to cisplatin. When the K562 resistant cell subline was grown in the absence of cisplatin, its amino acid transport properties, as well as cisplatin resistance, reverted to those of the K562 sensitive cell line. These data suggested that cellular membrane amino acid transport systems might be altered in cisplatin resistance. Recently, a 200-kD membrane glycoprotein was identified in a R1.1 murine lymphoma cell subline resistant to cisplatin, and was distinct from the multidrug resistance-associated P-glycoprotein (Kawai et al., 1990). The R1.1 subline was 40-fold resistant to cisplatin, but had only a 2-fold decrease in cisplatin accumulation. However, the levels of the 200-kD glycoprotein correlated with reduced cisplatin accumulation. The ultimate contribution of the 200-kD glycoprotein to cisplatin resistance awaits further characterization (Bernal, 1990).

Several *in vivo* studies of cisplatin resistance have been reported. The 2008 human ovarian carcinoma cells were made resistant to cisplatin as xenografts in athymic mice (Andrews et al., 1990). The cisplatin-resistant cells (2.2- to 1.4-fold) showed a 28% decrease in cisplatin accumulation, which might be associated with cisplatin resistance. Similar studies were performed with the A2780 human ovarian cell carcinoma (Rose and Basler, 1990), but the mechanisms of cisplatin resistance were not clarified.

Although many investigators have studied the uptake and accumulation of cisplatin, there is limited data on cisplatin efflux. In one study, the efflux of cisplatin from 2008 human ovarian carcinoma cells was biphasic, with a very rapid initial phase followed by a much slower terminal phase (Mann et al., 1990). The biphasic efflux was also observed in K562 human leukemia cells as measured by ^{195m}Pt-cisplatin retention (Shionoya et al., 1986). Cisplatin interacts with cellular glutathione (GSH), and the complex of 2:1 molar ratio of GSH/cisplatin has been detected in L1210 murine leukemia cells (Ishikawa and Ali-Osman, 1993). The transport of the GSH/cisplatin complex across the cell membrane was found to be an ATP-dependent process which is inhibited by vanadate, S-(2,4-dinitrophenyl)-glutathione, leukotriene C_4 and glutathione disulfide. Correlation between the ATP-dependent efflux and cisplatin accumulation by Na^+, K^+-ATPase (Andrews et al., 1991) is not known.

Sulfhydryl Peptides

Glutathione (GSH) is one of the most prevalent cellular sulfhydryl peptides, and has been shown to be involved in many cellular functions such as protection of oxidative stress, drug metabolism and intracellular detoxification (Meister and Anderson, 1983). Although levels of GSH are commonly increased in cisplatin-resistant tumor cell lines, its role in contributing to resistance remains controversial. Several investigators have reported a significant correlation between cellular GSH and cisplatin sensitivity; however, increases in GSH were less than increases in cisplatin resistance in human cell lines (Mistry et al., 1991; Godwin et al., 1992). The BE human colon cancer cell subline, resistant to cisplatin, showed a 3-fold increase in GSH which was associated with a 5-fold resistance to cisplatin and a significant decrease in DNA interstrand cross-link formation compared with the sensitive cell lines (Farm et al., 1990). DNA intrastrand cross-link formation was equivalent in BE resistant and sensitive cell lines. GSH may thus interfere with the conversion of DNA-cisplatin adducts to DNA interstrand cross-links.

Glutathione S-transferases (GST) are widely distributed enzymes that may participate in the metabolism and detoxification of environmental toxins and chemotherapeutic drugs (Pickett and Lu, 1989). Several investigators have reported a relationship between cisplatin resistance and the activity of GST. In one study, a human embryonal cell carcinoma subline resistant to cisplatin showed 1.5-fold increased GST activity as well as a 1.4-fold increased GSH level (Timmer-Bosscha et al., 1993). By contrast, the other studies revealed no remarkable correlation between GST and cisplatin resistance (Fujiwara et al., 1990a; Nakagawa et al., 1990).

Metallothioneins are small, thiol-rich proteins important in binding and detoxifying heavy metals (Hamer, 1986). Several reports have suggested that some, but not all, cell lines resistant to cisplatin may have increased expression for metallothioneins (Kelly et al., 1988; Schilder et al., 1990; Andrews and Howell, 1990). In one model system, transfected mouse C127 cells containing the human metallothionein-IIa gene were resistant to cisplatin, melphalan and chlorambucil (Kelly et al., 1988). Universal overexpression of metallothionein-IIa, compared with other metallothionein isoforms, was detected in the SCC25 human head-and-neck squamous cell carcinoma cell subline, and H69 and SW2 human small cell lung carcinoma cell sublines resistant to cisplatin (Yang et al., 1994). In another study, H69 cells were shown to have elevated levels of metallothionein, 1.6- and 2.3-fold in 6.2- and 10.0-fold cisplatin resistant cells, respectively (Kasahara et al., 1991). In addition, decreased levels of DNA interstrand cross-links correlated with levels of resistance to cisplatin in the H69 cells. By contrast, 48 patients were analyzed for changes in metallothionein levels in ovarian tumors before and after chemotherapy. The conclusion from these studies was that metallothionein content was not a major determinant of tumor sensitivity to chemotherapy (Murphy et al., 1991). Metallothionein and GST may play a role in cisplatin resistance, in concert with other mechanisms which may drive their expression (Scanlon et al., 1991a).

Repair of Cisplatin-DNA Adducts

Several studies indicate that the cellular toxicity of cisplatin occurs through its ability to covalently bind to DNA and prevent DNA replication and transcription. Cisplatin attacks the N7 position of guanine residues to form several types of adducts with DNA bases. The two major adducts are Pt-d(GpG) and Pt-d(ApG) intrastrand cross-links, and the remaining include Pt-(dG) monoadducts, Pt-d(GpNpG) intrastrand cross-links, and Pt(dG)$_2$ interstrand cross-links (Eastman, 1982, 1986; Fichtinger-Schepman et al., 1985; Corda et al., 1993). The cells exposed to cisplatin must either repair or tolerate the resulting DNA damage (i.e., cisplatin-DNA adducts) in order to survive. Several investigators have reported evidence of increased DNA repair (2- to 4-fold) in the total genomic DNA of cisplatin-resistant cells (Eastman and Schulte, 1988; Masuda et al., 1988, 1990; Lai et al., 1988; Parker et al., 1991). There also appears to be a correlation between repair of cisplatin-DNA damage *in vitro* and cytotoxicity (Roberts and Friedlas, 1987; Scanlon et al., 1990a), supported by data from clinical samples (Reed et al., 1987, 1990; Kashani-Sabet et al., 1990b).

In several model systems, it appears that DNA repair occurs preferentially in transcribed genes relative to the overall genome (Bohr, 1991). In a methotrexate-resistant Chinese hamster ovary cell line with elevated dihydrofolate reductase, cisplatin-DNA adducts were removed faster in the transcribed region of the dihydrofolate reductase and c-*myc* genes than in the non-coding region of the *fos* gene (Jones et al., 1991). It has also been reported that the gene-specific repair of cisplatin interstrand cross-links may be associated with cellular resistance in human ovarian cancer cell lines (Zhen et al., 1992).

A recent development concerns the identification of proteins that can recognize cisplatin-modified DNA (Toney et al., 1989; Chu and Chang, 1990; Fujiwara et al., 1990b). Three investigative groups have characterized 80-130 kDa proteins that bind specifically to cisplatin-modified DNA, but are not differentially expressed in cells that differ in resistance to cisplatin (Andrews and Jones, 1991; Bruhn et al., 1992; Pil and Lippard, 1992; Chao et al., 1991). The first group detected proteins which specifically bind to DNA damaged by platinum compounds of *cis* but not *trans* stereochemistry. The protein level has been similar in ovarian and kidney tubule cell lines with different sensitivities to cisplatin (Andrews and Jones, 1991). The second group reported the cloning of a previously identified structure-specific recognition protein SSRP1

(Bruhn et al., 1992). The cDNA sequence predicts an 81 kDa protein with a stretch of amino acids with 47% identity to human high mobility group 1 (HMG1). The binding of recombinant rat HMG1 protein to cisplatin-damaged DNA and specifically to intrastrand d(GpG) and d(ApG) adducts has been previously demonstrated (Pil and Lippard, 1992). A third group has reported that two DNA damage recognition proteins, approximately 130 and 95kDa, were induced after exposure of HeLa cells to cisplatin and were overexpressed in cisplatin-resistant HeLa cells (Chao et al., 1991).

DNA polymerases constitute some of the enzymes necessary to repair cisplatin-DNA damage (Lai et al., 1989; Scanlon et al., 1989a,b,c). Our studies have shown enhanced levels of DNA polymerase ß between 3 and 9 hours after cisplatin treatment (Scanlon et al., 1990b), suggesting transient expression in response to cisplatin. However, 2008 ovarian carcinomas did not have elevated mRNA levels for DNA polymerase α and ß 18 hours after cisplatin treatment (Katz et al., 1990). A second class of repair enzymes, ERCC1 and ERCC2, has been implicated in cisplatin resistance (Hoeijmakers and Bootsma, 1990). In a study which analyzed expression of ERCC1 and ERCC2 in tumor tissue from patients with ovarian cancer, a 2.6-fold higher expression level of the ERCC1 gene was observed in tumor tissues of patients clinically resistant to therapy, as compared to ERCC1 expression in tissues from patients who responded to therapy (Dabholkar et al., 1992). The relative levels of expression of ERCC2 did not differ significantly between responders and non-responders. Dihydrofolate reductase, dTMP synthase and topoisomerases have also been implicated in cisplatin resistance (Scanlon and Kashani-Sabet, 1988; Scanlon et al., 1990b, 1991a). The repair of damaged DNA likely includes several enzymatic steps; the above mentioned enzymes could exist as a multi-enzymatic complex that responds to nuclear oncogene expression and repairs the damaged chromosome (Reddy and Pardee, 1980; Pardee, 1987).

Using patient materials, tumors from ovarian or colon cancer patients failing to respond to cisplatin-based treatment have elevated gene expression of enzymes associated with DNA repair (Kashani-Sabet et al., 1988, 1990b), and these studies are consistent with data on ovarian and colon carcinoma cell lines in culture (Scanlon et al., 1989b).

Signal Transduction Pathway

Cell growth and differentiation can be initiated by signal cascades (Edelman et al., 1987; Hunter, 1991). Cancer chemotherapeutic agents have been shown to disrupt this signal transduction pathway which may contribute to the evolution of drug- resistant clones (Brunton and Workman, 1993; Tritton and Hickman, 1990).

Membrane signal transduction includes two major pathways; the first is through protein kinase C (PKC), and the second is through cAMP and protein kinase A (PKA). Both PKC and PKA are followed by nuclear signaling through a phosphorylation cascade. PKC is activated by growth factors, such as epidermal growth factor (EGF) and platelet-derived growth factor (PDGF), and the tumor promoter 12-O-tetradecanoylphorbol-13-acetate (TPA). It has been reported that EGF increased cisplatin sensitivity in human ovarian carcinoma cell lines (Christen et al., 1990). The sensitization to cisplatin was shown to be dependent on both EGF concentration and EGF receptor number; the results suggested that the signal pathway activated by EGF determined the sensitivity to cisplatin. A monoclonal antibody against the c-*erb*B-2 protein, a member of the EGF receptor family, also enhanced the cytotoxicity of cisplatin against a human breast cancer cell line (Hancock et al., 1991). TPA is a dynamic modulator of PKC (see the following section "Modulators of Cisplatin Resistance"). A PKC activator, bryostatin 1, sensitized human cervical carcinoma cells to cisplatin (Basu and Lazo, 1992), possibly by increasing cellular accumulation of cisplatin. Meanwhile, several ligands such as prostaglandins stimulate adenyl cyclase, resulting in increased intracellular cAMP levels. The increased cAMP activates PKA. In one study, a relationship between cAMP and cisplatin uptake has been described (Mann et al., 1991). Cisplatin uptake was correlated to cAMP levels in the human ovarian cell carcinoma cell line, while the uptake was not associated with cAMP levels in the resistant cell subline to cisplatin. This study showed that the signal pathway through cAMP and PKA could be modulated to enhance sensitivity to cisplatin.

Membrane tyrosine kinases associated with the EGF receptor family combine with *ras* p21 to activate a cascade which involves *raf*-1, MAP kinase kinase, and MAP kinase (Roberts, 1992). MAP kinase translocates to the nucleus and may phosphorylate Jun and Fos proteins. Activator protein 1 (AP-1) plays an important role in transcription of DNA. AP-1 is a complex of several different proteins, including the c-*jun* and c-*fos* proteins. c-*jun* expression was induced by treatment of human myeloid leukemia cells with cisplatin (Rubin et al., 1992). The increased c-*jun* expression could be associated with the PKC-dependent pathway because down-regulation of PKC by TPA decreased the cisplatin-induced c-*jun* expression. The oncogene *fos* showed increased expression in cisplatin resistant cells and with cisplatin treatment *in vitro* (Scanlon et al., 1988, 1989c; Hollander and Fornace, 1989) and in patients (Scanlon et al., 1988, 1989b). The c-*fos* oncogene has been shown to modulate the expression of AP-1 responsive genes such as dTMP synthase, topoisomerase I and metallothionein. A *fos* ribozyme has also been shown to completely reverse cisplatin resistance by downregulating these genes (Scanlon et al., 1991a; see the following section "The *fos* Oncogene in Drug Resistance"). Both nuclear oncogenes *jun* and *fos* may play a role in the cellular response to cisplatin-induced DNA damage and in the development of cisplatin resistance.

The p53 gene, which codes for a nuclear transcription factor, is known to play a crucial role in the regulation of DNA replication at the G1/S checkpoint (Kastan et al., 1991; Kuerbits et al., 1992). Wild-type p53 allows cells to arrest in G1 so as to provide an opportunity for DNA repair prior to commencement of replicative DNA synthesis. In contrast, mutant p53 proteins are unable to act in this manner; p53 mutations are now believed to be a major cause of genetic instability in many cancers (Raycroft et al., 1990). Elevated p53 protein levels were observed in both A2780/cp70 and OVPI/DDP cisplatin-resistant ovarian human tumor lines. The A2780 cell line had a wild-type p53 gene, while the OVIP/DDP had a heterozygous mutation at codon 126 (Brown et al., 1993). These data suggested the close correlation between cisplatin resistance and DNA repair ability conferred by the functioning p53 protein.

The role of DNA polymerase ß in the cell has been linked to DNA repair by gap-filling synthesis (Wang, 1991; see section "Repair of Cisplatin-DNA Adducts"). DNA polymerase ß, as well as metallothionein, has an H-*ras* responsive element that responds to changes in H-*ras* gene expression (Schmidt and Hamer, 1986; Kedar et al., 1990). Some reports show a correlation between cisplatin resistance and H-*ras* gene expression (Sklar, 1988; Niimi et al., 1991). These studies have been confirmed in cisplatin-resistant human cells *in vitro* and from patients (Scanlon and Kashani-Sabet, 1989; Scanlon et al., 1989b, c; Kashani-Sabet et al., 1990b). The H-*ras* oncogene has also been shown to influence the methionine requirement in H-*ras* transformed cells

(Vanhamme and Szpirer, 1987). These studies strengthen the link between methionine/folate metabolism, DNA repair systems and proto-oncogenes. H-*ras* may also enhance transcriptional activity of c-*jun* through specific changes in the phosphorylation of the Jun protein (Binetruy et al., 1991).

Topoisomerase I and II are nuclear enzymes involved in various DNA transactions such as replication, transcription, and recombination (Wang, 1985; Liu, 1989). The function of topoisomerase II is based on its ability to relax DNA in a two-step process involving the nicking and religation of both strands of the DNA double helix. Novobiocin, a topoisomerase II inhibitor, inhibited 73% of topoisomerase II activity in the nuclear extracts of HBT28 human glioblastoma cells; residual DNA cross-linking in the cells was increased by 3-fold in cells treated with cisplatin, compared with untreated cells (Ali-Osman et al., 1993). The data suggested that topoisomerase II could potentially affect the level of DNA interstrand cross-links induced by cisplatin.

Mitochondrial Membrane Potential

Alterations in membrane structure and function that affect resistance to cisplatin are not limited to the cell membrane, but also extend to the mitochondrial membrane. 2008 human ovarian carcinoma cell sublines resistant to cisplatin had a variety of mitochondrial defects; the defects increased sensitivity both to mitochondrial poisons and cisplatin (Andrew and Albright, 1992).

CIRCUMVENTING CISPLATIN RESISTANCE

Platin Analogs

Cisplatin has proven effective against testicular (Cavalli, 1983), ovarian (Wiltshaw et al., 1986), and small cell and non-small cell lung cancer (Evans et al., 1986; Bonomi, 1986). In recent years, the search for platin compounds with reduced toxicity and broad antitumor activity has been the main goal in development of the first generation of platin analogs. Carboplatin (Bradner et al., 1980; Connors et al., 1979) and iproplatin (Bradner et al., 1980) were initially developed and have been used in many *in vitro* studies and clinical trials. Although cisplatin and carboplatin are the only two platinum compounds in clinical use, and iproplatin has just started clinical trials (Sessa et al., 1990), they may not be as effective as cisplatin against a wide spectrum of tumors (Harstrick et al., 1989). In addition, these analogues are cross-resistant to cisplatin in ovarian cancer (Eisenhauer et al., 1990; Sessa et al., 1988). In the last few years, however, several new platin compounds have been synthesized and have shown promise in tissue culture and clinical trials against human tumors (Christian, 1992; Hamilton et al., 1993; Gordon and Hollander, 1993).

Ormaplatin [tetrachloro(D,L-*Trans*)1,2 diamino cyclohexane platinum (IV)] (formerly known as tetraplatin) is a second generation platin analog which displays a broad spectrum of antitumor activity against the L1210 murine leukemia cisplatin-resistant cell line (Anderson et al., 1986), human ovarian carcinoma cisplatin-resistant cell lines (Perez et al., 1991; Scanlon et al., 1987, 1989b), small cell lung carcinoma (Hospers et al., 1988), colon carcinoma, and breast carcinoma (Scanlon et al., 1989b). However, it is clearly not effective against all cisplatin-resistant cell lines (Schmidt and Chaney, 1993; Kelland et al., 1992a; Perez et al., 1991). In preclinical studies, ormaplatin is less nephrotoxic than cisplatin (Muller et al., 1991). A phase I clinical trial of ormaplatin was initiated by O'Rourke et al., (1991), and preliminary results show mild myelosuppression, nausea, vomiting and severe peripheral neuropathy in very few cases without nephrotoxicity (Petros et al., 1994; Plaxe et al., 1993).

Oxaliplatin, *trans*-1-diaminocyclohexane-platinum, shows effectiveness that is similar to that of cisplatin against several transplanted murine tumors (Boughattas et al., 1989), without the development of nephrotoxicity (Mathe et al., 1985). A phase I clinical trial of oxaliplatin was conducted by Mathe et al. (1986). In other phase I studies, oxaliplatin, at equally active doses of cisplatin, did not cause nephrotoxicity and had far less myelosuppression (Extra et al., 1990; Caussanel et al., 1990), but the dose-limiting toxicity was peripheral sensory neuropathy (Extra et al., 1990). Phase II studies are under way using high doses of oxaliplatin resulting from optimization of circadian rhythm-based strategies and in combination with 5-fluorouracil. Preliminary studies have shown clinical responses to oxaliplatin alone and in combination with 5-fluorouracil (Misset et al., 1991).

L-NDDP, *cis*-Bis-neodecanoato-*trans*-R,R-1,2-diaminohexane platinum(II), represents another attempt to improve the therapeutic index of platinum therapy by entrapping the drug in liposomes to reduce toxicity and by incorporating the diaminocyclohexane (DACH) moiety as a means of overcoming platinum resistance (Christian, 1992). L-NDDP is not cross-resistant to cisplatin in the A2780/CDDP ovarian carcinoma cell line and in L1210/CDDP leukemia cells (Han et al., 1993; Perez-Soler et al., 1987), and has shown greater efficacy than cisplatin *in vivo* against L1210 leukemia and liver metastases of M5076 reticulosarcoma (Perez-Soler et al., 1987).   The major toxicity in mice is myelosuppression and in dogs the lethal dose resulted in an acute and diffuse hemorrhagic syndrome involving mainly the gastrointestinal tract. However, nephrotoxicity is not observed (Perez-Soler et al., 1989). In a phase I study, the dose limiting toxicity is myelosuppression affecting all three blood cell lineages (Perez-Soler et al., 1990).

DWA2114R and CI-973(NK-121) are included in the cyclobutanedicarboxylato compound group. DWA2114R is active against cisplatin and carboplatin-resistant cell lines (Endo et al., 1992). CI-973 reveals cross resistance to cisplatin in the lower level of cisplatin-resistant ovarian carcinoma cell lines; conversely, the drug is active against higher levels of cisplatin resistance (Perez et al., 1991).   254-S (cis-diammine(glycolate)platinum II) is one of the other new platinum analogs and is active against a cisplatin-resistant murine leukemia (McKeage et al., 1991).   In a phase I study of DWA2114R, CI-973 and 254-S, no nephrotoxicity was observed, but myelosuppression was frequent though rarely severe (Majima, 1991).

Amine/amine dicarboxylate platinum (II or IV) compounds (e.g., JM216, JM221, JM244) are suitable for oral administration with activity against cisplatin-resistant tumors (McKeage et al., 1991, 1994a; Kelland et al., 1991, 1992a; Yoshida et al., 1994).   JM216 and JM221 are not cross-resistant to the A2780/CDDP ovarian carcinoma cell line (Schuring et al., 1991).   Both JM221 and JM244 also reveal no cross resistance to the 41M *cis*R ovarian carcinoma cell line with cisplatin resistance, and L1210/CDDP and L1210/ormaplatin-resistant leukemia cell lines (Kelland et al., 1992b; Orr et al., 1991).   Preclinical studies of JM216 show no nephrotoxicity compared to cisplatin and ormaplatin at the maximal tolerated dose in rats (McKeage et al., 1994b).

Modulators of Cisplatin Resistance

As we elucidate the mechanisms of action for cisplatin, rational strategies will emerge to exploit or circumvent the phenotypic properties of cisplatin-resistant cells. Several classes of biochemical modulators have been identified that modulate acquired cisplatin resistance (Timmer-Bosscha et al., 1992; Gately and Howell, 1993; and see section

"Mechanisms of Cisplatin Resistance").

Hyperthermia is a membrane modulator and has been shown to increase cisplatin uptake and cytotoxicity in both cisplatin sensitive and resistant cell lines (Wallner et al., 1986; Eichholtz-Wirth and Hietel, 1990); however, the cytotoxic and the drug-sensitizing effect of heat appears to vary significantly between cell lines (Eichholtz-Wirth and Hietel, 1986). Another mechanism shown to increase intercellular cisplatin accumulation concerns lowering extracellular pH and osmolarity (Andrews et al., 1987).

Amphotericin B (AmB), an antifungal agent, has been shown to reverse resistance to cisplatin (Masuda et al., 1991), possibly by decreasing intracellular potassium ion stores resulting from the modification of membrane permeability. In a recent study, amphotericin-induced increases in cisplatin-induced interstrand cross-link formation were observed, the magnitudes of which corresponded to the magnitudes of AmB-augmented cisplatin cytotoxicity. Increased intracellular cisplatin accumulation is observed in the presence of AmB in cisplatin-sensitive and resistant human lung cancer cell lines that are sensitized to cisplatin by AmB (Morikage et al., 1993).

Docosahexanenoic acid (DCHA) has been shown to change the lipid membrane composition of small cell lung carcinoma cells and enhance cisplatin activity in the cisplatin-resistant cells (Timmer-Bosscha et al., 1989). This three-fold increase in cisplatin cytotoxicity in the resistant cells was not associated with drug transport or changes in GSH levels, but with decreased ability to remove cisplatin-DNA adducts. These results suggest that DCHA may modify the signal transduction pathway and thus limit the cell's ability to repair damaged DNA.

Calcium channel blockers and calmodulin antagonists have been shown to have synergistic toxicity when either are combined with cisplatin. Verapamil, a calcium channel blocker, enhances the antitumor effect of cisplatin against transplanted neuroblastoma in BALB/c athymic mice (Ikeda et al., 1987). Naphthalenesulfonamide, a calmodulin antagonist, also enhances the synergistic effect, compared to treatment with naphthalenesulfonamide or cisplatin alone in BALB/c athymic mice bearing human ovarian carcinoma (Kikuchi et al., 1987). However, some experiments have shown no synergy using the aforementioned combinations (Hong et al., 1988; Onoda et al., 1989). Thus, the synergistic effect of the agents with cisplatin may depend on the individual cell lines, with the mechanism remaining uncertain at this time.

Protein kinases have been shown to play an important role in the signal transduction pathway, which involves membrane ion fluxes, modulation of AP-responsive elements and direct effects on DNA synthesis enzymes (see section "Signal Transduction Pathway"). Thus, it is not surprising that heavy metals (Zn^{2+}, Cd^{2+} and Hg^{2+}) have been shown to inhibit TPA binding and alter protein kinase activity (Speizer et al., 1989).

Forskolin, an adenyl cyclase antagonist which leads to the activation of PKA by increasing cAMP, has been shown to enhance the cellular accumulation and cytotoxicity of cisplatin in resistant 2008 cells. However, forskolin caused a marked increase in cAMP levels in both sensitive and resistant 2008 cells. Therefore, these findings suggest that there is a target downstream of PKA that is an important participant in cisplatin accumulation, and that this target is defective or missing in cisplatin-resistant cells (Mann et al., 1991).

TPA is a dynamic modulator of PKC, depending on the dose and length of exposure. TPA can act directly on responsive elements of DNA synthesis genes such as topoisomerase I (Pommier et al., 1990), the metallothionein IIA gene (Hamer, 1986) and the c-*fos* and c-*jun* oncogenes (Huang et al., 1991). If cells have a short term exposure to TPA, a transient level of increased PKC activity and gene expression is noted. In contrast, long term exposure to TPA results in decreased PKC activity and gene expression in the signal transduction pathway. TPA has been shown to transiently modulate cisplatin toxicity in human ovarian carcinoma cells (2.5-fold) after 1 hr and 24 hr but not 7 day exposures (Isonishi et al., 1990). TPA has also been shown to cause a 9-fold increase in cisplatin cytotoxicity in HeLa cells with a 24 hr exposure (Basu et al., 1990). Lyngbyatoxin A, a potent activator of PKC, is as effective as TPA in enhancing the sensitivity of HeLa cells to cisplatin (9-fold). Interestingly, inhibitors of PKC, such as quercetin, ilmofosine, and staurosporin (Hofmann et al., 1988; Basu et al., 1991) also affect cisplatin cytotoxicity. Thus, the mechanism of modulation of cisplatin sensitivity related to PKC remains uncertain. One clue may be provided by studies showing that the protein kinase inhibitor, H-7, inhibits c-*fos* mRNA accumulation and the transcriptional activation of c-*fos* (Shibanura et al., 1987).

Tamoxifen (TAM), which has the ability to inhibit the function of the estrogen receptor (ER), calmodulin and PKC, has also been shown to enhance the cytotoxicity of cisplatin in human melanoma cell lines (McClay et al., 1992b). The combination chemotherapy including TAM in patients with metastatic melanoma also reveals a marked response rate that is not seen in regimens excluding TAM (McClay et al., 1989). The synergy between TAM and cisplatin is not mediated by the effects of TAM on the ER, calmodulin, PKC, or cell cycle regulation (McClay et al., 1993).

EGF increases cisplatin sensitivity in the two human ovarian carcinoma cell lines 2008 and 316, and its effect depends on the EGF concentration and number of EGF receptors. However, EGF does not enhance sensitivity to cisplatin in the cisplatin-resistant 2008 cell line despite the presence of functional EGF receptors on these cells. This suggests that cisplatin cytoxicity may be associated with a defect in EGF signal transduction pathway (Christen et al., 1990).   Cyclosporin A (CSA), used primarily as an immunosuppressant in transplantation, has been shown to reverse resistance to a variety of chemotherapeutic agents, including cisplatin (Kashani-Sabet et al., 1990a). It is intriguing that CSA can restore sensitivity to cisplatin-resistant cells because of the potential clinical implications. It has been suggested that CSA interacts with either plasma membrane potentials (Damjanovich et al., 1986), calcium-calmodulin pathways (Colombiani et al., 1985), or acts by suppressing nuclear oncogene expression (Kashani-Sabet et al., 1990a; Scanlon et al., 1990b).

The role of GSH in resistance to cisplatin has been extensively studied (see section "Sulfhydryl Peptides") but the data remains inconclusive. BSO (D,L-buthionine-S-R-sulphoximine), a known irreversible inhibitor of the GSH synthesis enzyme gamma glutamyl cysteine synthetase, has been shown to modulate sensitivity of cisplatin in cisplatin-resistant cell lines (2- to 4-fold). Several investigators (Hamilton et al., 1985; Meijer et al., 1990, Meijer et al., 1992) examined the efficacy of pretreatment with BSO followed by treatment with several platin analogs in two cisplatin-resistant cell lines. In the GLC_4/CDDP cell line, GSH depleted by BSO increased sensitivity to cisplatin, carboplatin, zeniplatin, and enloplatin (1.7- to 3.2-fold) but not labaplatin, iproplatin, and tetraplatin. On the other hand, in the Tera-CP cell line, Tera-CP plus BSO increased sensitivity to cisplatin, carboplatin and zeniplatin (1.2- to 1.9-fold) but not other platin analogs (Meijer et al., 1992). This may reflect the specificity of various cell lines. BSO treatment may play a role in eliminating GSH from the cytosol and enhancing the formation of platin-DNA adducts. However, pretreatment with BSO has been shown to increase cellular platinum levels in both GLC_4 and GLC_4/CDDP cells while platinum-DNA binding remains unchanged (Meijer et al., 1992). Thus, BSO-mediated depletion of glutathione levels results in only partial reversal of cisplatin resistance, in contrast to that achieved by CSA or ribozymes (see Section "The *fos* Oncogene in Drug Resistance").

Aphidicolin (APC), a specific inhibitor of DNA polymerase α, can dramatically reduce the level of DNA synthesis (Sheaff et al., 1991) and inhibit DNA repair synthesis in cisplatin-sensitive and resistant A2780 cell lines (Lai et al., 1989). Hrubisko et al. have shown that APC itself demonstrated cytotoxicity in cisplatin-resistant L1210 cells (L1210RC). Moreover, the cytotoxicity of cisplatin was enhanced by APC (Hrubiski et al., 1993). Aphidicolin glycinate (AG), which was developed as a water-soluble salt of APC suitable for clinical study, and the combination of AG with cisplatin *in vivo* markedly increased the survival rate compared to the administration of cisplatin alone (O'Dwyer et al., 1994). The combination of BSO and APC has been shown to additively increase the cytotoxicity of cisplatin in human ovarian carcinoma cells (Lai et al., 1989).

Novobiocin a topoisomerase II inhibitor that has been shown to enhance the cytotoxicity of cisplatin in several cisplatin-resistant cell lines with increased topoisomerase II activity (De Jong et al., 1990). Novobiocin has also been shown to increase DNA interstrand cross-links (De Jong et al., 1991). Administration of 200µM of novobiocin alone shows no direct cytotoxicity in human glioblastoma multiforme cells, although it inhibits 73% of topoisomerase II activity (Ali-Osman et al., 1993). However, in this cell line, novobiocin also enhanced the cytotoxicity of cisplatin with increasing DNA interstrand cross-links (Ali-Osman et al., 1993).

The c-fos Oncogene in Drug Resistance

Several investigations in a variety of cisplatin-resistant cell lines have suggested the importance of the c-*fos* oncogene in drug resistance (Scanlon et al., 1989b). The A2780DDP cisplatin-resistant ovarian carcinoma cell line has been shown to exhibit c-*fos* overexpression, concomitant with overexpression of oncogenes (c-H-*ras*, c-*myc*), thymidine synthesis genes (TS, TK), DNA synthesis and repair genes (DNA polymerase ß, topoisomerases) and metallothionein II-A (hMTII-A) (Scanlon et al., 1990b, 1991a). *In vivo*, tumor cells derived from a patient with colon adenocarcinoma failing cisplatin/5-FUra treatment revealed a similar pattern of gene expression to the A2780DDP cells (Kashani-Sabet et al., 1990b). The hypothesis that some of these genes are induced by overexpression of c-*fos* can be supported by the following experiments: i) in A2780DDP cells, c-*fos* was rapidly expressed within 1 hr of cisplatin treatment. TS subsequently increased within 2 hr and DNA polymerase ß and topoisomerase I were expressed within 3 hr (Scanlon et al., 1990b). Thus, c-*fos*, an early response gene (Greenberg and Ziff, 1984), effectuates a cascade of gene expression. ii) The A2780S cisplatin sensitive cell line transfected with the c-*fos* gene showed overexpression of c-*fos*, TS, DNA polymerase ß, topoisomerase I and hMTII-A, and simultaneously demonstrated cisplatin resistance almost at the same magnitude as the A2780DDP cell line (Funato et al., 1992). iii) dTMP synthase (Takeishi et al., 1989), topoisomerase I (Kunze et al., 1990) and hMTII-A (Lee et al., 1987) contain AP-1 binding sequences in their 5' regulatory sequences. DNA polymerase ß contains a *ras*-responsive element (Kedar et al., 1990) and *fos* has been shown to operate downstream of H-*ras* in signal transduction pathway (Ledwith et al., 1990). These findings suggest that the c-*fos* oncogene can stimulate these AP-1 responsive genes.

Thus, as described above, c-*fos* plays an important role in the development of cisplatin resistance. Based on these studies, we have designed a *fos* ribozyme which selectively cleaves c-*fos* mRNA and uncouples the sequential expression of the genes necessary for DNA repair. Hammerhead ribozymes are catalytic RNAs that can cleave a specific RNA sequence and do not require an external energy source (Cech and Bass, 1986). Specificity of the cleavage reaction is accomplished by complementarity between the ribozyme and the sequences flanking the target RNA. *Trans*-acting catalytic RNAs use any GUX (X being A, C, or U) as the target for cleavage of the RNA (Haseloff and Gerlach, 1988). DNA encoding the c-*fos* ribozyme was cloned into the pMAMneo plasmid and transfected into cisplatin-resistant A2780DDP cells (Scanlon et al., 1991b; Funato et al., 1992). The transformants were shown to have restored sensitivity to cisplatin, as well as diminished c-*fos* expression and reversed cellular morphology. Moreover, the expression of TS, DNA polymerase ß, topoisomerase I and hMTII-A was suppressed with *fos* ribozyme action. In our current study, an actinomycin D-resistant A2780 cell line (A2780AD) which exhibits the multidrug resistance (MDR) phenotype but is not cross-resistant to cisplatin demonstrates the overexpression of c-*fos*, mdr-1, p53 and topoisomerase I genes. This A2780AD cell line which was transfected with the c-*fos* ribozyme also shows downregulation of these genes and restored sensitivity to actinomycin D (Scanlon et al., 1994). Therefore, the c-*fos* ribozyme can be an effective strategy for circumvention of drug resistance in cell cultures and possibly even in patients.

CSA has been shown to modulate cisplatin resistance (see section "Modulators of Cisplatin Resistance"). The A2780DDP cell line treated with CSA reveals dramatic reversal of cisplatin resistance as well as the overexpression of c-*fos*, c-H-*ras*, TS, DNA polymerase ß and topoisomerase I and II (Scanlon et al., 1990b). Overall, CSA has the potential to modulate cisplatin resistance similar to the c-*fos* ribozyme. Thus, the signal transduction pathway, including especially c-*fos*, plays an important role in cisplatin resistance processes and has been the target of strategies used to modulate gene expression and consequently reverse cisplatin resistance.

BIOCHEMICAL MODULATION OF CISPLATIN RESISTANCE

Given the involvement of certain important biochemical pathways in the development of cisplatin resistance, rational strategies can be devised to exploit these mechanisms and potentiate cytotoxicity of chemotherapeutic agents in cisplatin-resistant cells. These strategies include the use of the thymidylate synthase cycle, the thymidine salvage pathway, and nucleoside analogs.

The increased expression of enzymes involved in synthesis and phosphorylation of thymidine in cisplatin-resistant cells has led to intriguing observations regarding the biochemical modulation of drug cytotoxicity. Correlating with overexpression of thymidine kinase and DNA polymerase ß in cisplatin-resistant cells, HCT8DDP and A2780DDP cells are cross-resistant to azidothymidine (AZT). AZT is thought to achieve cytotoxicity at the cellular level by inhibition of DNA polymerase ß, as well as incorporation of AZTTP as a suicide substrate into DNA, causing chain termination. Therefore, the mechanism of cross-resistance to AZT in cisplatin-resistant cells is likely the overexpression of DNA polymerase ß (Scanlon et al., 1989c, 1990a). However, the upregulation of the aforementioned enzymes can be manipulated to render cisplatin-resistant cells sensitive to the action of AZT. For instance, in HCT8DDP cells, pretreatment with a suboptimal dose of cisplatin (EC_{50}) resulted in a 13-fold increase in AZT potency (Scanlon et al., 1989b). In A2780DDP ovarian carcinoma cells, which are inherently more cross-resistant to AZT than HCT8DDP cells, pretreatment with a suboptimal dose of cisplatin restored AZT cytotoxicity 50-fold, back to that of A2780S drug sensitive cells (Scanlon et al., 1990a). Interestingly, there is no effect of cisplatin pretreatment on AZT cytotoxicity in A2780S and HCT8S cells, suggesting that the cisplatin pretreatment utilizes an existing property of drug-resistant cells to restore AZT potency. In fact, with upregulation of the machinery for DNA synthesis and repair, A2780DDP cells are capable of rapid turnover of DNA with a 5.6-fold increased incorporation of labeled thymidine into DNA (Scanlon et al., 1990a). This corresponds to an almost 5-fold increased incorporation of labeled AZT into DNA when A2780DDP cells are pretreated with cisplatin (Scanlon et al., 1990a). This suggests that cisplatin-resistant cells respond to cisplatin administration by elevated expression of thymidine kinase (as part of the upregulation of the DNA repair pathway), thereby increasing formation of AZTTP and enhancing AZTTP chain termination of DNA, presumably leading to enhanced AZT cytotoxicity. Preliminary studies using carboplatin and AZT in platinum-resistant pediatric malignancies have shown partial responses in two out of four patients (Malogolowkin et al., 1994).

Thymidine selectivity in cisplatin-related processes is evident in a negative manner i.e., cisplatin does not form adducts with thymidine (Eastman, 1982). Interestingly, iododeoxyuridine (IdUrd), a thymidine analog, has been utilized to chemosensitize 647V human bladder carcinoma cells to cisplatin (Chi et al., 1994) by forming IdUrd-Pt-guanine analogs. Therefore, substitution of IdUrd for dThd seemingly creates a new target for cisplatin-DNA interactions. These studies were carried out in drug-sensitive cells. It would be intriguing to analyze the effect of IdUrd in cisplatin-resistant cells which have increased capacity to repair cisplatin-DNA adducts and investigate whether this synergy would still remain operative.

Cisplatin is also an important modulator of the thymidylate synthase cycle both at the molecular level by increasing expression of dTMP synthase (Kashani-Sabet et al., 1990a) and at the biochemical level by perturbing folate pools (Scanlon et al., 1986). These interactions likely account for the biochemical basis of cisplatin-5-fluorouracil synergy (Scanlon et al., 1986) which has been described in different human cancer cell lines (Scanlon et al.,1986; Tsai et al., 1994) and has been noted clinically, as the combination of cisplatin and 5-fluorouracil is actively utilized in chemotherapy of head and neck, cervical, and upper digestive tract neoplasms (Etienne et al., 1991; Khansur and Kennedy, 1991; Decker et al., 1983). Recently, the addition of leucovorin to the aforementioned regimen has proved synergistic in a variety of human non-small cell lung cancer lines (Tsai et al., 1994). However, given the upregulation of dTMP synthase cycle genes upon cisplatin resistance (Scanlon and Kashani-Sabet, 1988; Kashani-Sabet et al., 1990b), and the concomitant development of cross-resistance to 5-fluorouracil, it is unlikely that further biochemical modulation will restore drug sensitivity to this combination in drug-resistant human tumors.

Finally, the development of DNA chain terminating analogs as antiviral agents has led to investigation of their efficacy in treating human cancer. Similar to AZT, these analogs require phosphorylation prior to their activation as potential suicide substrates for DNA polymerases and in DNA synthesis. Therefore, overexpression of thymidine kinase in cisplatin-resistant cells may be utilized, as in the case with AZT, to overcome drug resistance. For instance, cisplatin pretreatment has also been shown to potentiate dideoxycytodine (ddC) cytotoxicity in A2780S and HCT8DDP cells. Interestingly, ddC appears to have less activity on A2780DDP cells after cisplatin pretreatment than does AZT (Scanlon et al., 1991b). Moreover, ganciclovir, which may act through inhibition of DNA polymerase α, is almost 4 times more effective in A2780DDP cells than in A2780S cells (Scanlon et al., 1989b).

AraC (1-ß-D-arabinofuranocylcytosine, cytarabine) has also been heavily investigated as a potential modulator of drug resistance in human cancers, though its role is less clear at this time. This may be partly due to the multifactorial   mechanism of its cytotoxicity, which is more complex than the inhibition of DNA polymerase ß alone (Zittoun et al., 1989). Synergy of the cisplatin-ara-C combination has been demonstrated in some (Swinnen et al., 1989; Kingston et al., 1989), but not all human carcinoma cell lines (Howell and Gill, 1986). For this regimen to be effective, sequencing ara-C prior to cisplatin is a demonstrated requirement (Kern et al., 1988). Finally, ara-C and hydroxyurea have been utilized in tandem to increase cisplatin cytotoxicity in a human colon cancer line (Swinnen et al., 1989). The postulated mechanism of action is inhibition of the excision repair system. This study did demonstrate higher levels of DNA interstrand cross-links when cisplatin was coupled with hydroxyurea and ara-C, even though intrastrand cross-links constituted the majority of platinum-DNA adducts (Eastman, 1986). Early studies suggest the potential clinical utility of this approach (Albain et al., 1990).

CLINICAL RESISTANCE

Clinical studies of Cisplatin Resistance

Cisplatin and its analogs are widely used in the treatment of several types of malignancies. This is especially true in human ovarian cancer, where platinum is most commonly used as the first line chemotherapeutic agent. Approximately 50% of initially treatment-sensitive tumors are ultimately resistant to conventional chemotherapy. Based on the numerous experiments attempting to elucidate the mechanisms of cisplatin resistance at the cellular level, many clinical trials of novel approaches have been attempted to improve the response rate in cisplatin-refractory cancer patients.

Cisplatin analogs, such as carboplatinum, were developed primarily to reduce the clinical toxicities of cisplatin. Recently, ormaplatin, a novel analogue representing minimum cross-resistance to cisplatin or carboplatin *in vitro*, has emerged as a potentially important agent in the chemotherapy of cisplatin-resistant disease (Perez et al.,1993). Phase I studies have demonstrated that this second-generation analog showed reduced nephrotoxicity compared to that seen with cisplatin (Plaxe et al., 1993; Petros et al., 1994). However, additional studies should be carried out to determine the maximally tolerated dose and clinical toxicities, as well as *in vivo* response rate in refractory patients.

Several chemical modulators may also have clinical usefulness in the treatment of cisplatin-resistant cancer. In recent reports, dose-intense Taxol produced a 48% response rate in patients with advanced platinum-resistant ovarian cancer (Kohn et al., 1994; Rowinsky et al., 1991). Seventy-two percent of platinum-resistant ovarian cancer patients experienced disease progression with administration of 5-FU and leucovorin (Reed et al., 1992). The combination of platinum and etoposide (VP16) has also improved the response rate whether by oral or intraperitoneal administration (Hoskins and Swenerton, 1994; Bajorin et al., 1993; Howell et al., 1990; Muggia et al., 1993; Willemse et al., 1992)). In other tumor types, newly-developed modulators have been evaluated in Phase I trials. Such agents have included APC for non-small cell lung cancer and adenocarcinoma of the colon (Sessa et al., 1991), and tamoxifen for malignant melanoma (McClay et al., 1992a,b; 1993).

Despite the appearance of novel strategies, new drugs and new drug regimens, any clinical advantage of novel combinations over classical cisplatin-based therapy remains to be determined. Still, these trials are potentially important and will permit the development of more effective approaches to platinum-refractory diseases.

The Evaluation of Clinical Drug Resistance

In the clinical context, the patterns of resistance may be expected to vary widely in different patients, even with similar histological parameters, clinical stage, and history of treatment. Not only the clinical data but molecular biological information directly from tumor tissue may be very important to evaluate and predict the drug resistance individually. However, it is not clinically practical to obtain sufficient quantities of patient tumor material for conventional blotting techniques at regular intervals during cancer treatment.

The polymerase chain reaction (PCR), currently a routinely used laboratory tool, enabled us to overcome this significant limitation. In fact, for the past several years, drug-resistant gene expression in patient material has been actively investigated by using this technique (Kramer et al., 1993; Holzmayer et al., 1992). So far, however, little is known about the altered expression of DNA damage/repair-related genes in large series of cisplatin-resistant patients. Recently, multiple tumor samples from a patient with clinically cisplatin-resistant disease have shown increased expression of oncogenes and enzymes associated with DNA synthesis and repair, such as dihydrofolate reductase, dTMP synthase and DNA polymerase ß (Scanlon and Kashani-Sabet, 1989; Miyachi et al., 1991; Horikoshi et al., 1992). This study has shown the PCR assay to be an effective device in detecting early failure of patients treated with chemotherapy.

Regarding the mechanisms of action of cisplatin on DNA, a series of studies demonstrated the overall correlation between high DNA adduct levels measured by the cisplatin-DNA ELISA and a positive clinical response (Poirier et al., 1992a,b; Reed et al., 1990, 1993). Although this positive correlation might support the possibility of a parallel between malignant and non-malignant rapidly dividing tissues within the same individual, more clinical studies, especially prospective, will be necessary before we can evaluate whether cisplatin-DNA adducts can be a useful parameter in predicting cisplatin resistance. A newly developed PCR-based method for detecting the cisplatin adducts in a specific gene might represent another approach to elucidate the relationship between cisplatin adducts and clinical response (Jennerwein and Eastman, 1991).

Recently, it has been recognized that multiple mechanisms of resistance can evolve in established malignancies. Therefore, the appropriate detection of alteration of several genes related to DNA damage/repair should be helpful clinically. In the future, altered patterns of gene expression during treatment may provide us with useful information and guide the rationale for choosing and changing chemotherapy regimens.

CONCLUSIONS

We have hereby attempted to review the molecular mechanisms of cisplatin resistance in a coherent manner by discussing potential associations between seemingly unrelated processes. We have also discussed the rational approaches utilized to modulate and/or overcome cisplatin resistance both in cultured cell lines as well as in clinical trials. The key to understanding the molecular determinants of drug resistance likely lies in the elucidation of signal transduction processes, which mediate the cellular response to extracellular agents. In our model system, common signalling pathways (i.e., those involving H-*ras*, protein kinase C, and c-*fos*/c-*jun*) become activated in response to diverse stimuli such as growth factors and chemotherapeutic agents. The activation of the Fos/Jun complex in the nucleus may represent the hallmark of this response, which typically occurs in a transient fashion. These transient increases in gene expression then result (through transcriptional activation of AP-1 responsive genes) in long term phenotypic changes. However, there is also specificity within the system. Therefore, Fos/Jun activation by cisplatin may lead to induction of genes involved in DNA synthesis and repair, metallothionein, and glutathione-S-transferase, whereas its activation by actinomycin D or etoposide, compounds known to be in the classical multidrug-resistant phenotype, may lead to induction of the mdr-1 and topoisomerase II genes. Thus, even though the cell uses similar nuclear oncoproteins to respond to different stimuli, it has the ability to differentiate between them by its differential activation of genes further downstream in the signal transduction cascade. The use of ribozyme technology has allowed the uncoupling of downstream events after administration of diverse chemotherapeutic agents, and has clarified the correlation between the signal transduction pathway and the effects of chemotherapeutic agents including cisplatin. This represents a potent tool for inhibition of gene-specific expression with dramatic results not only on the drug resistant-phenotype (Scanlon et al., 1991a, 1994), but on the transformed phenotype as well (Kashani-Sabet *et al.*, 1992, 1994). Therefore, there may be a role for anti-oncogene ribozymes not only in gene therapy of cancer, but potentially also in the re-sensitization of resistant tumors to chemotherapy and radiotherapy.

REFERENCES

Albain KS, Swinnen LJ, Erickson LC, Stiff PJ, Fisher RI (1990): Cisplatin preceded by concurrent cytarabine and hydroxyurea: A pilot study based on an *in vitro* model. *Cancer Chemother Pharmacol* 27:33-40

Ali-Osman F, Berger MS, Rajagopal BS, Spence A, Livingston RB (1993): Topoisomerase II inhibition and altered kinetics of formation and repair of nitrosourea and cisplatin-induced DNA interstrand cross-links and cytotoxicity in human glioblastoma cells. *Cancer Res* 53:5663-5668

Anderson WK, Quagliato DA, Haugwitz RD, Narayanan VL, Wolpert-DeFilippes MK (1986): Synthesis, physical properties, and antitumor activity of tetraplatin and related tetra-chloroplatinum (IV) stereoisomers of 1,2-diaminocyclohexane. *Cancer Treat Rep* 70:997-1002

Andrews PA, Mann SC, Velury S, Howell SB (1987): Cisplatin uptake mediated cisplatin-resistance in human ovarian carcinoma cells. In: *Platinum and Other Metal Coodination Compounds in Cancer Chemotherapy*. Nicolini M, ed. Padua, Italy:Martius Nijhoff Publishing

Andrews PA, Howell SB (1990): Cellular pharmacology of cisplatin: Perspective on mechanisms of acquired resistance. *Cancer Cells* 2:35-43

Andrews PA, Jones JA, Varki NM, Howell SB (1990): Rapid emergence of acquired *cis*-diamminedichloroplatinum(II) resistance in an *in vivo* model of human ovarian   carcinoma. *Cancer Comm* 2:93-100

Andrews PA, Jones JA (1991): Characterization of binding proteins from ovarian carcinoma and kidney tubule cells that are specific for cisplatin-modified DNA. *Cancer Comm* 3:93-102

Andrews PA, Mann SC, Huynh HH, Albright KD (1991): Role of the Na^+, K^+-adenosine triphosphatase in the accumulation of *cis*-diamminedichloroplatinum (II) in human ovarian carcinoma cells. *Cancer Res* 51:3677-3681

Andrews PA, Albright KD (1992): Mitochondrial defects in *cis*-diamminedichloroplatinum (II)-resistant human ovariancarcinoma cells. *Cancer Res* 52:1895-1901

Bajorin DF, Sarosdy MF, Pfister DG, Mazumdar M, Motzer R, Scher HI, Geller
    NL, Fair WR, Herr H, Sogani P, Sheinfeld J, Ruso P, Vlamis V, Carey R,
    Vogelzang NJ, Crawford ED, Bosl GJ (1993): Randomized trial of etoposide
    and cisplatin in patients with good-risk germ cell tumors: a multi institutional
    study. *J Clin Oncol* 11:598-606
Basu A, Teicher BA, Lazo JS (1990): Involvement of protein kinase C in
    phorbol   ester-induced   sensitization   of   HeLa   cells   to   cis-
    diaminedichloroplatinum(II). *J Biol Chem* 265:8451-8457
Basu A, Kozikowski AP, Sato K, Lazo JS (1991): Cellular sensitization to cis-
    diaminedichloroplatinum(II) by novel analogs of the protein kinase C
    activator lyngbyatoxin A. *Cancer Res* 51:2511-2514
Basu A, Lazo JS (1992): Sensitization of human cervical carcinoma cells to *cis*-
    diamminedicholorplatinum(II) by bryostatin 1. *Cancer Res* 52:3119-3124
Bernal SD, Speak JA, Boeheim K, Dreyfuss AI, Wright JE, Teicher BA,
    Rosowsky A, Tsao S-W, Wong Y-C (1990): Reduced membrane protein
    associated with resistance of human squamous carcinoma cells to
    methotrexate and *cis*-platinum. *Mol Cell Biochem* 95:61-70
Binetruy B, Smeal T, Karin M (1991): Ha-Ras augments c-Jun activity and
    stimulates phosphorylation of its activation domain. *Nature* 351:122-127
Boguski MS, McCormick F (1993): Proteins regulating *ras* and its relatives.
    Nature 366:643-654
Bohr VA (1991): Gene specific DNA repair. *Carcinogenesis* 12:1983-1992
Bonomi P (1986): Brief over view of combination chemotherapy in non-small
    cell lung cancer. *Semin Oncol 13* (Suppl 3):89-91
Boughattas, NA, Levi F, Fournier C, Lemaigre G, Roulon A, Hecquet B, Mathe
    G, Reinberg A (1989): Circadian rhythm in toxicities and tissue uptake of
    1,2-diamino-cyclohexane(*trans*-1)oxalatoplatinum(II) in mice. *Cancer Res*
    49:3362-3368
Bradner WT, Rose WC, Huftalen JB (1980): Antitumor activity of platinum
    analogs. In: *Cisplatin: Current Status and New Developments*, Prestayko
    AW, Crooke ST, Carter SK, eds. San Diego: Academic
Brown R, Clugston C, Burns P, Edlin A, Basey P, Vojtesek B, Kay SB (1993):
    Increased accumulation of p53 protein in cusokatub-resistant ovarian cell
    lines. *Int J Cancer* 55:678-684
Bruhn SL, Pil PM, Essigman JM, Housman DE, Lippard SJ (1992): Isolation
    and characterization of human cDNA clones encoding a high mobility group
    box protein that recognizes structural distortions to DNA caused by binding
    of the anticancer agent cisplatin. *Proc Natl Acad Sci USA* 89:2307-2311
Brunton VG, Workman P (1993): Cell-signalling targets for antitumor drug
    development. *Cancer Chemoth Pharm* 32:1-19

Caussanel JP, Levi F, Brienza S, Misset JL, Itzhaki M, Adam R, Milano G,Hecquet B, Mathe G (1990): Phase I trial of 5-day continuous venous infusion of oxaliplatin at circadian rhythm-modulated rate compared with constant rate. *J Natl Cancer Inst* 82:1046-1050

Cavalli F (1983): Chemotherapy of testicular cancer: from palliation to cure. In: *Cancer Chemotherapy*, Muggia RF, ed. Boston: M. Nijhoff

Cech TR and Bass BL (1986): Biological catalysis by RNA. *Ann Rev Biochem* 55:599-629

Chao CC, Huang SL, Lee LY, Lin-Chao S (1991): Identification of inducible damage-recognition proteins that are overexpressed in HeLa cells resistant to *cis-*   diamminedichloroplatinum (II). *Biochem J* 277:875-878

Chi K-H, Kunugi KA, Kinsella TS (1994): Iododeoxyuridine chemosensitization of cis-diamminedichloroplatinum(II) in human bladder cancer cells. *Cancer Res* 54:2701-2706

Christen RD, Hom DK, Porter DC, Andrews PA (1990): Epidermal growth factor regulates the *in vitro* sensitivity of human ovarian carcinoma cells to cisplatin. *J Clin Invest* 86:1632-1640

Christian MC (1992): The current status of new platinum analogs. *Semin Oncol* 19:720-733

Chu G, Chang E (1990): Cisplatin-resistant cells express increased levels of a factor that recognizes damaged DNA. *Proc Natl Acad Sci USA* 87:3324-3327

Colombiani PM, Robb A, Hess AD (1985): Cyclosporin A binding to calmodulin: A possible site of action on T lymphocyte. *Science* 228:337-339

Connors TA, Cleare MJ, Harrap KR (1979): Structure activity relationships of the antitumor platinum coordination complexes. *Cancer Treat Rep* 63:1499-1502

Corda Y, Job C, Anin MF, Leng M, Job D (1993): Spectrum of DNA-platinum adduct recognition by prokaryotic and eukaryotic DNA-dependent RNA polymerases. *Biochemistry* 32:8582-8588

Dabholkar M, Bostick-Burton F, Weber C, Bohr V , Egwuagu C, Reed E (1992): ERCC1 and ERCC2 expression in malignant tissues from ovarian cancer patients. *J Natl Cancer Inst* 84:1512-1517

Damjanovich S, Aszalos A, Mlhern S, Balazs M, Mtyus L (1986): Cytoplasmic membrane potential of mouse lymphocytes is decreased by cyclosporins. *Mol Immun* 23:175-180

Decker DA, Drelichman A, Jacobs J, Hoschner J, Kinzie J, Loh JJ-K, Weaver A, Al-Sarraf M (1983): Adjuvant chemotherapy with *cis-*diamminedichloroplatinum II and 120-hr infusion 5-fluorouracil in stage III and IV squamous cell carcinoma of the head and neck. *Cancer* 51:1353-1355

De Jong S, Timmer-Bosscha H, de Vries EGE, Mulder NH (1990): Increased topoisomerase II activity in a cisplatin resistant cell line. *Proc Am Assoc Cancer Res* 31:337

De Jong S, Timmer-Bosscha H, de Vries EGE, Mulder NH (1991): Topoisomerase II, nuclear matrix proteins and formation of interstrand cross-links in a CDDP resistant human small cell carcinoma cell line. *Proc Am Assoc Cancer Res* 32:361

Eastman A (1982): Separation and characterization of products resulting from the reaction of *cis*-diamminedichloroplatinum (II) with deoxyribonucleosides. *Biochemistry* 21:6732-6736

Eastman A (1986): Reevaluation of interaction of *cis*-dichloro(ethylenediammine)platinum (II) with DNA. *Biochemistry* 25:3912-3915

Eastman A, Schulte N (1988): Enhanced DNA repair as a mechanism of resistance to *cis*-diamminedichloroplatinum(II). *Biochemistry* 27:4730-4734

Edelman AM, Blumenthal DK, Kreb EG (1987): Protein serine/threonine kinases. *Ann Rev Biochem* 56:567-613

Eichholtz-Wirth H and Hietel B (1986): The relationship between cisplatin sensitivity and drug uptake into mammalian cells *in vitro*. *Br J Cancer* 54:239-243

Eichholtz-Wirth H and Hietel B (1990): Heat sensitization to cisplatin in two cell lines with different drug sensitivities. *Int J Hyperthermia* 6:47-55

Eisenhauer E, Swerton K, Sturgeon J, Fine S, O'Reilly S, Canetta R (1990): Carboplatin therapy for recurrent ovarian carcinoma: National Cancer Institute of Canada experience and a review of the literature. In: *Carboplatin: Current Perspectives and Future Directions*, Bunn P, Canetta R, Ozols R, Rozencweig eds. Philadelphia: W.B. Saunders Co.

Endo K, Akamatsu K, Matsumoto T, Morikawa K, Koizumi M, Mitsui H, Koizumi K (1992): Comparison of DWA2114R with cisplatin and carboplatin. *Anticancer Res* 12:49-58

Etienne MC, Bernard S, Fischel JL, Formento P, Gioanni J, Santini J, Demard F, Schneider M, Milano G (1991): Dose reduction without loss of efficacy for 5-fluorouracil and cisplatin combined with folinic acid. *In vitro* study on human head and neck carcinoma cell lines. *Br J Cancer* 63:372-377

Evans WK, Feld R, Murray N, Pater J, Shelley W, William A, Osoba D, Levitt M, Coy P, Hodson I, Payne DG, MacDonald AS (1986): The use of VP-16 plus cisplatin during induction chemotherapy for small cell lung cancer. *Semin Oncol* 13 (suppl 3):10-16

Extra JM, Espie M, Calvo F, Ferme C, Mignot L, Marty M (1990): Phase I study of oxaliplatin in patients with advanced cancer. *Cancer Chemother Pharm* 25:299-303

Farm RJ, Woda BA, Woda JM, Robichaud N (1990): Characterization of acquired resistance to cis-diamminedichloroplatinum (II) in BE human colon carcinoma cells. *Cancer Res* 50:72-77

Farrell N (1993): Nonclassical platinum antitumor agents: Perspectives for design and development of new drugs complementary to cisplatin. *Cancer Invest* 11:578-589

Fichtinger-Schepman AMJ, van der Veer JL, den Hartog JHJ, Lohman PHM, Reedijk J (1985): Adducts of the antitumor drug cis-diamminedichloroplatinum(II). *Biochemistry* 24:707-713

Fram RJ (1992): Cisplatin and platinum analogues: recent advances. *Curr Opin Oncol* 4:1073-1079

Fujiwara Y, Kasahara K, Sugimoto Y, Nishio K, Ohmori T, Saijo N (1990a): Detection of proteins that recognize platinum-modified DNA using gel mobility shift assay. *Jpn J Cancer Res* 81:1210-1213

Fujiwara Y, Sugimoto Y, Kasahara K, Bungo M, Yamakido M, Tew KD, Saijo N (1990b): Determinants of drug response in a cisplatin-resistant human lung cancer cell line. *Jpn J Cancer Res* 81:527-535

Funato T, Yoshida E, Jiao L, Tone T, Kashani-Sabet M, Scanlon KJ (1992): The utility of an anti-*fos* ribozyme in reversing cisplatin resistance in human carcinomas. *Adv Enz Reg* 32:195-209

Gale GR, Morris CR, Atkins, LM, Smith AB (1973): Binding of an antitumor platinum compound to cells as influenced by physical factors and pharmacologically active agents. *Cancer Res* 33:813-818

Gately DP, Howell SB (1993): Cellular accumulation of the anticancer agents cisplatin: A review. *Br J Cancer* 67:1171-1176

Godwin AK, Meister A, O'Dwyer PJ, Huang CS, Hamilton TC, Anderson, ME (1992): High resistance to cisplatin in human ovarian cancer cell lines in association with marked increase of glutathione synthesis. *Proc Natl Acad Sci USA* 89:3070-3074

Gordon M, Hollander S (1993): Review of platinum anticancer compounds. *J Med* 24:209-265

Gottesman MM, Pastan I (1993): Biochemistry of multidrug resistance mediated by the multidrug transporter. *Ann Rev Biochem* 62:385-427

Greenberg ME and Ziff EB (1984): Stimulation of 3T3 cells induces transcription of the c-*fos* proto-oncogene. *Nature* 311:433-438

Hamer DH (1986): Metallothionein. *Ann Rev Biochem* 55:913-951

Hamilton TC, Winker MA, Louie KG, Batist G, Behrens BC, Tsuruo T, Grotzinger KR, McKoy WM, Young RC, Ozols RF (1985): Augmentation of adriamycin, melphalan and cisplatin cytotoxicity in drug-resistant and -sensitive human ovarian carcinoma cell lines by buthionine sulfoximine mediated glutathione depletion. *Biochem Pharmacol* 34:2583-2586

Hamilton TC, O'Dwyer PJ, Ozols RF (1993): Platinum analogues in preclinical and clinical development. *Cur Opin Oncol* 5:1010-1016

Han I, Ling YH, Al-Baker S, Khokhar AR, Perez-Soler R (1993): Cellular pharmacology of liposomal cis-Bis-neodecanoato-*trans*-R,R-1,2-diamino-cyclohexaneplatinum(II) in A2780/DDP cells. *Cancer Res* 53:4913-4919

Hancock MC, Langton BC, Chan T, Toy P, Monahan JJ, Mischak RP, Shawver LK (1991): A monoclonal antibody against the c-*erb*B-2 protein enhances the cytotoxicity of *cis*- diamminedichloroplatinum against human breast and ovarian tumor lines. *Cancer Res* 51:4575-4580

Harstrick A, Casper J, Guba R, Wilke H, Poliwoda H, Schmoll HJ (1989): Comparison of the antitumor activity of cisplatin, carboplatin and iproplatin against established human testicular cancer cell lines *in vivo* and *in vitro*. *Cancer* 63:1079-1083

Haseloff J and Gerlach WL (1988): Simple RNA enzymes with new and highly specific endoribonuclease activities. *Nature* (*London*) 334:585-591

Hoeijmakers JHJ, Bootsma D (1990): Molecular genetics of eukaryotic DNA excision repair. *Cancer Cells* 2:311-320

Hofmann J, Doppler W, Jakob A, Maly K, Posch L, Uberall F, Grunicke HH (1988): Enhancement of the antiproliferative effect of cis-diamminedichloroplatinum(II) and nitrogen mustard by inhibitors of protein kinase C. *Int J Cancer* 42:382-388

Hollander MC, Fornace AJ Jr (1989): Induction of *fos* RNA by DNA-damaging agents. *Cancer Res* 49:1687-1692

Holzmayer TA, Hilsenbeck S, Von Hoff DD, Roninson I (1992): Clinical correlates of MDR1 (P-glycoprotein) gene expression in ovarian and small-cell lung carcinomas. *J Natl Cancer Inst* 84:486-1491

Hong WS, Saijo N, Sasaki Y, Minato K, Nakano H, Nakagawa K, Fujiwara Y, Nomura K, Twentyman PR (1988): Establishment and characterization of cisplatin-resistant sublines of human lung cancer cell lines. *Int J Cancer* 43:462-467

Horikoshi T, Danenberg KD, Stadlbauer THW, Volkenandt M, Shea LCC, Aigner K, Gustavsson B, Leichman L, Frosing R, Ray M, Gibson GW, Spears P, Danenberg PV (1992): Quantification of thymidylate synthase, dihydrofolate reductase, and DT-diaphorase gene expression in human tumors using the polymerase chain reaction. *Cancer Res* 52:108-116

Hoskins PJ, Swenerton KD (1994): Oral etoposide is active against platinum-resistant epithelial ovarian cancer. *J Clin Oncol* 12:60-63

Hospers GAP, Mulder NH, De Jong B, De Ley L, Uges DRA, Fichtinger-Schepman AMJ, Scheper RJ, De Vries EGE (1988): Characterization of a human small cell lung carcinoma cell line with acquired resistance to *cis*-diamminedichloroplatinum(II) *in vitro*. *Cancer Res* 48:6803-6807

Howell SB, Gill S (1986) Lack of synergy between cisplatin and cytarabine against ovarian carcinoma *in vitro*. *Cancer Treat Rep* 70:409-410

Howell SB, Kirmani S, Lucas WE, Zimm S, Goel R, Kim S, Horton MC, McVey L, Morris J, Weiss RJ (1990): A phase 2 trial of intraperitoneal cisplatin and etoposide for primary treatment of ovarian epithelial cancer. *J Clin Oncol* 8:137-145

Hrubisko M, McGown AT, Fox BW (1993): The role of metallothionein, glutathione, glutathione S-transferases and DNA repair in resistance to platinum drugs in a series of L1210 cell lines made resistant to anticancer platinum agents. *Biochem Pharmacol* 45:253-256

Huang TS, Lee SC, Lin JK (1991): Suppression of c-Jun/AP-1 activation by an inhibitor of tumor promotion in mouse fibroblast cells. *Proc Natl Acad Sci USA* 88:5292-5296

Hunter T (1991): Cooperation between oncogenes. *Cell* 64:249-270

Ikeda H, Nakano G, Nagashima K, Sakamoto K, Harasawa N, Kitamura T, Nakamura T, Nagamachi Y (1987): Verapamil enhancement of antitumor effect of cis-diamminedichloroplatinum (II) in nude mouse-grown human neuroblastoma. *Cancer Res* 47:231-234

Ishikawa T, Ali-Osman F (1993): Glutathione-associated *cis*-diamminedichloroplatinum(II) metabolism and ATP-dependent efflux from leukemia cells. *J Biol Chem* 268:20116-20125

Isonishi S, Andrews PA, Howell SB (1990): Increased sensitivity to *cis*-diamminedichloroplatinum (II) in human ovarian carcinoma cells in response to treatment with 12-*O* -tetradecanoylphorbol 13-acetate. *J Biol Chem* 265:3623-3627

Jennerwein MM, Eastman A (1991): A polymerase chain reaction-based method to detect cisplatin adducts in specific genes. *Nucleic Acids Res* 19:6209-6214

Johnson SW, Ozols RF, Hamilton TC (1993): Mechanisms of drug resistance in ovarian cancer. *Cancer* 71:644-649

Johnson SW, Perez RP, Godwin AK, Yeung AT, Hardel LM, Ozols RF, Hamilton TC (1994): Role of platinum-DNA adduct formation and removal of cisplatin resistance in human ovarian cancer cell lines. *Biochem Pharm* 47:689-687

Jones JC, Zhen W, Reed E, Parker RJ, Sancar A, Bohr VA (1991): Gene-specific formation and repair of cisplatin intrastrand adducts and interstrand cross-links in Chinese hamster ovary cells. *J Biol Chem* 266:7101-7107

Kasahara K, Fujiwara Y, Nishio K, Ohmori T, Sugimoto Y, Komiya K, Matsuda T, Saijo N (1991): Metallothionein content correlates with the sensitivity of human small cell lung cancer cell lines to cisplatin. *Cancer Res* 51:3237-3242

Kashani-Sabet M, Rossi JJ, Lu Y, Ma JX, Chen J, Miyachi H, Scanlon KJ (1988): Detection of drug resistance in human tumors by *in vitro* enzymatic amplification. *Cancer Res* 48:5775-5778

Kashani-Sabet M, Wang W, Scanlon KJ (1990a): Cyclosporin A suppresses cisplatin-induced c-*fos* gene expression in ovarian carcinoma cells. *J Biol Chem* 265:11285-11288

Kashani-Sabet M, Lu Y, Leong L, Haedicke K, Scanlon KJ (1990b): Differential oncogene amplification in tumor cells from a patient treated with cisplatin and 5-fluorouracil. *Eur J Cancer* 26:383-390

Kashani-Sabet M, Funato T, Tone T, Jiao L, Wang W, Yoshida E, Wu AM, Moreno JG, Traweek ST, Ahlering T, Scanlon KJ (1992): Reversal of the malignant phenotype by an anti-*ras* ribozyme. *Antisense Res Dev* 2:3-15

Kashani-Sabet M, Funato T, Florenes VA, Fodstad O, Scanlon KJ (1994): Suppression of the neoplastic phenotype *in vivo* by an anti-*ras* ribozyme. *Cancer Res* 54:900-902

Kastan MB, Onyekwere O, Sidransky D, Vogelstein B, Craig RW (1991): Participation of p53 protein in the cellular response to DNA damage. *Cancer Res* 51:6304-6311

Katz EJ, Andrews PA, Howell SB (1990): The effect of DNA polymerase inhibitors on the cytotoxicity of cisplatin in human ovarian carcinoma cells. *Cancer Comm* 2:59-164

Kawai K, Kamatani N, George E, Ling V (1990): Identification of a membrane glycoprotein overexpressed in murine lymphoma sublines resistant to *cis*-diamminedichloroplatinum(II). *J Biol Chem* 265:13137-13142

Kedar PS, Lowy DR, Widen SG, Wilson SH (1990): Transfected human beta-polymerase promoter contains a *ras*-responsive element. *Mol Cell Biol* 10:3852-3856

Kelland LR, Abel G, Murrer BA, Abrams MJ, Giandomenico C, Wyer S, Harrap KR (1991): A novel class of platinum compounds exhibiting selective cytotoxicity against cisplatin-resistant human ovarian carcinoma cell lines. *Anticancer Drug Design* 6:218

Kelland LR, Mistry P, Abel G, Loh YL, O'neill CF, Murrer BA, Harrap KR (1992a): Mechanism-related circumvention of acquired *cis*-diamminedichloroplatinum(II) resistance using two pairs of human ovarian carcinoma cell lines by ammine/ammine platinum(IV) dicarboxylates. *Cancer Res* 52:3857-3864

Kelland LR, Murrer BA, Abel G, Giandomenico CM, Mistry P, Harrap KR (1992b): Ammine/ammine platinum(IV) dicarboxylates: A nobel class of platinum complex exhibiting selective cytotoxicity to intrinsically cisplatin-resistant human ovarian carcinoma cell lines. *Cancer Res* 52:822-828

Kelly SL, Basu A, Teicher BA, Hacker MP, Hamer DH, Lazo JS (1988): Overexpression of metallothionein confers resistance to anticancer drugs. *Science* 241:1813-1815

Kern DH, Morgan CR, Hildebrand-Zanki SU (1988): *In vitro* pharmacodynamics of 1-ß-D-arabinofuranosylcytosine: Synergy of antitumor activity with *cis*-diamminedicholoroplatinum (II). *Cancer Res* 48:117-121

Khansur Y, Kennedy A (1991): Cisplatin and 5-fluorouracil for advanced locoregional and metastatic squamous cell carcinoma of the skin. *Cancer* 67:2030-2032

Kikuchi Y, Oomori K, Kizawa I, Hirata J, Kita T, Miyauchi M, Kato K (1987): Enhancement of antineoplastic effects of cisplatin by calmodulin antagonists in nude mice bearing human ovarian carcimnoma. *Cancer Res* 47:6459-6461

Kingston RE, Sevin B-U, Ramos R, Saks M, Donato D, Jarrell MA, Averette HE (1989): Synergistic effects of *cis*-platinum and cystosine arabinoside on ovarian carcinoma cell lines, demonstrated by dual-parameter flow cytometry. *Gyn Oncol* 32:282-287

Kohn EC, Sarosy G, Bicher A, Link C, Christian M, Steinberg SM, Rothenberg M, Adamo DO, Davis P, Ognibene FP, Cunnion RE, Reed E (1994): Dose-intense taxol: high response rate in patients with platinum-resistant recurrent ovarian cancer. *J Natl Cancer Inst* 86:18-24

Kramer R, Weber TK, Morse B, Arceci R, Staniunas R, Steele G, Summerhayes IC (1993): Constitutive expression of multidrug resistance in human colorectal tumors and cell lines. *Br J Cancer* 67:959-968

Kuerbits SJ, Plunkett BS, Walsh WV, Kastan MB (1992): Wild-type p53 is a cell cycle checkpoint determinant following irradiation. *Proc Natl Acad Sci USA* 89:7491-7495

Kunze N, Klein M, Richter A, Knippers R (1990): Structural characterization of the human DNA topoisomerase I gene promotor. *Eur J Biochem* 194:323-330

Lai G-M, Ozols RF, Smyth JF, Young RF, Hamilton TC (1988): Enhanced DNA repair and resistance to cisplatin in human ovarian cancer. *Biochem Pharm* 37:4597-4600

Lai G-M, Ozols RF, Young RC, Hamilton TC (1989): Effect of glutathione on DNA repair in cisplatin-resistant human ovarian cancer cell lines. *J Natl Cancer Inst* 81:535-539

Ledwith BJ, Manam S, Kraynak AR, Nichols WW, Bradley MO (1990): Antisense-*fos* RNA causes partial reversion of the transformed phenotypes induced by the c-Ha-*ras* oncogene. *Mol Cell Biol* 10:1545-1555

Lee W, Haslinger A, Karin M, Tjian R (1987): Activation of transcription by two factors that bind promoter and enhancer sequences of the human metallothionein gene and SV40. *Nature (London)* 325:368-372

Liu LF (1989): DNA topoisomerase poisons as antitumor drugs. *Ann Rev Biochem* 58:351-375

Majima H (1991): Clinical studies with cisplatin analogues, 254-S, DWA2114R and NK121. In: *Platinum and Other Metal Coordination Compounds in Cancer Chemotherapy*, Howell S, ed. New York:Plenum

Malogolowkin, MH, Steele, DA, Ortega JA, Rowland J, Scanlon (1994): Circumvention of platinum resistance by azidothymidine (AZT) in childhood malignancies. *Proc Amer Assoc Cancer Res* 35:2802

Mann SC, Andrews PA, Howell SB (1990): Short-term *cis*-diamminedichloroplatinum(II) accumumulation in sensitive and resistant human ovarian carcinoma cells. *Cancer Chemother Pharm* 25:236-240

Mann SC, Andrews PA, Howell SB (1991): Modulation of *cis*-diamminedicholoroplatinum(II) accumulation and sensitivity by forskolin and 3-isobuthyl-l-methylxanthine in sensitive and resistant ovarian carcinoma cells. *Int J Cancer* 48:866-872

Masuda H, Ozols RF, Lai G-M, Fojo A (1988): Increased DNA repair as a mechanism of acquired resistance to *cis*-diamminedichloroplatinum (II) in human ovarian cancer cell lines. *Cancer Res* 48:5713-5716

Masuda H, Tanaka T, Matsuda H, Kusaba I (1990): Increased removal of DNA-bound platinum in a human ovarian cancer cell line resistant to *cis*-diamminedichloroplatinum(II). *Cancer Res* 50:1863-1866

Masuda H, Tanaka T, Kido A, Kusaba I (1991): Potentiation of cisplatin against sensitive and resistant human ovarian cancer cell lines by amphotericin B. *Cancer J* 4:119-124

Mathe G, Kidain Y, Noji M, Maral R, Bourut C, Chenu E (1985): Antitumor activity of 1-OHP in mice. *Cancer Lett* 27:135-143

Mathe G, Kidain Y, Triana K, Brienza S, Ribaud P, Goldschmidt E, Esctein E, Despax R, Musset JL (1986): A phase I trial of *trans*-1-diaminocyclohexane oxalatoplatinum (1-OHP). *Biomed Pharmacother* 40:372-376

McClay EF, Mastrangelo MJ, Bellet RE, Berd D (1989): The importance of tamoxifen to a cisplatin containing regimen in the treatment of malignant melanoma. *Cancer* 63:1292-1295

McClay EF, Mastrangelo MJ, Berd D, Bellt RE (1992a): Effective combination chemo/hormonal therapy for malignant melanoma: Experience with three consecutive trials. *Int J Cancer* 50:553-556

McClay EF, Albirght KD, Jones JA, Eastman A, Christen RD, Howell SB (1992b): Modulation of cisplatin resistance in human malignant melanoma cells. *Cancer Res* 52:6790-6796

McClay EF, Albright KD, Jones JA, Christen RD, Howell SB (1993): Tamoxifen modulation of cisplatin sensitivity in human malignant melanoma cells. *Cancer Res* 53:1571-1576

McKeage MJ, Higgins JD, 3rd Kelland LR (1991): Platinum and other metal coordination compounds in cancer chemotherapy. A commentary on the sixth international symposium: San Diego, California, 23-26th January 1991. *Brit J Cancer* 64:788-792

McKeage MJ, Abel G, Kelland LR, Harrap JR (1994a): Mechanisms of action of an orally administered platinum complex [ammine bis butyrato cyclohexylamine dichloroplatinum(IV)(SM221)] in intrinsically cisplatin-resistant human ovarian carcinoma *in vitro. Br J Cancer* 69:1-7

McKeage MJ, Boxall FE, Jones M, Harrap KR (1994b): Lack of neurotoxicity of oral bisacetatoamminedichlorocyclohexylamine-platinum(IV) in comparison to cisplatin and tetraplatin in the rat. *Cancer Res* 54:629-631

Meijer C, Mulder NH, Hospers GAP, Uges DRA, de Vries EGE (1990): The role of glutathione in resistance to cisplatin in human small cell lung cancer cell line. *Br J Cancer* 62:72-77

Meijer C, Mulder NH, Timmer-Bosscha HT, Sluiter WJ, Meersma GJ, de Vries EGE (1992): Relationship of cellular glutathione to the cytotoxicity and resistance of seven platinum compounds. *Cancer Res* 52:6885-6889

Meister A, Anderson ME (1983): Glutathione. *Ann Rev Biochem* 52:711-760

Misset JL, Kidani Y, Gastiaburu J, Jasmin C, Levi F, Boughattas N, Lemaigre, G, Caussanel JP, Brienza S, Triana BK, Goldschmidt E, Musset M, Mauvernay RY, Mathe G (1991): Oxalatoplatin (1-OHP) Experimental and clinical studies. In: *Platinum and Other Metal Coordination Compounds in Cancer Chemotherapy*, Howell S, ed. New York:Plenum

Mistry P, Kelland L, Abel G, Sidhar S, Harrap K (1991): The relationships between glutathione, glutathione-S-transferase, and cytotoxicity of platinum drugs and melphalan in eight human ovarian carcinoma cell lines. *Br J Cancer* 64:215-220

Miyachi H, Han H, Scanlon KJ (1991): Dihydrofolate reductase gene expression characterized by the PCR assay in human leukemia cells. *In Vivo* 5:7-12

Morikage T, Ohmori T, Nishino K, Fujiwara Y, Takeda Y, Saijo N (1993): Modulation of cisplatin sensitivity and accumulation by amphotericin B in cisplatin-resistant human lung cancer cell lines. *Cancer Res* 53:3302-3307

Muggia FM (1993): Platinum resistance: Laboratory findings and clinical implications. *Stem Cells* 11:182-193

Muggia FM, Groshen S, Russell C, Jeffers S, Chen S-C, Schlaerth J, Curtin J, Morrow CP (1993): Intraperitoneal carboplatin and etoposide for persistent epithelial ovarian cancer: Analysis of results by prior sensitivity to platinum-based regimens. *Gynecol Oncol* 50:232-238

Muller MR, Wright KA, Twentyman PR (1991): Differential properties of cisplatin and tetraplatin with respect to cytotocity and perturbation of cellular glutathione levels. *Cancer Chemother Pharmacol* 287:273-276

Murphy D, Mc Gown AT, Criwther D, Mander A, Fox BW (1991): Metallothionein levels in ovarian tumors before and after chemotherapy. *Br J Cancer* 63:711-714

Nakagawa N, Saijo N, Tsuchida S, Sakai M, Tsunokawa Y, Yokota J, Muramatsu M, Sato K, Terada M, Tew KD (1990): Glutathione-S-transferase π as a determinant of drug resistance in transfectant cell lines. *J Biol Chem* 265:4296-4301

Niimi S, Nakagawa K, Yokota J, Tsunokawa Y, Nishio K, Terashima Y, Shibuya M, Terada M, Saijo N (1991): Resistance to anticancer drugs in NIH3T3 cells transfected with c-*myc* and/or c-H-*ras* genes. *Br J Cancer* 63:237-241

O'Dwyer PJ, Moyer JD, Suffness M, Harrison SD, Cysyk JR, Hamilton TC, Plowman J (1994): Antitumor activity and biochemical effects of aphidicolin glycinate (NSC 303812) alone and in combination with cisplatin *in vivo*. *Cancer Res* 54:724-729

Ogawa M, Gale GR, Keirn SS (1975): Effects of *cis*-diamminedichloroplatinum (NSC 119875) on murine and human hemopoietic precursor cells. *Cancer Res* 35:1398-1401

Onoda JM, Nelson KK, Taylor JD, Hohn KV (1989): *In vitro* characterization of combination antitumor chemotherapy with calcium channel blockers and cis-diamminedichloroplatinum (II). *Cancer Res* 49:2844-2850

O'Rourke T, Rodgriques G, Cagnola J, von Hoff D (1991): Phase I trial of tetraplatin(NSC 363812) administered daily for 5 consecutive days every 25 days. *Anti-Cancer Drug Des* 6:285

Orr RM, O'Neill CF, Nicolson MC, Murrer BA, Vollano JF, Wyer SB, Phillips RL, Harrap KR (1991): Platinum-resistant L1210 cell lines in new platinum drug development *Anti-Cancer Drug Des* 6:308

Pardee AB (1987): Molecules involved in proliferation of normal and cancer cells: Presidential address. *Cancer Res* 47:1488-1491

Parker RJ, Eastman A, Bostick-Burton F, Reed E (1991): Acquired cisplatin resistance in human ovarian cancer cells is associated with enhanced repair of cisplatin-DNA lesions and reduced drug accumulation. *J Clin Invest* 87:722-777

Perez RP, O'Dwyer PJ, Handel LM, Ozols RF, Hamilton TC (1991): Comparative cytotoxicity of CI-973,cisplatin, carboplatin and tetroplatin in human ovarian carcinoma cell lines. *Int J Cancer* 48:265-269

Perez RP, Hamilton TC, Ozols RF, Young RC (1993): Mechanisms and modulation of resistance to chemotherapy in ovarian cancer. *Cancer* 71:1571-1580

Perez-Soler R, Khokhar AR, Lopez-Berestein G (1987): Treatment and prophylaxis of experimental liver metastases of M5076 reticulosarcoma with *cis*-bis-neodecanoato-*trans*-R,R-1,2-diaminocyclohexaneplatinum(II) encapsulated in multilamellar vesicles. *Cancer Res* 47:6462-6466

Perez-Soler R, Lautersztain J, Stephens LC, Wright K, Khokhar AR (1989): Preclinical toxicity and pharmacology of lipo-entrapped *cis*-bis-neodecanoato-*trans*-R,R-1,2 diaminocyclohexane-platinum(II). *Cancer Chemother Pharmacol* 24:1-8

Perez-Soler R, Lopez-Berestein G, Lautersztain J, Al-Baker S, Francis K, Macias-Kiger D, Raber MN, Khokhar AR (1990): Phase I clinical and pharmacological study of liposome-entrapped cis-bis-neodecanoato-trans-R,R-1,2 diaminocyclohexaneplatinum (II). *Cancer Res* 50:4254-4259

Petros WP, Chaney SG, Smith DC, Fangmeier J, Sakata M, Brown TD, Trump DL (1994): Pharmacokinetic and biotransformation studies of ormaplatin in conjunction with a phase 1 clinical trial. *Cancer Chemother Pharmacol* 33:347-354

Pickett CB, Lu AYH (1989): Glutathione S-transferases: Gene structure, regulation, and biological function. *Ann Rev Biochem* 58:743-764

Pil PM, Lippard SJ (1992): Specific binding of chromosomal protein HMG1 to DNA damaged by the anticancer drug cisplatin. *Science* 256:234-237

Plaxe SC, Braly PS, Freddo JL, McClay E, Christen RD, Kirmani S, Kim S, Heath D, Howell SB (1993): Phase 1 and pharmacokinetic study of intraperitoneal ormaplatin. *Gynecol Oncol* 51:72-77

Poirier MC, Reed E, Litterst CL, Katz D, Gupta-Burt S (1992a): Persistence of platinum-ammine-DNA adducts in gonad and kidney of rats and multiple tissues from cancer patients. *Cancer Res* 52:149-153

Poirier MC, Shamkhani H, Reed E, Tarone RE, Gupta-Burt S. (1992b): DNA adducts induced by platinum drug chemotherapeutic agents in human tissues. Relevance of animal studies to the evaluation of human cancer risk. *Prog Clin Biol Res* 374:197-212

Pommier Y, Kerrigan D, Hartman KD, Glazer RI (1990): Phosphorylation of mammalian DNA topoisomerse I and activation by protein kinase C. *J Biol Chem* 265:9418-9422

Ransone LJ, Verma IM (1990): Nuclear proto-oncogenes *Fos* and *Jun*. *Ann Rev Biol* 6:539-557

Raycroft L, Wu HY, LozanoG (1990): Transcriptional activation by wild-type but not transforming mutants of the p53 anti-oncogene. *Science* 249:1049-1051

Reddy GPV, Pardee AB (1980): Multienzyme complex for metabolic channeling in mammalian DNA replication. *Proc Natl Acad Sci USA* 77:3312-3316

Reed E, Ozols RF, Tarone R, Yuspa SH, Poirier MC (1987): Platinum-DNA adducts in leukocyte DNA correlate with disease response in ovarian cancer patients receiving platinum-based chemotherapy. *Proc Natl Acad Sci USA* 84:5024-5028

Reed E, Ostchega Y, Steinberg SM, Yuspa SH, Young RC, Ozols RF Poirier MC (1990): Evaluation of platinum-DNA adduct levels relative to known prognostic variables in a cohort of ovarian cancer patients. *Cancer Res* 50:2256-2260

Reed E, Jacob J, Ozol RF, Young RC, Allegra C (1992): 5-Fluorouracil (5-FU) and leucovorin in platinum-refractory advanced stage ovarian carcinoma. *Gynecol Oncol* 46:326-329

Reed E, Parker RJ, Gill I, Bicher A, Dabholkar M, Vionnet JA, Bostick-Bruton F, Tarone R, Muggia FM (1993): Platinum-DNA adduct in Leukocyte DNA of a Cohort of 49 patients with 24 different types of malignancies. *Cancer Res* 53:3694-3699

Roberts J, Friedlas F (1987): Quantitative estimation of cisplatin-induced DNA interstrand cross-links and their repair in mammalian cells: Relationship to toxicity. *Pharm Ther* 34:215-246

Roberts TM (1992): A signal chain of events. *Nature* 360:534-535

Rose WC, Basler GA (1990): *In vivo* model development of cisplatin-resistant and -sensitive A2780 human ovarian carcinomas. *In Vivo* 4:391-396

Rosenberg B (1985): Fundamental studies with cisplatin. *Cancer* 55:2303-2316

Rowinsky EK, Gilbert MR, McGuire WP, Noe DA, Grochow LB, Forastiere AA, Ettinger DS, Lubejko BG, Sartorius SE, Cornblath DR, Hendricks CB, Donehower RC (1991): Sequences of taxol and cisplatin: a phase 1 and pharmacologic study. *J Clin Oncol* 9:1692-1703

Rubin E, Kharbanda S, Gunji H, Weichselbaum R, Kufe D (1992): *cis*-diammine-dichloroplatinum(II) induces c-*jun* expression in human myeloid leukemia cells: Potential involvement of a protein kinase C-dependent signalling pathway. *Cancer Res* 52:878-882

Scanlon KJ, Newman EM, Lu Y, Priest DG (1986): Biochemical basis for cisplatin and 5-fluorouracil synergism in human ovarian carcinoma cells. *Proc Natl Acad Sci USA* 83:8923-8925

Scanlon KJ, Kashani-Sabet M, Cashmore AR, Pallai M, Moroson BA, Saketos M (1987): The role of methionine in methotrexate-sensitive and methotrexate-resistant mouse leukemia L1210 cells. *Cancer Chemother Pharmacol* 19:25-29

Scanlon KJ, Kashani-Sabet M (1988): Elevated expression of thymidylate synthase cycle genes in cisplatin-resistant human ovarian carcinoma A2780 cells. *Proc Natl Acad Sci USA* 85:650-653

Scanlon KJ, Lu Y, Kashani-Sabet M, Ma Jx, Newman E (1988): Mechanisms for cisplatin-FUra synergism and cisplatin resistance in human ovarian carcinoma cells both *in vitro* and *in vivo*. *Adv Exp Med Biol* 244:127-135.

Scanlon KJ, Kashani-Sabet M (1989): Utility of the polymerase chain reaction in detection of gene expression in drug-resistant human tumors. *J Clin Lab Anal* 3:323-329

Scanlon KJ, Kashani-Sabet M, Miyachi H (1989a): Differential gene expression in human cancer cells resistant to cisplatin. *Cancer Invest* 7:581-587

Scanlon KJ, Kashani-Sabet M, Miyachi H, Sowers LC, Rossi JJ (1989b): Molecular basis of cisplatin resistance in human carcinomas: Model systems and patients. *Anticancer Res* 9:1301-1312

Scanlon KJ, Kashani-Sabet M, Sowers LC (1989c): Overexpression of DNA replication and repair enzymes in cisplatin-resistant human ovarian carcinoma cells. *Cancer Comm* 1:269-275

Scanlon KJ, Funato T, Pezeshki B, Tone T, Sowers LC (1990a): Potentiation of azidothymidine cytotoxicity in cisplatin-resistant human ovarian carcinoma cells. *Cancer Comm* 2:339-343

Scanlon KJ, Wang W, Han H (1990b): Cyclosporin A suppresses cisplatin-induced oncogene expression in human cancer cells. *Cancer Treat Rev* 17:27-35

Scanlon KJ, Jiao L, Funato T, Wang, W, Tone T, Rossi JJ, Kashani-Sabet M (1991a): Ribozyme-mediated cleavage of c-*fos* mRNA reduces gene expression of DNA synthesis enzymes and metallothionein. *Proc Natl Acad Sci USA* 88:10591-10595

Scanlon KJ, Kashani-Sabet M, Tone T, Funato T (1991b): Cisplatin resistance in human cancers. *Pharm Ther* 52:385-406

Scanlon KJ, Ishida H, Kashani-Sabet M (1994): Ribozyme-mediated reversal of the multi-drug resistant phenotype. Submitted, *Proc Natl Acad Sci USA*

Schilder RJ, Hall L, Monks A, Handel LM, Fornace AJ, Ozols RF, Fojo AT, Hamilton TC (1990): Metallothionein gene expression and resistance to cisplatin in human ovarian cancer. *Int J Cancer* 45:416-422

Schmidt CJ, Hamer DH (1986): Cell specificity and an effect of *ras* on human metallothionein gene expression. *Proc Natl Acad Sci USA* 83:3346-3360

Schmidt W, Chaney SG (1993): Role of carrier ligand in platinum resistance of human carcinoma cell lines. *Cancer Res* 53:799-805

Schurig JE, Crosswell AR, Trail PA, Johnson KA, Henderson AJ, Jones M, Giandomenico C, Murrer BA, Cassaza AM (1991): Platinum analogs active against a cisplatin-resistant cell line. *Anti-Cancer Drug Des* 6:277

Sessa C, Vermorken J, Renanrd J, Kaye S, Smith D, Ten Bokkel Huinink W, Cavalli F, Pinedo H (1988): A phase II study of iproplatin in advanced ovarian carcinoma. *J Clin Oncol* 6:98-105

Sessa C, Cerny T, Kaye S, Monfardini S, Renald J, Cavilli F (1990): A phase II study of iproplatin in advanced metastatic stomach cancer. *Eur J Cancer* 26:61-62

Sessa C, Zucchetti M, Davoli E, Califano R, Cavalli F, Frustaci S, Gumbrell L, Sulkes A, Winograd B, D'Inacalci M (1991): Phase 1 and clinical pharmacological evaluation of aphidicolin glycinate. *J Natl Cancer Inst* 83:1160-1164

Sheaff R, Ilsley D, Kuchta R (1991): Mechanism of DNA polymerase α inhibition by aphidicolin. *Biochemistry* 30:8590-8597

Shibanura M, Kuroki T, Nose K (1987): Inhibition of proto-oncogene c-*fos* transcription by inhibitors of protein kinase C and ion transport. *Eur J Biochem* 164:15-19

Shionoya S, Lu Y, Scanlon KJ (1986): Properties of amino acid transport systems in K562 cells sensitive and resistant to *cis*-diamminedichloroplatinum(II). *Cancer Res* 46:3445-3448

Sklar MD (1988): Increased resistance to *cis*-diamminedichloroplatinum (II) in NIH3T3 cells transformed by *ras* oncogene. *Cancer Res* 48:793-737

Speizer LA, Watson MJ, Kanter JR, Brunton LL (1989): Inhibition of phorbol ester binding and protein kinase C activity by heavy metals. *J Biol Chem* 264:5581-5585

Swinnen LJ, Barnes DM, Fisher SG, Albain KS, Fisher RI, Erickson LC (1989): 1-ß-D-arabinofuranosylcytosine and hydroxyurea production of cytotoxic synergy with *cis*-diamminedichloroplatinum(II) and modification of platinum-induced DNA interstrand cross-linking. *Cancer Res* 49:1383-1389

Takeishi K, Kaneda S, Ayusawa D, Shimizu K, Gotoh O, Seno T (1989): Human thymidylate synthase gene: Isolation of phage clones which cover a functionally active gene and structural analysis of the region upstream from the translation initiation codon. *J Biochem* 106:575-583

Timmer-Bosscha H, Hospers GAP, Meijer C, Mulder NH, Muskiet FAJ, Martini IA, Uges DRA, de Vries EGE (1989): Influence of docosahexaenoic acid on cisplatin resistance in human small cell lung carcinoma cell line. *J Natl Cancer Inst* 81:1069-1075

Timmer-Bosscha, Mulder NH, de Vries EGE (1992): Modulation of cis-diamminedichloroplatinum(II) resistance: a review. *Br J Cancer* 66:227-238

Timmer-Bosscha H, Timmer A, Meijer C, de Vries GE, de Jong B, Oosterhuis JW, Mulder N (1993): *cis*-Diamminedichloroplatinum(II) resistance *in vitro* and *in vivo* in human embryonal carcinoma cells. *Cancer Res* 53:5707-5713

Toney JH, Donahue BA, Lellett PJ, Bruhn SL, Essigmann JM, Lippard SJ (1989): Isolation of cDNA encoding a human protein that binds selectively to DNA modified by the anticancer drug *cis*-diamminedichloroplatinum(II). *Proc Natl Acad Sci USA* 86:8328-8332

Tritton TR, Hickman JA (1990): How to kill cancer cells: Membranes and cell signaling as targets in cancer chemotherapy. *Cancer Cells* 2:95-105

Tsai C-M, Hsiao S-H, Frey CM, Chang K-T, Perng R-P, Gazdar AF, Kramer BS (1994): Combination cytotoxic effects of *cis*-diamminedichloroplatinum(II) and 5-fluorouracil with and without leucovorin against human non-small cell lung cancer cell lines. *Cancer Res* 53:1079-1084

Vanhamme L, Szpirer C (1987): Methionine metabolism defect in cells transfected with an activated HRAS1 oncogene. *Exp Cell Res* 169:120-126

Wallner KE, De Gregorio MW, Li GC (1986): Hyperthermic potential of *cis*-diamminedichloroplatinum(II) cytotoxicity in Chinese hamster ovary cells resistant to the drug. *Cancer Res* 46:6242-6245

Wang JC (1985): DNA topoisomerases. *Ann Rev Biochem* 54:665-697

Wang TS-F (1991): Eukaryotic DNA polymerases. *Ann Rev Biochem* 60:513-552

Weinberg RA (1989): Oncogenes, antioncogenes, and the molecular bases of multistep carcinogenesis. *Cancer Res* 49:3713-3721

Willemse PHB, Sleijfer DT, de Vries EGE, Boonstra H, Bouma J, Julder N.H. (1992): A phase 1-2 study with intraperitorneal cisplatin plus systemic etoposide in patients with minimal residual ovarian cancer. *Eur J Cancer* 28:479-481

Wiltshaw E, Evans B, Rustin G, Gilbey E, Baker J, Barker G (1986): A prospective randomized trial comparing high-dose cisplatin with low-dose cisplatin and chlorambucil in advanced ovarian carcinoma. *J Clin Oncol* 4:722-729

Yang Y-Y, Woo ES, Reese CE, Bahnson RR, Saijo N, Lazo JS (1994): Human metallothionein isoform gene expression in cisplatin-sensitive and resistant cells. *Mol Pharm* 45:453-460

Yoshida M, Khokhar AR, Siddik ZH (1994): Biochemical pharmacology of homologous alicyclic mixed amine platinum(II) complexes in sensitive and resistant tumor cell lines. *Cancer Res* 54:3468-3473

Zhen W, Link CJ Jr, O'Conner PM, Reed E, Parker R, Howell SB, Bohr VA (1992): Increased gene-specific repair of cisplatin interstrand cross-links in cisplatin-resistant human ovarian cancer cell lines. *Mol Cell Biol* 12:3689-3698

Zittoun J, Marquet J, David JC, Maniey D, Zittoun R (1989): A study of the mechanisms of cytotoxicity of ara-C on three human leukemic cell lines. *Cancer Chemother Pharm* 24:251-255

PERSPECTIVES

John A. Kellen

No man sees far; the most see no
farther than their noses.

Thomas Carlyle

Forecasting gives you a comfortable feeling of some control over an uncontrollable world. This is not meant to negate progress and predictability. Both are unmistakably part of our life and if we disregard little faddish swings such as the recent butter/margarine controversy, we clearly steer somewhere. Once a goal is set, we can evaluate our success in reaching it; when the goal is highly elusive, our approach is at best asymptotic and eventually, we come as close as our capacity for abstraction permits to understand the mechanisms of nature. In cancer research, we are imbued with horror of agnosticism and satisfactory answers must translate into measurable improvement of a patient's conditions, as final proof of "being right".

To start with a rhetorical question: how does this all apply to multidrug resistance and its reversal, or, in trivial terms: does our understanding of a resistance mechanism contribute to more effective chemotherapy with the introduction of efficient circumventive measures? The logic of this approach is indisputable, but logic is now increasingly considered as fuzzy, at least in real life. We can still take solace in the Italian saying: if it is not true, at least it is well invented.

Resistant cells, single or in tissues, inhabit today's world with thousands of species and trillions of individuals. Resistance is the result of clonal dominance; in neoplastic cells, new variations continuously come into existence, increase their presence and evade in growing numbers chemotherapy and other types of treatment (Kaiser, 1994). The rising tide of information related to resistance and its mechanisms is getting difficult to sift and starts to clog our mental arteries with databits; what we are lacking is not facts, but meaning (Goodman, 1993). It is popular to choose a model (with the least possible variables), expose it to clinically unrealistic conditions, observe with sophisticated methods drug responses or the lack of them, evaluate all with increasingly complex statistical methods and pronounce the result as truism. Next, correlations with single variables are sought and found; a limit is set at which such correlations are considered to be significant. Even such limits may be exceeded by chance. It is well known that correlations never actually prove causality, as illustrated by the humorous bon mot: there is a strong correlation between the decline of birthrates and the number of stork's nests in Central Europe (Levy, 1994). In brief: there are many reliable data on various aspects of MDR but few which can be generalized and used in a clinical setting. Enthusiasts who expect an answer to all resistance questions, past, present and future, from reversing MDR and sensitizing resistant cancer cells, should soberly consider the very general and by no means exhaustive listing of promising avenues of therapy in Table 1. One learns *ex post facto* that some work better than others.

If we accept that decreased (and therefore insufficient) drug accumulation in the intracellular space of target cells is the basic cause of MDR, the logical point of attack should be the drug transport mechanisms. Any efflux pump which is protein-mediated and functions as an active transport (as opposed to gradient-caused) is open to interference (by virtue of it's energy dependence) and to competitive inhibition by structurally similar compounds. Energy deprivation, specifically targeted at cancer cells only, is difficult to envisage; competition by "fooling" the system is relatively simple and is limited only by the necessity to achieve high local saturation of the competitor, which might be toxic to the host. When examining the various prospects for sensitization by manipulation of efflux mechanisms, the perhaps best understood and even clinically successful target (at least in hematological malignancies) is the P-glycoprotein. Interference with this efflux system is not always synonymous with competition; the inhibitory effect of some drugs such as Verapamil and its analogues is non-competitive. Attempts to modify the activity of P-glycoprotein have been extensively reviewed

Table 1. Future Directions of Cancer Therapy
    Chemoprevention
    New chemotherapeutic agents
    Modulators of drug resistance
    Immunotherapy
    Hematopoietic growth factors
    Autologous bone marrow/peripheral-blood stem-cell support
    Accelerated hyperfraction radiation therapy
    Interdigitation of radiation therapy and chemotherapy
    Genetic modulation and interference

by Fan et al. (1994) and many others. In general, "resistance modifying" agents (a nicely vague term, which does not promise too much!) are less effective in the non-P-glycoprotein mediated MDR models.

The identification of the MDR mechanism or mechanisms does not provide instant remedies. Single mechanisms can vary in intensity and are almost never entirely responsible for resistance. There is a fundamental difference between MDR defined in cell cultures and what really takes place at the clinical level (i.e. what happens to measurable tumor masses, their response or further growth during treatment, Cazin et al., 1992). A frequently neglected factor is prior drug treatment for benign or chronic disorders which may trigger alterations in drug metabolism and "prepare" subclinical malignancies for MDR (Umeda et al., 1994).

Many other factors, independent from the MDR mechanisms *per se*, come into play. As tumors grow larger, local hypoxia, acidosis and the proportion of the non-cycling cell population increase, while drug delivery decreases (Lee et al., 1994). Different sites of growth of the same tumor influence morphology, doubling times and drug sensitivity (Kal et al., 1994). In relapsed patients, a more homogeneous cell population may exist, with narrowed diversity and increasingly effective MDR mechanisms (Fojo et al., 1994). Prolonged periods of treatment may trigger new efflux mechanisms (Marsh et al., 1986). Perhaps the drug dose should more intensive to avoid drug resistance developing because of increased treatment time (Carl and Tropé, 1993). In some treatment modalities, recessive but functional resistance arises which can block drug uptake, as opposed to an increase in efflux (Weber et al., 1989).

A solid tumor is a complex, dynamic association, composed of cells in various stages of growth and dying, heterogeneous genetic make-up and varying degrees of vascular supply. With increase of tumor size, some of these cell populations grow or decline in numbers. It is impossible to create an *in vitro* model which would faithfully reflect these changing conditions; at best, extrapolations from cell cultures or tumor samples allow for rough estimates of reality; when the successful treatment of a patient depends on such data, they are not good enough. If response to cytostatics could be predicted with confidence, the so identified drug(s) would have a high probability of patient benefit and reduce unnecessary toxicity from ineffective therapeutic modalities. The potential advantages of individualized chemotherapy must be emphasized; the human tumor clonogenic assay (HTCA) has proven to be a clinically useful test, at least in predicting drug resistance (Parchment et al., 1992). However, in view of the above, studies comparing HTCA results with clinical response leave much to be desired. The *in vitro* identification of pleiotropic drug resistance (in cell clones derived from early detected growth) may serve as an indicator of the *ad hoc* situation only (Schadendorf et al., 1994). Advances in methods which would predict clinical response based on *in vitro* measurement of DNA damage can be expected to provide realistic guidance to innovative cytotoxic drug strategies (Epstein, 1990).

Again, to play the role of the devil's advocate: very successful interference with MDR mechanisms necessarily is unphysiological; it harbours the potential danger that MDR reversal would significantly increase the mutagenicity of other compounds in our environment (Ferguson et al., 1993). Resistance of tumor cells to drugs is not accompanied by increased resistance of normal host cells (Bertino, 1990).

Apart from numerous, theoretically well-founded efforts to contravene the P-glycoprotein efflux pump, the increasing awareness of many other resistance mechanisms triggers new approaches to reverse MDR. It is too soon to predict which direction holds promises; in every such study, it is imperative to keep in mind that the gap between experimental data from cell cultures and the clinical situation in an individual patient is enormous. Furthermore, it is necessary to establish that, in each case where the therapeutic response has been unsatisfactory (which is unfortunately *post factum*), the factual presence of MDR in the remaining, recurring or metastasizing malignancy needs to be established. At present, this is a formidable task. Even in the best case scenario, in which excellent, sensitive and specific methods for MDR "markers" were available, many other factors would need to be considered. The determination of drug metabolites, drug-metabolizing enzymes and drug availability would help to completize the highly individual picture *ad hoc*, for each tumor, in each patient. Recently, a valuable means of studying intracellular metabolic processes has become available by NMR spectroscopy. Steady-state ^{31}P NMR spectra of wild type and resistant Ehrlich ascites tumor cells were found to differ (Rasmussen et al., 1993).

Again and again, it must be emphasized that the bulk of our knowledge about MDR mechanisms and their modulation is based in results obtained in cell cultures. While *in vitro* studies offer the advantage of clean experiments with few and controlled variables, it is difficult to extrapolate such data and apply them to a clinical situation. There is obviously a lack for ideal models and for simple, highly sensitive *in vivo* detection methods for the various "markers" of MDR. The P388/VMDRC.04 (mouse leukemic) cell line has been suggested as a perfect model for studying P-glycoprotein antagonists; it displays the MDR phenotype, over-expresses P-glycoprotein but no other recognized mechanisms of resistance and can be grown in animals (Yang et al., 1994).

There is much progress in the development of detection methods for different facets of MDR. The soft agarose clonogenic assay shows that tumor cell lines, established from untreated SCLC patients, are often sensitive to cytotoxic drugs *in vitro*, while cell lines from relapsed patients are typically MDR. The microculture tetrazolium assay (MTT) in viable cells shows a correlation between *in vitro* results and the clinical response to chemotherapy and survival (Doyle, 1993). However, in leukemias, *in vitro* sensitivity to drugs determined by the MTT assay predicted poorly the clinical response to combination chemotherapy (Phillips, 1990). Another promising approach may be the rapid screening and characterization of different resistance mechanisms to hydrophilic and lipophilic antifolates by flow cytometry, using fluorescein labelling (Assaraf, 1993). The dynamics (i.e. in- and efflux) of intracellular drugs can be monitored by a highly sensitive and convenient method, by matrix-assisted laser desorption/ionization mass spectrometry (MALD-MS). This may prove a rapid, superior alternative to existing methods for analysis of drugs and their metabolites in tissues and cells. The application for MDR cells is obvious (Rideout et al., 1993).

There is a flurry of activity in the general direction of reversal or circumvention of MDR. Some more established (and even tested in clinical trials) have been reviewed by Fan et al. (1994). In general, many approaches to "overcome" MDR are being developed, ranging from heroic dosages (with simultaneously protection or restitution of the bone marrow) to alternating drug combinations and some novel intracellular targets. Promising aspects have been covered in the previous chapters. As this point in time, success of any of these modalities is unpredictable. To recapitulate a few:

MRP may be a future target for pharmacological chemosensitization (Schneider et al., 1994). The use of transferrin as a drug carrier increases doxorubicin toxicity in resistant cells (Lemieux et al., 1994). Several light-activated drugs lyse cancer cells independently of their resistance status (Gulati et al., 1994). Inhibition of topoisomerase II may provide potentially effective clinical sensitization of human brain tumors (Ali-Osman et al., 1993) and many others (Zijlstra et al., 1990). In a different vein: drugs that target cell division (such as cytarabine) could be delivered in a circadian-adjusted schedule to expose potentially resistant cell populations in their most vulnerable phase (Haus, 1989).

In cancer, multiple clonal deletions or mutations are common; there are about 60 enzymes which effect biotransformation (both activation or inactivation) of established chemotherapeutic agents - which opens the possibility of "negative" gene deletion targets for cancer therapy, resulting in selective cytotoxicity. Further knowledge of the cellular regulation of topoisomerases should lead to more effective selection of chemotherapy, treatment modalities and hopefully prevention or circumvention of drug resistance (Ziljstra et al., 1990). In altered or mutated topo II (causing MDR in the human ovarian cancer cell line A2780 DX3), tumor necrosis factor was found to potentiate topo II-targeted drugs and thus aid in the reversal of MDR (Cimoli et al., 1994).

Encapsulation in liposomes may change pharmacokinetic and pharmacodynamic properties of some drugs, increase tolerance to greater doses and thus overcome drug resistance (Sharma et al., 1993). Taxol may be administered in better tolerated formulations, for ex. taxol-phospholipid complexes (liposomes). Similarly, nanoparticles of PIBCA (polyisobutylcyanoacrylate) and PIHCA (polyisohexylcyanoacrylate), loaded with doxorubicin, are able to reverse resistance in P388 cells (Némati et al., 1994).

DNA transfection combined with a masking technique (surface-epitope masking, SEM) should be useful in providing monoclonal antibodies which identify genes associated with important processes, such as multidrug resistance (Shen et al., 1994). Finally, entirely novel pharmacological approaches, such as self-assembling antineoplastic drugs ("covalent modulation") show inherent advantages in overcoming MDR by building up higher intracellular concentrations in cancer cells as compared with normal tissue (Rideout, 1994).

All these efforts are difficult to evaluate; they reflect the recognized necessity of action and the importance of multidrug resistance. There is only one perspective which leaves no place for doubt: unless this problem (together with all other aspects of malignant growth) is vigorously pursued, our chances to improve the overall record in our fight with cancer are questionable.

REFERENCES

Ali-Osman F, Berger MS, Rajagopal S, Spence A, Livingston RG (1993): Topoisomerase II Inhibition and Altered Kinetics of Formation and Repair of Nitrosourea and Cisplatin-induced DNA Interstrand Cross-Links and Cytotoxicity in Human Glioblastoma Cells. *Cancer Res* 53:5663-5668

Assaraf YG (1993): Characterization by flow cytometry and fluorescein-methotrexate labeling of hydrophilic and lipophilic antifolate resistance in cultured mammalian cells. *Anti-cancer Drugs* 4:535-544

Bertino JR (1990): "Turning the Tables" - Making Normal Marrow Resistant to Chemotherapy. *JNCI* 82:1234-1235

Carl J, Tropé C (1993): Gestational trophoblastic tumors: cytostatic treatment response evaluated from hCG modeling. *Int J Gynecol Cancer* 3:265-270

Cazin J-L, Gosselin P, Cappelaere P, Robert J, Demaille A (1992): Drug resistance in oncology: from concepts to applications. *J Cancer Res Clin Oncol* 119:76-86

Cimoli G, Valenti M, Parodi S, De Sessa F, Russo P (1994): Circumvention of Atypical Multidrug Resistance with Tumor Necrosis Factor. *Jpn J Cancer Res* 85:155-138

Doyle LA (1993): Mechanisms of Drug Resistance in Human Lung Cancer Cells. *Sem Oncol* 20:326-337

Epstein RJ (1990): Drug-Induced DNA Damage and Tumor Chemosensitivity. *J Clin Oncol* 8:2062-2084

Fan D, Beltran PJ, O'Brian CA (1994): Reversal of Multidrug Resistance. In: *Reversal of Multidrug Resistance in Cancer* (ed. JA Kellen), pp. 93-125. Boca Raton: CRC Press

Ferguson LR, Baguley BC (1993): Multidrug resistance and mutagenesis. *Mut Research* 285:79-90

Fojo T, Scala S, Zhan Z, Mickley L (1993): Heterogeneity of Drug Resistance. In: *Heterogeneity of Cancer Cells*, vol. 95 (eds. M D'Incalci, A Mantovani and S Farattini), pp. 27-39. New York: Raven Press

Goodman E (1993): Will the Information Highway Turn Out to Be Another Dead End? *Philadephia Enquirer*, 23 Oct

Gulati SC, Lemoli RM, Igarashi T, Atzpodien J (1994): Newer Opinions for Treating Drug-Resistant (MDR+) Cancer Cells using Photoradiation Therapy. *Leuk & Lymphoma* 12:427-433

Haus E (1989) in: NEWS, *JNCI* 81:1769

Kaiser HE (1994): Neoplastic Autonomy: A Fundamental Phenomenon (Introduction). *In vivo* 8:1-2

Kal HB, Van Berkel AH, Goedoen HH (1994): Growth Rate, Morphology and Drug Responses of Rat Lung Tumours Growing at Different Sites. *Anticancer Res* 14:495-500

Lee KE, Fujioka T, Kubota T, Hoffman R (1994): The Relationship between Tumor Size and Chemosensitivity of Murine Bladder Cancer. *Anticancer Res* 13:465-468

Lemieux P, Page M (1994): Sensitivity of Multidrug-Resistant MCF-7 Cells to a Transferrin-Doxorubicin Conjugate. *Anticancer Res* 13:397-404

Levy GB (1994): Another red herring perchance? *American Lab* 6:312-314

Marsh W, Sicheri D, Center MS (1986): Isolation and Characterization of Adriamycin-resistant HL-60 Cells Which Are Not Defective in the Initial Interacellular Accumulation of Drug. *Cancer Res* 46:4053-4057

Némati F, Dubernet C, de Verdière AC, Poupon MF, Treupel-Acar L, Puisieux F, Couvreur P (1994): Some parameters influencing cytotoxicity of free doxorubicin and doxorubicin-loaded nanoparticles in sensitive and multidrug resistant leucemic murine cells: incubation time, number of nanoparticles per cell. *Int J Pharmaceutics* 102:55-62

Parchment RE, Soleimanpour K, Petrose S, Murphy MR Jr (1992): Pharmacologic Validation of Human Tumor Clonogenic Assays Based on Pleiotropic Drug Resistance: Implications for Individualized Chemotherapy and New Drug Screening Programs. *Int J Cell Cloning* 10:359-368

Phillips JK (1990): Use of the MTT assay to assess drug resistance patterns in acute myeloid leukaemia. *Brit J Ca* 61:559

Rasmussen J, Hansen LL, Friche E, Jaroszewski JW (1993): ^{31}P and ^{13}CNMR Spectroscopic Study of Wild Type and Multidrug Resistant Ehrlich Ascites Tumor Cells. *Oncology Res* 5:119-126

Rideout D, Bustamante A, Siuzdak G (1993): Cationic drug analysis using matrix-assisted laser desorption/ionization mass spectrometry: Application to influx kinetics, multidrug resistance and intracellular chemical change. *Proc Natl Aca Sci USA* 90:10226-10229

Rideout D (1994): Self-Assembling Drugs: A New Approach to Biochemical Modulation in Cancer Chemotherapy. *Cancer Invest* 12:189-202

Schadendorf D, Worm M, Algermissen B, Kohlmus CM, Czarnetzki B (1994): Chemosensitivity Testing of Human Malignant Melanoma. *Cancer* 73:103-108

Schneider E, Yamazaki H, Sinha BK, Cowan KH (1994): Chemosensitization of drug-sensitive and -resistant human breast cancer MCF7 cells expressing the multidrug-associated protein (MRP). *Proc AACR* 35:359

Sharma A, Mayhew E, Straubinger RM (1993): Antitumor Effect of Taxol-containing Liposomes in a Taxol-resistant Murine Tumor Model. *Cancer Res* 53:5877-5881

Shen R, Su Z-Z, Olsson CA, Goldstein NI, Fisher PB (1994): Surface-Epitope Masking: a Strategy for the Development of Monoclonal Antibodies Specific for Molecules Expressed on the Cell Surface. *JNCI* 86:91-98

Umeda Y, Yamauchi K, Sugawara I, Arimore S, Nagao T (1994): Relationship between expression of P-glycoprotein and use of noncytotoxic drugs before chemotherapy in acute leukemia. *Cancer Jrnl* 7:39-43

Weber JW, Sircar S, Horvath J, Dion P (1989): Atypical multidrug resistance in adenovirus transformed revertant rat cells selected for resistance to MGBG. *Proc AACR* 30:532

Yang JM, Goldenberg S, Gottesman MM, Hait WN (1994): Characteristics of P388/VMDRC.04, a Simple, Sensitive Model for Studying P-Glycoprotein Antagonists. *Cancer Res* 54:730-737

Zijlstra JG, De Jong S, De Vries EGE, Mulder NH (1990): Topoisomerases, new targets in cancer chemotherapy. *Med Oncol & Tumor Pharmacother* 7:11-18

CONCLUSIONS

John A. Kellen

Preoccupation with cause and effect
helps to expand the intellect,
but it limits as well to facts
which will be writ in proper tracts.
Samuel Sterns

Some general rules appear to apply to multidrug resistance; some of these only confirm that very much is left to be explained and done. So far, no single parameter accounts totally for the spectrum of MDR. The mechanisms involved are, at least in part, elements of a global, non-specific protection system which ensures survival. Undesirable compounds (which encompass antineoplastic agents, unfortunately) are transported by a variety of mechanisms, some of which are switched on or amplified by the agents themselves. Even profound understanding of such mechanisms is not offering perfect solutions: individual patients show very different patterns of MDR, with none, few or several resistance mechanisms active at any one time. There is continuous adaptation to timing, dosage and targets of drug administered, both within the tumor and in secondary growth. Metastases of solid tumors are notoriously difficult to erradicate by chemotherapy. It is to be expected that the number of cell generations reached by a metastatic growth to be clinically detectable exceeds 100, which allows for a large number of mutations. Adaptation, in response to injury from chemotherapy, leads to a predominantly MDR cell population, which requires radical new approached in treatment. So far, all new modalities do not achieve even the modest goal of longer growth suppression without toxicity (Israel, 1990). Every individual cancer case probably requires the setting up of its own "resistance profile" (Volm et al., 1994).

Some forms of resistance, such as to platinum compounds, develop rapidly, with clinically significant levels present after three or four exposures to the drug (Los and Muggia, 1994). Other may take years and many courses of therapy to develop. Some mechanisms maintain full efficiency even during prolonged absence of drugs, others fade away rapidly (only to re-awake on repeated stimuli). Perhaps the only general rule is that there is no apparent rule at all.

The information gathered from our systematic search for MDR mechanisms should help to achieve the pragmatic goal: circumvent, prevent or reverse the process. Forewarned is not, as yet, forearmed. The main target for MDR modulation remains P-glycoprotein; apart from the numerous drugs which interfere with efflux pump action in various (still poorly understood) ways, some more recent monoclonal antibodies (265/F4, MRK 16, HYB 612) show promise, at least in cell cultures. Inhibition of P-glycoprotein expression is not limited to tumor cells, but also affects normal cells; cell lines with low amounts of P-gp were found to be less affected (Efferth et al., 1993). The effects of various MDR modulators on antineoplastic drug pharmacokinetics and pharmacodynamics, in clinical trials, have been extensively reviewed (Lum et al., 1993). Only modulators with modest side effects at effective plasma concentrations are suitable for realistic treatment of patients (Pommerenke et al., 1994).

In vivo, reversal of MDR by co-administration of non-cytotoxic drugs is fraught with numerous problems: it is often impossible to achieve adequate drug concentrations (equivalent to the levels effective *in vitro*) because of toxicity; drug interactions are still unknown and may cause undesirable pharmacokinetic consequences, the bioavailability of both chemotherapeutic agents and MDR modulators *in vivo* might be questionable, proper controls in trials are difficult to establish and finally, interference with one MDR mechanism might not influence other mechanisms simultaneously or subsequently present in the tumor (Leyland-Jones et al., 1993).

On the positive side: administration of modulating agents able to preclude defensive and evasive maneuvres by cancer cells, together with chemotherapeutic cocktails simultaneously aimed at various vulnerable chinks in the armour of these cells should lead to destruction of such specificity, magnitude and speed that all recuperative mechanisms are too litte, too late. This is a plausible, but reductionist scenario.

If these maximalistic expectations can not be met (for ex. such optimal combinations might be too toxic for the patient himself), there are still "second best" situations. A successful "sensitizer" might increase the number of lethal kills in the first rounds of treatment, decreasing the prospects of future regrowth or postponing it considerably. The time gained might even allow for the introduction of new chemotherapeutic agents or other treatment regimens. Finally, such a treatment might significantly improve the quality of life, by allowing for shorter and fewer treatment courses. In sum, an ideal futuristic chemotherapy would consist of detailed, pretreatment investigations of sensitivity or resistance of the tumor in each individual patient, followed by a custom-tailored treatment combination, with follow-up testing for MDR and further therapy adapted to fit changing circumstances. This would resemble a chess-game, where the opponent's tactics are out-guessed and rendered ineffectual by appropriate measures.

Now, to play the role of devil's advocate: if we accept that drug resistance is an integral part of the general survival capacity (of every life form, large or small), the endless variety and adaptability of this capacity should eventually overcome every effort for selective cytotoxicity - because all cells, good or "bad", are alike - only some more than others. To evoke the spectre of the chess-game again: this time our adversary outguesses the chemotherapist and there will be just the right, albeit minute, number of cells able to withstand any attack and come back with a vengeance. Unfortunately, recent world-wide developments of resistance in microorganisms seem to support this pessimistic extreme.

There are, of course, other tremendous obstacles in the way of a successful sensitization of drug resistance in cancer. Even in the case of clear understanding of the cause of resistance and the method of circumvention, a new therapeutic modality needs to be tested in clinical trials with adequate numbers of patients, appropriate controls and sufficient duration of follow-up. Needless to say, setting up meaningful control groups, randomized (for ethical and scientific reasons), can be a formidable problem. Tumors are not only heterogeneous in their cell population, but subpopulations change in their relative proportions with time and treatment. These dynamics are unpredictable and probably different in individual patients. At present, we have no reliable methods to define and determine such changes.

If the treated group is large enough, results with resistance modifiers may cause modest, incremental advances over the traditional treatment protocol and the improvement achieved may not be statistically convincing (even if very successful in a small number of patients within the group). If the group was initially small (usually for lack of suitable patients, available for the particular protocol), the results will be unacceptable, according to traditional statistics. The "Icarus principle" applies: we fly with gossamer wings to reach the sun and when we err, our wings melt and we fall back to earth, only to try and try again.

REFERENCES

Efferth T, Volm M (1993): Modulation of P-Glycoprotein-Mediated Multidrug Resistance by Monoclonal Antibodies, Immunotoxins or Antisense Oligonucleotides in Kidney Carcinoma and Normal Kidney Cells. *Oncology* 50:303-308

Israel L (1990): Accelerated genetic destabilization and dormancy; two distinct causes of resistance in metastatic cells; clinical magnitude, therapeutic approaches. *Clin Expl Metastasis* 8:1-11

Leyland-Jones B, Dalton W, Fisher GA, Sikic BI (1993): Reversal of Multidrug Resistance to Cancer Chemotherapy. *Cancer* 72:3484-3488

Los G, Muggia FM (1994): Platinum Resistance. *Hematol/Oncology Clin North America* 8:411-429

Lum BL, Fisher GA, Brophy NA, Yahanda AM, Adler KM, Kaubisch S, Halsey J, Sikic BI (1993): Clinical Trials of Modulation of Multidrug Resistance. *Cancer* 72:3502-3514

Pommerenke E, Mattern J, Volm M (1994): Modulation of doxorubicin toxicity by tamoxifen in multidrug-resistant tumour cells in vitro and in vivo. *J Cancer Res Clin Oncol* 129:422-426

Volm M, Efferth (1994): Resistenzueberwindung bei Tumoren. *Dtsch Med Wschr* 119:475-479

Index

Very frequently occuring terms,such as MDR (Multidple Drug Resistance) have not been indexed.